Speech and Language Disorders in Bilinguals

SPEECH AND LANGUAGE DISORDERS IN BILINGUALS

ALFREDO ARDILA
AND
ELIANE RAMOS
EDITORS

Nova Science Publishers, Inc.
New York

LIBRARY OF CONGRESS CATALOGING-IN-PUBLICATION DATA

Available upon request.

ISBN 978-1-60021-560-5

Published by Nova Science Publishers, Inc. ✣ New York

CONTENTS

PREFACE

During the last years a significant number of papers, books, and monographs devoted to speech and language impairments in bilingual children have been published. Different aspects and questions have been approached and, today, we have a relatively good understanding of the specific characteristics of the speech and language difficulties observed in bilingual and multilingual children. This interest has significantly resulted from the potential developmental and educational consequences of bilingualism.

Our understanding of communication disorders in adult populations is notoriously limited, even though over 50% of the adult population can speak at least one language in addition to his/her native language. That simply means that over 50% of the communication disorders observed in adults are bilingual speech and language disorders: bilingual aphasias, bilingual dementias, bilingual stuttering, etc. This collection of papers was written with the specific purpose of filling this gap. The major purpose of this book is to present the state of the art knowledge on the different aspects of communication disorders observed in adult bilinguals.

The book is organized in such a way that an integrated perspective of bilingualism is presented: from the normal conditions to the pathologies; from the clinical descriptions to the rehabilitation issues; from the biological factors to the cultural variables. Initially, a general overview of the importance of bilingualism in the contemporary world ("Bilingualism in the contemporary world") is introduced, emphasizing that bilingualism represents a most significant human phenomenon. The following chapter reviews the question of the similarities and differences in the brain organization of language ("Brain organization of language in bilinguals"). The chapter "Psycholinguistics of bilingualism and multilingualiism" continues the analysis of the different systems participating in the bilinguals with a major emphasis in the models of bilingual language representation.

Code-switching and code-mixing, probably the two extensively examined expressive phenomena in bilinguals, are discussed in the following chapter ("Code-switching and code-mixing"). This chapter is followed by an analysis on the lexicons and the meanings of the two languages and how they are organized in bilinguals ("Lexical and semantic organization and retrieval").

The following two chapters analyze two specific pathologies as they are manifested in bilinguals: aphasia and stuttering in bilinguals. The following chapter ("Bilingualism across the life-span under normal and abnormal conditions") extends the analysis of pathology in bilinguals, referring to other conditions, such as dementia in bilinguals.

Language and speech skills present certain variability according to the specific cultural conditions. Realistic assessment and treatment of bilingual speakers must acknowledge the various factors, including linguistic and sociocultural experiences, impacting on these individuals communication competence, as discussed in the following chapter ("Cultural and linguistic diversity in language impairments").

The following two chapters approach the questions of the assessment of communication disorders in bilinguals ("Speech and language assessment in bilinguals") and the complexities of the rehabilitation process when dealing with bilingual populations ("Considerations for an ethnopsycholinguistic framework for aphasia intervention with bilingual speakers"). The book closes with a rather psychologically oriented chapter: the relationships between bilingualism and cognition. It is emphasized that bilingualism, regardless of its potentially interfering and challenging properties, can result in significant cognitive advantages under certain conditions. Language represents the major instrument of cognition and using two or more different languages provides additional strategies in different intellectual tasks.

We sincerely hope that this book will contribute to a better understanding of the speech and language disorders observed in adult bilingual populations and that it will encourage research in this area.

Alfredo Ardila
Eliane Ramos

In: Speech and Language Disorders in Bilinguals
Editors: Alfredo Ardila and Eliane Ramos, pp. 1-19
ISBN 978-1-60021-560-5

Chapter 1

BILINGUALISM IN THE CONTEMPORARY WORLD

Alfredo Ardila
Department of Communication Sciences and Disorders
Florida International University
Miami, Florida 33199, USA

LANGUAGES IN THE CONTEMPORARY WORLD

How Many Languages and Speakers are there for Each One?

Contemporary man (~ 6 billon people) speaks about 6,800 different languages (www.ethnologe.com). It means, on average every language has less than one million speakers. An enormous disparity, however, exists in the number of speakers. Just about 347 (or approximately 5%) of the world's languages have one million speakers or over and account for 94% of the world's population. Out of these 347 languages, there are only eight or nine languages with over 100 million speakers; they are spoken by about 40% of the world population. By contrast, 95% of languages are spoken by only 6% of the world's people. About 3,500 languages (half of the total number of languages) have less than 100,000 speakers. These figures point to a very uneven distribution of world languages with regard to the number of speakers. Table 1 presents the distribution of languages by number of first-language speakers.

A small number of languages, including English, Spanish, French, Arabic, Russian, Hindi, Malay, German, Mandarin, Portuguese, and Russian frequently serve as *lingua franca*. They are frequently considered as international languages, and used for wider communication among people from different countries. Often, they represent the official languages of the international organizations, not only in politics, but also in commerce, and science. Sometimes these languages are used as official languages in countries having a diversity of native languages, such as in Nigeria. Quite often, they are languages spoken as a second or third language.

Table 1. Distribution of languages by number of first-language speakers (*http://www.ethnologue.com/ethno_docs/distribution.asp?by=size*)

Population range	living languages			number of speakers		
	Number	%	Cumulative	Number	%	Cumulative
100,000,000 to 999,999,999	8	0.1	0.1%	2,301,423,372	40.20753	40.20753%
10,000,000 to 99,999,999	75	1.1	1.2%	2,246,597,929	39.24969	79.45723%
1,000,000 to 9,999,999	264	3.8	5.0%	825,681,046	14.42525	93.88247%
100,000 to 999,999	892	12.9	17.9%	283,651,418	4.95560	98.83807%
10,000 to 99,999	1,779	25.7	43.7%	58,442,338	1.02103	99.85910%
1,000 to 9,999	1,967	28.5	72.1%	7,594,224	0.13268	99.99177%
100 to 999	1,071	15.5	87.6%	457,022	0.00798	99.99976%
10 to 99	344	5.0	92.6%	13,163	0.00023	99.99999%
1 to 9	204	3.0	95.5%	698	0.00001	100.00000%
Unknown	308	4.5	100.0%			
Totals	6,912	100.0		5,723,861,210	100.00000	

The most influential languages of international communication have been changing throughout history; e.g., Greek, Latin, French, etc. Today, the most important international language is English. Estimating how many people speak a particular language is not easy, and figures may be quite variable (Crystal, 1987). For example, English estimates vary from 275 to 450 million, Spanish from 200 to over 400 million, Hindi from 150 to 350 million, and Russian from 150 to 200 million. To define who really is a speaker of a language may not be so simple. Many people world-wide speak a second or third language with highly variables degrees of mastery, and to establish a cut-off criterion of bilingualism is not easy. To partially overcome this difficulty, some surveys of languages give information on native speakers only. Others count both native speakers and *secondary* speakers (those who use the language regularly or primarily even though it is not their native language).

The Summer Institute for Linguistics (SIL) Ethnologue Survey (1999) (*www.ethnologue.com/show_serial.asp?name=886*) lists the following as the top languages by population (number of native speakers in parentheses):

1. Chinese (937,132,000)
2. Spanish (332,000,000)
3. English (322,000,000)
4. Bengali (189,000,000)
5. Hindi/Urdu (182,000,000)
6. Arabic (174,950,000)
7. Portuguese (170,000,000)
8. Russian (170,000,000)
9. Japanese (125,000,000)

Weber (1997) considers that the largest languages according to the number of speakers are:

1. Mandarin Chinese (1.1 billion)
2. English (330 million)
3. Spanish (300 million)
4. Hindi/Urdu (250 million)
5. Arabic (200 million)
6. Bengali (185 million)
7. Portuguese (160 million)
8. Russian (160 million)
9. Japanese (125 million)
10. German (100 million)

If adding secondary speaker populations to the primary speaker populations, approximately the following distribution would be found:

1. Mandarin Chinese (1.1 billion)
2. English (480 million)
3. Spanish (350 million)
4. Russian (285 million)
5. French (265 million)
6. Hindi/Urdu (250 million)
7. Arabic (221 million)
8. Portuguese (188 million)
9. Bengali (185 million)
10. Japanese (133 million)
11. German (109 million)

An important distinction should be introduced between *individual bilingualism* (i.e., individuals speaking two languages) and *geographic bilingualism* (i.e., areas where two different languages are spoken). Not only the population (number) of language speakers, but also the geographic distribution of these languages is important. Some languages have relatively large populations of native speakers but are used almost exclusively in one country (e.g., Japanese). Other languages are used in many different countries as an official or national language (e.g., Spanish).

The following is a list of these languages in terms of the number of countries where each is spoken. The number that follows is the total number of countries that use that language (Weber, 1997):

1. English (115)
2. French (35)
3. Arabic (24)
4. Spanish (20)

5. Russian (16)
6. German (9)
7. Mandarin (5)
8. Portuguese (5)
9. Hindi/Urdu (2)
10. Bengali (1)
11. Japanese (1)

Nonetheless, in a particular country a language can be the official and most spoken language, whereas in other one, it can be spoken by a limited number of people, and it is not the official language. French is the official language in France, but also a diversity of regional languages is spoken in France, including Basque, Catalan, Franco-Provençal, etc., are spoken. The number of countries includes *core countries* (where the language has full legal or official status), *outer core countries* (where the language has some legal or official status and is an influential minority language, such as English in India or French in Algeria), and *fringe countries* (where the language has no legal status, but is an influential minority language in trade, tourism, or the preferred foreign language of the young people, such as English in Japan or French in Romania). Some languages do not have a core country, even though they are the primary language for a significant amount of people; the best example may be Romany (Gipsy language), with estimates between 6 and 11 millions of speakers.

Additionally, it is noteworthy that there are many interlanguages (Crystal, 1987; Siguan, 2001). When two languages come in close contact (French and German, Spanish and Portuguese, etc.), an interlanguage may emerge.

Official and National Languages

Table 2 presents the world languages with over 50 millions speakers, the language family, the writing system, and the areas where it is spoken. Some languages have a specific geographical location and are linked to one specific country (e.g., Turkish), whereas others are spoken in rather scattered areas (e.g., English).

Some countries do not have an official language (e.g., USA). Most countries in the world recognize only one official language (e.g., Costa Rica). Fewer than 25% of the world's approximately 200 countries recognize two or more official languages (e.g., Bolivia, India, Luxembourg, Nigeria). In some countries, official languages vary according to the region. In Peru Spanish is the official language but Quechua, Aymara and other regional languages are also recognized in the areas where they are predominant.

Interesting to note, there are many more children throughout the world who have been and continue to be educated through a second or a later-acquired language -at least for some portion of their formal education, than there are children educated exclusively using the first language (see, e.g., Dutcher, 1994; World Bank, 1995). Frequently, in many countries bilingualism or multilingualism constitutes the normal everyday experience.

Table 2. Major world languages (*http://www.krysstal.com/spoken.html*)

	Language	Family	Script(s) Used	Speakers (Millions)	Where Spoken (Major)
1	Mandarin	Sino-Tibetan	Chinese Characters	885	China, Malaysia, Taiwan
2	Spanish	Indo-European	Latin	332	South America, Central America, Spain
3	English	Indo-European	Latin	322	USA, UK, Australia, Canada, New Zealand
4	Arabic	Afro-Asiatic	Arabic	235	Middle East, Arabia, North Africa
5	Bengali	Indo-European	Bengali	189	Bangladesh, Eastern India
6	Hindi	Indo-European	Devanagari	182	North and Central India
7	Portuguese	Indo-European	Latin	170	Brazil, Portugal, Southern Africa
8	Russian	Indo-European	Cyrillic	170	Russia, Central Asia
9	Japanese	Altaic	Chinese Characters and 2 Japanese Alphabets	125	Japan
10	German	Indo-European	Latin	98	Germany, Austria, Central Europe
11	Wu	Sino-Tibetan	Chinese Characters	77	China
12	Malay, Indonesian	Malayo-Polynesian	Latin	76	Indonesia, Malaysia, Singapore
13	Korean	Altaic	Hangul	75	Korean Peninsula
14	French	Indo-European	Latin	72	France, Canada, West Africa, Central Africa
15	Turkish	Altaic	Latin	69	Turkey, Central Asia
16	Vietnamese	Austroasiatic	Based on Latin	68	Vietnam, China
17	Telugu	Dravidian	Telugu	67	Southern India
18	Cantonese	Sino-Tibetan	Chinese Characters	66	Southern China
19	Marathi	Indo-European	Devanagari	65	Western India
20	Tamil	Dravidian	Tamil	63	Southern India
21	Italian	Indo-European	Latin	59	Italy, Central Europe
22	Urdu	Indo-European	Nastaliq	58	Pakistan, India

A *national language* is a language (or dialect) which represents the national identity of a nation or country. An *official language* is the language used for political and legal issues, and is designated by a country's government. National languages are often also official languages. Some countries claim to have more than one national language. Spain, for example, recognizes Galician as one of Spain's four official languages, the others being Castilian (also called Spanish), Catalan, and Basque. Galician is spoken by more than 3 million people, but geographically is rather limited to the autonomous community of Galicia. It is the national language in Galicia, and it is also the national language for the Galicians living in different South American countries. A national language is transmitted from parents to children during several generations. Chinese can be regarded as a national language for the Chinese-Canadian community in Canada, and Romany is a national language in many countries. Yiddish is a national language for many Jews.

The national languages of stateless nations are often not official languages in any country (e.g., Romany language). Some have no government recognition, while others may enjoy a high degree of official recognition. Examples of national languages that are not official languages are Cherokee and Navajo (and other living Amerindian languages). In Colombia, on the other hand, there is only one official language (Spanish), but a diversity of Amerindian languages are recognized in different Indian communities. Tagalog is recognized as the official language in the Phillipines (English is also recognized), but in the country there are more than 170 spoken languages. These are national languages for the different Philippine communities.

Degree of Bilingualism in Different Countries

The degree of bilingualism is highly variable across different countries. There are countries with hundreds of different languages, and there are countries with just a few languages. The extreme examples are Papua New Guinea (about 5 million inhabitants) with 820 different languages, and Cuba (about 11 million inhabitants) with only one language. Cuba indeed might be regarded as the only monolingual country in the world. In Cuba, as a matter of fact three languages are listed (Spanish, Lucumi and Cuban sign language) (*http://www.ethnologue.com/show_country.asp?name=CU*). However, Lucumi (or Yoruba) is a sacred language used only for ritual purposes in the Santeria religion. There are no native speakers. There are no estimates about the users of Cuban sign language. So, strictly speaking, in Cuba only one language is *spoken*.

Frequently the Greenberg's diversity index (Lieberson, 1981) is used to describe the level of linguistic diversity in a country. This index indicates the probability that any two people of the country randomly selected would have different native languages. The highest possible value, 1, indicates total diversity (that is, no two people have the same native language) while the lowest possible value, 0, indicates no diversity at all (that is, everyone has the same native language). The computation of the diversity index is based on the population of each language as a proportion of the total population. This index refers to the language diversity simultaneously considering the total country population and the number of speakers of the different languages; in consequence, it is not equivalent to the number of languages that are spoken in that particular country. Some examples of linguistic diversity are presented in Table 3

Who is a Bilingual?

Bilingualism can be defined in different ways. Bilingualism is understood as involving two languages: a person who can communicate using two different languages. Bilingual individuals are all those people who use two or more languages or dialects in their everyday life (Fabbro, 1999). According to Grosdjean (1982) over 50% of the world population is bilingual. Some authors estimate the number of bilinguals even as high as 80% of the world population (Porch and Berkeley-Wykes, 1985).

Table 3. Index of linguistic diversity and number of anguages spoken in some selected countries

Country	Index	Number of languages
Papua New Guinea	0.990	820
Ethiopia	0.843	86
Thailand	0.753	83
Belize	0.693	12
Bolivia	0.680	39
Israel	0.665	48
Canada	0.549	145
Spain	0.438	20
USA	0.353	311
France	0.272	95
Mexico	0.135	297
Colombia	0.030	83
Portugal	0.022	8
Cuba	0.001	3

However, bilinguals represent a tremendously heterogeneous group. If the two languages are used in the everyday life, the term *active* bilingualism can be applied, contrasting with *passive* (*dormant*) bilingualism, when one of the languages is not used. The terms bilingual and trilingual are used to describe comparable situations in which two or three languages are involved. A person who speaks more than two languages is called *multilingual*. For simplicity, frequently the term bilingualism is used to refer to the ability to speak more than one language (two, three or more languages)

Bilingual speakers have acquired at least one language during childhood, the so-called mother tongue, or native language, or first language (L1). Bilingual speakers have the ability to use an extra language. This extra language can be referred to as L2.

Causes of Bilingualism

People may become bilingual either by acquiring two languages at the same time in childhood (*simultaneous bilingualism*) or by learning a second language sometime after acquiring their first language (*successive bilingualism*).

There are different social and personal reasons to become bilingual: because of migrating to another country, because temporarily living in a different linguistic environment, because of living in areas between two countries of mixed languages (e.g., the Mexican-American frontier), because parents each speak a different language, or because of living in bilingual society. A person can decide to learn a second language becoming bilingual. Some specific schools, activities, and jobs may require the person to learn a second and even a third language.

Many bilingual people grow up speaking two languages. This is a common situation in cases of immigrants' children; it is not uncommon to speak one language at school or work and another language at home. Children can also become bilingual if their parents speak more than one language to them or if someone else in the immediate social environment (such as the grandparents or babysitter) speaks another language. Sometimes a child grows up in a household in which each parent speaks a different language; in that case, the child may learn to speak to each parent in that parent's language; e.g., to the father in Chinese and to the mother in French. In short, a child exposed to two languages early in life will most likely become a fluent native speaker of both languages.

It is also possible to learn a second language sometime after early childhood, but the older you are, the harder it is to learn to speak a new language as well as a native speaker. Many linguists believe there is a 'critical period' (lasting roughly from birth until puberty) during which a child can easily acquire any language to which s/he is regularly exposed (Lennenberg, 1967). This simply means that it is much easier to learn a second language during childhood than as an adult.

In some countries, nearly everybody is bilingual or multilingual. In parts of India, for example, a small child usually knows several languages. In many European countries (e.g., the European Union), children are encouraged to learn a second and even a third language. Some countries clearly reinforce the ability to speak several languages (e.g., Israel). In many countries world wide speaking a second language implies certain social prestige and increases the likelihood to perform some qualified activities and jobs.

Types of Bilingualism

Some variables are considered crucial to pinpoint the degree of bilingualism: age and sequence of acquisition, method of acquisition, language of schooling, contexts of the two languages, patterns of use of the two languages, personal and social attitudes toward each language (e.g., Albert and Obler, 1978; Manuel-Dupont et al., 1992; Kilborn, 1994; Paradis, 1978; Vaid, 1986), and, it could be added, individual differences in verbal abilities. However, these are only general variables, and many variations can be found such was: (1) The age, sequence and method of acquisition are not necessarily correlated with the degree of mastery of each language.. (2) Language of schooling may indeed be a highly significant variable. (3) Personal and social attitudes toward the two languages can present significant variations. (4) Individual differences in the ability to learn a second language have rarely been addressed in the literature on bilingualism. But evidently, very significant differences are observed in the ability to learn and use not only a first, but also a second language (Ardila, 1998).

Bilingualism can be divided according to different criteria, such as mastery of the two languages, and age of acquisition of the second language.

Mastery of the Two Languages

A frequently used distinction in bilingualism refers to the mastery of both languages (Weinreich, 1953). Three situations can be distinguished:

Coordinate bilingualism: the linguistic elements (words, phrases) are all related to their own unique concepts. That means, an English-Spanish bilingual speaker of this type possesses different associations for 'table' and for 'mesa'. There are in consequence two lexical and two semantic systems

Compound bilingualism: speakers of this type attach their linguistic elements (words, phrases) to the same concepts. For them, a 'table' and a 'mesa' are two words for the same concept. There are in consequence two lexical systems but only one semantic system

Subordinate bilingualism: the linguistic elements of one of the speaker's languages are only available through elements of the speaker's other language. This type is typical of, but not restricted to, beginning L2-learners. “mesa” means “table” and table has a certain meaning. There is one semantic system, and lexicon in the second language is accessed using the first language lexicon.

Important to note, a bilingual can simultaneously be classified in more than one category. When learning a second language, its mastery progressively increases.

Time of Acquisition of the Second Language

Bilinguals can be distinguished according to the time of acquisition of the second language (e.g., Bialystok and Hakuta, 1999; Birdsong, 1992; Genesee, and Nicoladis, 1995; DeKeyser, 2000; Flege, 1999)

1. *Simultaneous bilingualism* (some times also named as *authentic bilingualism*). Learning two languages as "first languages" (two native languages). Infants who are exposed to two languages from birth will become simultaneous bilinguals. If exposure to the second language occurs after age 3-5, the term *sequential* bilingual is used.
2. *Early bilingualism*. The second language is acquired before completing the acquisition of the first one; it means, before the age of about 12 years.
3. *Late bilingualism.* The second language is acquired after completing the acquisition of the first one. Second language is learned mediated by the first language. Some times the term *consecutive or successive* bilingualism is used to refer that learning one language after already knowing another.

Some Additional Distinctions

Frequently, some additional distinctions are used in bilingual literature (e.g., Crystal, 1987; Fabbro, 1999; Paradis, 2004; Romaine, 1966).

*Balanced bilingualism***.** Equal proficiency in two languages across a range of contexts. This term usually describes a native-like competence in two languages.

Dominant language. Preferred and best spoken language. Language dominance varies according to the context where those languages are used and even across time

Receptive bilingualism. Being able to understand two languages but express oneself in only one.

Elective, or elitist bilingualism. Persons who choose to study a second language.

Natural, folk or circumstantial bilingualism. People who grow up in communities where several languages are spoken.

Distractive bilingualism. When acquisition of the first language is interrupted and insufficient, or unstructured language input follows from the second language.

*Subtractive bilingualism.*The addition of a second language leads to gradual erosion of competence in the first language.

Additive bilingualism. The speaker adds a second language without any loss of competence to the first language.

Semilingualism. An individual who lacks full competence in either language

Diglossia. A specific relationship between two or more varieties of the same language in use in a speech community in different functions.

Ambilinguism. An individual with native competency in two languages. Some times the term *balanced* bilingualism is used; the latter emphasizes the similar competence in both languages.

Individual multilingualism. An individual who has access to more than one linguistic code as a means of social communication.

Societal multilingualism. Refers to the state of a linguistic community in which two languages are in contact, with the result that two codes can be used in the same interaction and that a number of individuals are bilingual.

Pidgin is a communication system developed among people that do not share the same language, but need to talk for some reason.

Creole language is a pidgin that has become the native language of a community. Pidgin and Creole represent in consequence two steps in the same process (Crystal, 1987).

Dialect refers to a variation (usually -but not only, geographical) in a language that is understandable by other speakers of the same language.

Two Proposed Additional Classifications of Bilingualism

Strong vs. weak bilingualism (i.e. degree of similarity between the two languages). Most of the research on bilingualism has not distinguished the specific languages involved. However, the degree of linguistic similarity or difference between the two languages may be significant. The "*interlinguistic distance*" (James, 1979) between the two languages may also be included as a classification criterion in bilingualism. The linguistic distance between Spanish and Italian is minimal, whereas the linguistic distance between Spanish and Chinese is enormous. I am proposing to name the Spanish-Italian bilingualism as a "weak bilingualism" and to name the Spanish-Chinese bilingualism as a "strong bilingualism". When learning Italian, a Spanish speaker is acquiring just a little bit of new language, whereas when learning Chinese, s/he is learning a lot of new language. Of course, any degree of similarity could exist and "weak" and "strong" bilingualism refers to a continuum. Furthermore, the relative distance could be applied to different levels of the language:

phonology, lexicon, grammar and even prosody. For instance, the phonological distance between Spanish and Greek is mild, but the grammatical distance is large. Conversely, the phonological distance between Spanish and Portuguese is larger than the grammatical distance.

This similarity between the two languages may impact the cerebral representation. It has been suggested that the similarity between both languages can affect the relative rate of language recovery in cases of aphasia (Galloway, 1978; Lebrun, 1976; Whitaker, 1978). It has been proposed that the proximity of structurally similar languages may require additional effort to avoid interference, leading to more separate neural structures (Albert and Obler, 1978). The opposite point of view has also been suggested: the less two languages have in common, the more they are represented separately (Paradis, 1987).

Context-dependent vs. context-independent bilingualism. Any human activity is carried out in a particular context and is associated with a specific type of cognition. Language is the major instrument of cognition. Playing chess, solving a mathematical problem or presenting a lecture about bilingualism, is associated with some perceptual information (spatial, visual, auditory, tactile and even olfactory), some specific motor acts (moving the chess pieces, using a calculator, or writing on the blackboard), and certain cognition. The language used is one of the elements (or the instrument) of the cognition required to carry out that activity. Quite frequently, the bilingual learns to use L1 or L2 in a specific context (e.g., for solving mathematical problems L1 is used, but for teaching L2 is the appropriate language). L1 may be the family language, and for talking about family and home issues L1 is used; conversely, for working, L2 is the required one. Many bilinguals can use L1 or L2 mainly (and even only) within a specific context, but they have difficulties in using it in a context where usually the other language is the appropriate one. It means that quite frequently bilingualism is context-dependent. Rarely, a bilingual is equally capable of using either language in exactly the same contexts. For instance, few bilinguals are equally capable of solving mathematical problems in either language. Simultaneous translators may be an example of bilinguals using two languages in exactly the same context. This distinction is obvious a matter of degree and not a dichotomous distinction. This distinction could be named as "Context-dependent" vs. "context-independent bilingualism" or simple "*dissociated*" (context-dependent) vs. "*associated*" (context-independent) bilingualism. Of course, a particular individual can behave as a context independent bilingual for some activities (both languages can be used in that situation) and context-dependent for some other activities (s/he can use only one language in that situation). Different degrees of context dependency can be found.

Bilingualism Frequency

Most of the world's population is bilingual or multilingual. Grosjean (1982) stated that, bilingualism is present in practically every country in the world, in all social classes, and in all age groups. Just considering that there are about 200 different countries and 6,800 different languages, it is easy to conclude that many people have to be bilingual.

It is difficult to establish a clear criterion for bilingualism. A bilingual individual is not necessarily an ambilingual (an individual with native competency in two languages) but a bilingual of a specific type who, along with other bilinguals of many other different types, can be classified along a continuum. Some bilinguals possess very high levels of proficiency in both oral and spoken language. Others display varying degrees of proficiency in understanding and/or speaking skills, or reading/writing skills, depending on the immediate area of experience in which they are required to use their two languages.

A person able to read in a second language (e.g. French) but unable to use the spoken language is considered to be a particular type of bilingual. That individual has certain receptive competence in a second language. By the same token, a person able to understand a spoken second language but unable to speak or to read/write also represents a specific type of bilingual. Diverse types of bilinguals could be distinguished, emphasizing the heterogeneity of bilingualism.

Bilingualism in the USA

In the United States over 300 different languages are spoken of which 176 are indigenous languages (www.ethnologue.com). Interestingly, the United States does not have an official language; nevertheless, American English is the language used for legislation, regulations, executive orders, federal court rulings, and all other official pronouncements. Many individual states have adopted English as their official language, and several states are officially bilingual: Louisiana (English and French), New Mexico (English and Spanish), Hawaii (Hawaiian English and Hawaiian), and the associate state of Puerto Rico (Spanish and English). Until the 1950s, Pennsylvania was officially bilingual in English and German. Native American languages are official or co-official on many of the US Indian reservations (www.ethnologue.com). In the 2000 Census 46,951,595 persons (17.9%) reported that they speak a language other than English at home (population 5 years and over), and in the 2004 Census the number was 49,632,925 (18.7%).

The *English-Only* movement seeks to establish English as the only official language of the entire nation. However, almost one out of five people in the USA speak a language different than English at home. As observed, this percentage has been progressively increasing during recent years, due very specifically to the migration of Latin American Spanish speakers. Spanish is the second most important language in the USA.

As mentioned, 18.7% (about 50 million people) speak another language -instead of or in addition to English. Spanish-speakers represent about 75% of this group. Simply speaking, 37.5 million people speak Spanish and 12.5 million people speak languages other than English and Spanish. To estimate the number of Spanish-speakers is extremely difficult because of the significant illegal migration: it is calculated that in the country there are some eight million illegal immigrants; Mexicans represent six million; if counting immigrants from other Spanish speaking countries, the number of illegal Spanish-speaking immigrants may be around seven million. So, 37.5 million Spanish speakers may very likely be an underestimate. According to the Census Bureau 2004 in USA there were 40.459.196 people considered Hispanics (about 14% of the total population), and it is assumed that some 90% of Hispanics speak at least some Spanish, Indeed, the United States can be regarded as the fifth most important Spanish speaking country in the world after Mexico (~106 million), Colombia (~44 million), Spain (~43 million), and Argentina (~38 million).

The English and Spanish languages have been in contact for a long time and an interlanguage usually referred to as Spanglish has developed. Spanglish, however, has been rarely approached from the linguistic point of view (Ardila, 2002, 2005). Diverse studies have been devoted to the contact between Spanish and other languages (e.g., Roca and Jensen, 1996; Siguan, 2001; Silva-Corvalán, 1995; Zentella, 1997). Thus, Morales (1995) pointed out that the Spanish particle *se* (reflexive, indeterminate subject) has tended to disappear in Puerto Rican Spanish-English bilinguals, particularly with those who had their primary and secondary schooling in the United States, and those who went to the United States to study or to live after completing their schooling in Puerto Rico. García (1995) refered to the use of the Spanish preposition *en* (in, on) in San Antonio (Texas) under the influence of English. Gutierrez (1995) analyzed the future tense in Spanish of the Southwest American states. He concluded that the morphological form is still used by the speakers to refer to future events in the monolingual variety, but in the bilingual variety the temporal use of this form has been much reduced in favor of the extension of its modal use. Elías-Olivares (1995) observed in Mexican-origin speakers who had resided in Chicago for more than a decade that, despite speakers' weak proficiency in English or their null knowledge of that language, they already exhibit certain phenomena representative of language contact situations, such as loanwords, and semantic extensions. Smead and Clegg (1996) studied the English calques in Chicano Spanish. They concluded that the amount of lexical innovations in the Chicano lexicon English derived would probably be in the range of 7-9%.

Nonetheless, Spanish is not the only language to have contact with English. According to Ethnologue (*http://www.ethnologue.com/show_country.asp?name=US*) in the USA (population 300,000,000) there are 1,900,000 American Indians, not all speaking indigenous languages (1990 census). Spoken languages also include: Adyghe (3,000), Armenian (1,100,000), Assyrian Neo-Aramaic (80,000), Bahamas Creole English, Bahnar, Balkan Romani, Basque (8,108), Belarusan (70,808), Belize Kriol English (40,000), Bengali, Breton (32,722), Bukharic (50,000), Bulgarian, Burmese (1,581), Cajonos Zapotec, Carpathian Romani (18,000), Catalan-Valencian-Balear (40,000), Cebuano, Central Khmer (50,000), Chaldean Neo-Aramaic (80,000), Chru, Corsican, Crimean Turkish, Czech (1,452,812), Danish (194,000), Eastern Cham, Eastern Frisian, Eastern Kanjobal, Eastern Mnong, Eastern Panjabi (100,000), Eastern Yiddish (1,250,000), El Nayar Cora, Estonian (26,610), Fijian Hindustani, Finnish (266,096), French (1,100,000), Garifuna (65,000), Georgian (757), Gheg Albanian (79,829), Greek (458,699), Gujarati, Guyanese Creole English, Haitian Creole French (200,000), Hakka Chinese, Hebrew, Hiligaynon, Hindi (26,253), Hmong Daw (70,000), Hmong Njua (100,000), Hulaulá, Hungarian (447,497), Icelandic (9,768), Ilocano, Indonesian, Irish Gaelic, Italian (906,000), Iu Mien (24,000), Japanese (804,000), Jarai, Judeo-Tunisian Arabic, Kabardian (2,000), Kabuverdianu (400,000), Kalmyk-Oirat, Karachay-Balkar, Khmu, Khuen, Klao, Koho, Korean (1,800,000), Ladin, Ladino, Lahu Shi (2,000), Lao (171,577), Latvian (50,000), Laven, Laz, Lithuanian, Lombard, Luxembourgeois (20,618), Mal, Malay (6,253), Maltese, Mandarin Chinese, Mezquital Otomi, Min Nan Chinese, Mixtepec Mixtec, Najdi Spoken Arabic (193,520), Northern Kurdish, Northern Uzbek, Nung, Parsi (75,000), Peñoles Mixtec, Phu Thai, Piemontese, Pingelapese (500), Polish (3,398,763), Pontic, Portuguese (1,313,424), Rade, Rapa Nui, Romanian (56,590), Samoan (63,104), San Juan Guelavía Zapotec (500), Scottish Gaelic, Senaya (400), Serbian (169,938), Shelta (50,000), Sherpa (500), Silacayoapan Mixtec, Sindhi, Slovak, Slovenian (82,321), South Azerbaijani, Southwestern Caribbean Creole English, Standard German (6,093,054), Swahili (3,991), Swedish (626,102), Sylheti, Tagalog (377,000), Tai Daeng, Tai Dam (3,000), Tatar (7,000), Tày, Thai (14,416), Tibetan (3,000), Tokelauan, Tondano, Tongan (3,000), Tosk Albanian, Traveller Scottish, Turkish (24,123), Turkmen, Turoyo

(5,000), Ukrainian (844,026), Upper Guinea Crioulo (156,000), Upper Ta'oih, Uyghur, Vietnamese (859,000), Vlax Romani (650,000), Western Bru, Western Cham (3,000), Western Farsi (900,000), Western Kanjobal, Western Panjabi, Yalálag Zapotec, Yatzachi Zapotec, Yoruba, Yue Chinese, Zoogocho Zapotec (400), Arabic (3,000,000), Chinese (1,645,000), from the Philippines (1,405,000), South Asians (634,000), speakers of other African, Asian, European, Latin American, and Pacific languages. Approximately 1,000,000 Gypsies use a variety of Romany as a first or second language.

Considering that, (1) in the 2004 Census almost 50 million persons reported that at home they spoke a language different from English; and (2) many native English speakers (data not available) have learned a second language and can speak it at the level to maintain a simple conversation, it could be conjectured that the number of bilinguals in the USA may be significantly over 50 million, may be approaching the level of 80 million (supposing the 10% of the native English speakers have learned a second language to the level of maintaining a simple conversation. This percentage does not seem excessive, considering that in Europe about 45% of the people report that they can speak a second language at the level of maintaining a simple conversation). It can be conjectured in a conservative way that the number of bilinguals in the USA may be estimated between 50 and 80 millions, possible higher.

Policies with regard to bilingualism have changed. During the 18th and 19th centuries bilingualism was common, and there were bilingual education programs pertained to German, French, and the Scandinavian languages. At the mid XX century both under the influence of two World Wars and decreased European immigration, such programs disappeared (Castellanos, 1983).

Bilingual programs devoted to Spanish flourished and then tended to disappear during the mid and late XX century. In the early 1960s the revolution in Cuba brought many Spanish-speaking immigrants to southern Florida. Beginning in 1959, public schools introduced bilingual programs. By 1963, the practice drew national notice for its effectiveness (Gonzalez, 1979). Soon Spanish began to be taught again in the Southwest states. These successful experiences--first in Miami and later in Texas, New Mexico, and California--set the stage for more interest in bilingual education at the federal level (Castellanos, 1983).

In 1968 the Title VII Bilingual Education Act was passed and a new provision of the Elementary and Secondary Education Act of 1965 authorized funds for local school districts. These funds were specifically intended for programs with students who spoke languages other than English. Title VII funded 76 bilingual programs in its first year, and served students who spoke 14 different languages (Blanco, 1978).

Title VII encouraged the development of bilingual education in general. By 1968, 14 states had enacted statutes that permitted bilingual programs, and 13 others passed legislation that mandated them (National Clearinghouse, 1986).

In the 1980s, federal policy toward bilingual education changed. In 1982, lawmakers amended the Title VII legislation to give school districts more flexibility in implementing the goals of bilingual programs, and to offer Title VII projects the option of using English exclusively, if they so chose.

At the state level there have also been changes. Many states with large numbers of Mexican American students whose command of English is limited have repealed (Colorado, in 1984, and California in 1987) or revised (Texas and Illinois in 1983) their bilingual statutes.

The "English-only" movement has affected viewpoints of bilingual education around the whole country. The movement "English-only" seeks to make English the official language of the country and of the various states. Supporters of "English only" argue that many immigrants refuse to learn English, leaving them isolated from mainstream society and dependent on social services. In their view, bilingual education encourages such tendencies among immigrants.

Living with Multiple Languages: The Example of the European Union

Europe is a mosaic of cultures and languages. Creating an European community involved not only a big political, economical and social challenge, but also a major linguistic effort. Currently (2006) European Union has 27 member states. Bulgaria and Rumania joined in 2007, and Turkey is also a candidate and may also become a member in the near future. The proposed European Constitution is officially available in the 23 official languages, and the language of the candidate country (Turkish).

The languages of the European Union are languages used by people within the member states of the European Union. They include the 23 official languages of the European Union plus many others. European Union policy encourages all its citizens to be multilingual; specifically, it encourages them to be able to speak two languages in addition to their mother tongue. A number of European Union funding programs actively promote language learning and linguistic diversity, but the European Union has very limited influence in this area as the content of educational systems remains the responsibility of individual Member States.

The official languages of the European Union are: Bulgarian, Czech, Danish, Dutch, English, Estonian, Finnish, French, German, Greek, Hungarian, Irish (from 1 January 2007), Italian, Latvian, Lithuanian, Maltese, Polish, Portuguese, Romanian, Slovak, Slovene, Spanish and Swedish. All decisions by the institutions are translated into all official languages, and European citizens may contact the institutions and receive a reply in any official language. For top-level meetings, interpreting into any official language is arranged as needed. Simultaneous interpreting between all official languages is always arranged for sessions of the European Parliament and the European Council. Away from these formal meetings, a more flexible language régime is followed. The primary working languages of the institutions are English, French and to some extent German, but other languages are used as befits the situation and the language skills of the people involved. The 1995 and 2004 expansion of the Union to countries where French is less used have strengthened the position of English and German as working languages.

There has been a suggestion in an official briefing that the implicit principle for official languages of the European Union is that each member state can put forward at most one official language ('one member state, one language'). This has not been confirmed in documents.

The Spanish and Irish governments have sought the status of 'official' EU languages for Basque, Catalan, Galician and Irish. The 2667th Council Meeting of the Council of the European Union in Luxembourg on 13 June 2005 decided to authorize limited use at EU level languages recognized by Member States other than the official working languages. Besides making Irish the 21st official language, the council also granted recognition to "languages other than the languages referred to in Council Regulation No 1/1958 whose status is recognised by the Constitution of a Member State on all or part of its territory or the use of which as a national language is authorized by law." The official use of such languages will be authorized on the basis of an administrative arrangement between the Council and the requesting Member State

Besides the languages of Spain, there are other regional languages spoken within the European Union that do not have official recognition at EU level (although they may have some official status within the member state). Some of these have many more speakers than some of the lesser-used official languages. These include: Esperanto, the regional languages of France, Frisian, Ladin, Limburgisch language, Low German, Luxembourgish, Mirandese, Russian, Sami languages, Sorbian languages, Minority languages in Sweden, Languages in the United Kingdom (Scottish, Gaelic, Welsh, Scots, Ulster Scots) and Walloon language (http://en.wikipedia.org/wiki/Languages_of_the_European_Union)

Some interesting facts should be highlightened. English is the language which is most widely "spoken" in the European Union. While it is the mother tongue for 16% of the European population, a further 31% of the European Union citizens speak it well enough to hold a conversation. French is spoken by 28% of the population, of which more than half are native speakers. Italian is the fourth most widely known language - it has as many native speakers as French, while the proportion of non-native speakers is significantly smaller (2%). Fefteen percent of the European Union population speaks Spanish (11% as mother tongue and 4% as a foreign language). Forty-five percent of European citizens can take part in a conversation in a language other than their mother tongue The proportion who can take part in a conversation in a language other than their mother tongue ranges from 77% of students to only 19% of people who left school by the age of 15 or younger (average = 45%).

CONCLUSION

Bilingualism is represented throughout the human history and continues to be represented in the contemporary world as a most important cultural, social and psychological phenomenon. At least half of the population with speech and language disorders is bilingual.

Bilingualism, however, has a tremendous variability from the geographical and individual point of view. In some countries dozens (even hundreds) of different languages are used, but linguistic diversity is notoriously heterogeneous across the different countries. There is barely one single monolingual country in the world. Individual mastery of a second language is also highly variable, and bilingual individuals can be classified according to different criteria (e.g., mastery of the second language, age of acquisition, etc.). Socially and individually, variability represents a core issue in bilingualism.

Social attitude toward bilingualism is also highly variable. Whereas some countries strongly encourage bilingualism (e.g., European Union countries), some other countries try to move to the use of a single language (e.g., the USA).

REFERENCES

Albert, M. and Obler, L. (1978). *The bilingual brain*. New York: Academic Press.

Ardila, A. (1998). Bilingualism: A neglected and chaotic area. *Aphasiology, 12*, 131-134.

Ardila, A. (2002). Spanish-English bilingualism in the United States of America. In F. Fabbro (Ed*), Advances in the neurolinguistics of bilingualism. Essays in honor of Michel Paradis*, pp. 47-69. Udine (Italy): Forum

Ardila, A. (2005). Spanglish: An anglicized Spanish dialect. *Hispanic Journal of Behavioral Sciences, 27,* 60-81

Bialystok, E., and Hakuta, K. (1999). Confounded age: Linguistic and cognitive factors in age differences for second language acquisition. In D. Birdsong (Ed.), *Second language acquisition and the Critical Period Hypothesis* (pp. 161-181). Mahwah, NJ: Erlbaum.

Birdsong, D. (1992). Ultimate attainment in second language acquisition. *Language, 68,* 706-755.

Blanco, G. (1978). The implementation of bilingual/bicultural programs in the United States. In B. Spolsky (Ed.), *Case studies in bilingual education* (pp. 457-468). Rowley, MA: Newbury House.

Castellanos, D. (1983). *The best of two worlds: Bilingual-bicultural education*. Trenton, NJ: New Jersey State Department of Education.

Crystal, D. (1987). *The Cambridge encyclopedia of language*. Cambridge, MA: Cambridge University Press.

DeKeyser, R. M. (2000). The robustness of critical period effects in second language acquisition. *Studies in Second Language Acquisition, 22,* 499-533.

Dupont, S., Ardila, A., Rosselli, M. and Puente, A. Neuropsychological assessment in bilinguals. In: A.E. Puente, and R.J. McCaffrey (eds), *Handbook of Neuropsychological Assessment: A Biopsychosocial Perspective* (pp. 193-210). New York: Plenum Press.

Dutcher, N.(1994). *The use of first and second languages in education: A review of educational experience*. Washington, DC: World Bank, East Asia and the Pacific Region, Country Department III.

Elías-Olivares, L. (1995). Discourse strategies of Mexican American Spanish. In C. Silva-Corvalán (ed) *Spanish In four continents. Studies on language contact and bilingualism*, pp. 227-240. Washington, DC: Georgetown University Press *en.wikipedia.org/wiki /Languages_of_the_European_Union*

Fabbro, F. (1999). *The neurolinguistics of bilingualism.* Hove, UK: Psychology Press.

Flege, J. E. (1999). Age of learning and second-language speech. In D. Birdsong (Ed.), *Second language acquisition and the Critical Period Hypothesis* (pp. 101-131). Mahwah, NJ: Erlbaum.

Galloway, L. (1978). Language impairment and recovery in polyglot aphasia: A case of a heptaglot. In: M. Paradis (ed), *Aspects of bilingualism* (pp. 139-148) Columbia, SC: Hornbeam Press

García, M.E. (1995) *En los sábados, en la mañana, en veces:* A look at *en* in the Spanish of San Antonio. In C. Silva-Corvalán (ed) *Spanish In four continents. Studies on language contact and bilingualism*, pp. 196-213. Washington, DC: Georgetown University Press.

Genesee, F., and Nicoladis, E. (1995). Language development in preschool bilingual children. In E. Garcia and B. McLaughlin (Eds), *Meeting the Challenge of Linguistic and Cultural Diversity in Early Childhood Education*. New York: Teachers College Press.

Gonzalez, J. (1979). Coming of age in bilingual education: A historical perspective. In H. Trueba and C. Barnett-Mizrahi (Eds.), *Bilingual-multicultural education and the professional* (pp. 7-10). Rowley, MA: Newbury House.

Grosjean, F. 1982. *Life with two languages*. Cambridge, MA: Harvard University Press.

James, C.V. (1979). Foreign languages in school curriculum. In G.E. Perren (ed), *Foreign language in education* (pp. 7-28). London: CILT

Kilborn, K. (1994). Learning a language late: Second language acquisition in adults. In M.A. Gernsbacher (Ed.), *Handbook of psycholinguistics* (pp. 917-944). New York: Academic Press.

Lebrun, Y. (1976). Recovery in polyglots aphasics. In: Y. Lebrun and R. Hoops (eds), *Recovery in aphasics* (pp. 96-108). Amsterdam: Swets and Zeitlinger

Lenneberg, E. H. (1967). *Biological foundations of language*. New York: Wiley

Lieberson, S. (1981). *Language Diversity and Language Contact*. Stanford, California: Stanford University Press.

Morales, A. (1995). The loss of the Spanish impersonal particle *se* among bilinguals: A descriptive profile. In C. Silva-Corvalán (ed) *Spanish In four continents. Studies on language contact and bilingualism*, pp. 148-162. Washington, DC: Georgetown University Press.

National Clearinghouse for Bilingual Education. (1986, March). The status of state statutes for language minority students. Forum, pp.1-3.

Paradis, M. (Ed.). (1978). Aspects of bilingualism. Columbia, SC: Hornbeam Press.

Paradis, M. (1987). The assessment of bilingual aphasia. Hillsdale, NJ: Lawrence Erlbaum Associates.

Paradis, M. (2004) *Neurolinguistic Theory of Bilingualism*. Amsterdam: John Benjamins

Porch, B and Berkeley-Wykes, J. (1985). Bilingual aphasia and its implications for cerebral organization and recovery. *Clinical Aphasiology, 15*, 107-112.

Roca, A. and Jensen, B.J. (1996). *Spanish in contact: Issues in bilingualism*. Sommerville: Cascadilla Press.

Romaine, S. (1989). *Bilingualism*. Oxford: Basil Blackwell.

Siguan, M. (2001). *Bilingüismo y lenguas en contacto* [Bilingualism and languages in contact]. Madrid: Alianza Editorial.

Smead, R.N and Clegg, J.H. (1996). English calques in Chicano Spanish. In A. Roca and B.J. Jensen, B.J. *Spanish in contact: Issues in bilingualism*, pp. 123-130. Sommerville: Cascadilla Press.

Silva-Corvalán, C. (1995). (ed) *Spanish In four continents. Studies on language contact and bilingualism*. Washington, DC: Georgetown University Press.

Vaid, J. (Ed.). (1986). Language processing in bilinguals: Psycholinguistic and neuropsychological perspective. Hillsdale, NJ: Lawrence Erlbaum Associates.

United States Census Bureau. (2000). *United States population*. Washington, DC: US Census Bureau

United States Census Bureau. (2004). *United States population*. Washington, DC: US Census Bureau

Weber, G. (1997). *Top Languages: The World's 10 Most Influential Languages Language Today*, 3, 12-18,

Weinreich, U. (1953) *Languages in contact: Findings and problems*. New York: Linguistic Circle of New York

Whitaker, H.A. (1978). Bilingualism: A neurolinguistics perspective. In W.C. Ritchie (ed), *Second language acquisition research. Issues and implications* (pp. 21-32). New York: Academic Press.

World Bank. (1995). *Priorities and strategies for education.* Washington, DC: The International Bank for Reconstruction and Development.

www.ethnologue.com/show_serial.asp?name=886

www.ethnologue.com/ethno_docs/distribution.asp?by=size

www.ethnologe.com

www.krysstal.com/spoken.html

www.ethnologue.com/show_country.asp?name=US

www.ethnologue.com/show_country.asp?name=CU

Zentella, A.C. (1997). *Growing up bilingual.* Malden, MA: Blackwell Publishers Inc

In: Speech and Language Disorders in Bilinguals
Editors: Alfredo Ardila and Eliane Ramos, pp. 21-46
ISBN 978-1-60021-560-5

Chapter 2

BRAIN ORGANIZATION OF LANGUAGE IN BILINGUALS

Loraine K. Obler, Jung Moon Hyun, Peggy S. Conner, Barbara O'Connor and Inge Anema
Doctoral Program in Speech and Hearing Sciences
City University of New York Graduate Center, 365 Fifth Avenue
New York City, New York, 10016, USA

I. INTRODUCTION

Several streams of research provide us information about the brains of bilinguals: direct *localizationist* studies, studies that focus on *individual differences*, and studies that focus on specific *languages' structures*. The localizationist approaches ask relatively direct questions about brain organization in bilinguals. We treat those in two sections here: the first, section II, on pre-imaging localizationist approaches, the second, section IV, on localizationist approaches within the past two decades that employ current brain-imaging techniques.

The strictly localizationist approaches to understanding the bilingual brain are complemented by an interesting set of studies that we cover in section III. These focus on *behavioral* studies that identify individual-difference parameters, such as age of L2 acquisition, that, one can assume, reflect factors in brain organization in ways we cannot yet fully understand. Indeed, as we will demonstrate in section IV, the imaging studies incorporate several of these behavioral categories (most notably age of L2 acquisition and proficiency) in their designs as well. Thus it is not always easy to separate out how these localizationist and individual-difference factors interrelate, but we attempt to keep them somewhat separate in this paper, for purposes of exposition.

In the following section of the paper, section V, we discuss the somewhat smaller set of studies of linguistic structures specific to the languages a bilingual speaks that, too, appear to engage differences in brain organization and/or processing, even if we do not know yet precisely what these are.

II. Pre-Imaging Localizationist Approaches

As Fabbro (2001b) reminds us, the scientific debate regarding the localization of language in bilinguals and multilinguals[1] began when localizationism was succeeding phrenology. In 1867, Scoresby-Jackson postulated that a patient's mother tongue was represented in Broca's area, while subsequently learned languages were represented in cortical sites anterior to Broca's area. Scoresby-Jackson's theory of language localization in bilinguals was rejected when Veyrec (1931) reported that the post-mortem brain study of a multilingual speaker revealed no evidence that brain tissue anterior to Broca's area was atypical in formation. However, as Fabbro points out, just because no difference was evidenced upon neuroanatomical inspection, neurofunctional differences that may have operated in Broca's areas, or elsewhere, in bilinguals' brains are not precluded.

In addition to the *post-mortem data*, the bulk of theorizing about bilinguals' brains after this early debate arose from observing cases or series of cases of *aphasia* in bilinguals, and inferring what factors operate in determining brain organization in the two languages. Here we review only those points necessary to understand how aphasia studies addressed questions of bilinguals' brain-organization for language; the reader interested in further information should see Fabbro's chapter (this volume).

As Albert and Obler (1978) pointed out, the patterns of impairment and recovery across the numerous papers on bilinguals with aphasia are so varied that it is not possible to glean a single understanding of either the locations of language processing in 'the' bilingual, or the factors that 'determine' the differing patterns of impairment or recovery seen across bilingual individuals with aphasia. Paradis (1987, 1995), however, articulated the implications of the patterns of recovery from bilingual aphasia that he had identified in 1977 (Paradis, 1977 and in subsequent papers) for pre-morbid language organization in bilinguals' brains. He observed that two hypotheses regarding how language is organized in the brain of bilingual speakers are suggested by the six main patterns of recovery.

The first hypothesis the data support is the " *Extended System Hypothesis,*" which presupposes that subsequently learned languages are superimposed over the same cortical language areas as the patient's first language. The common pattern of *parallel* recovery from aphasia , in which the patient shows equal impairment and parallel recovery of all known languages, is an example of this. The second hypothesis is the " *Dual System Hypothesis,*" which supposes that elements of each language are stored separately and independently, at every possible level: "two independently represented sets of phonemes, morphemes, syntactic rules, etc." (Paradis, 1987, p. 8). This hypothesis, therefore, suggests distinct cortical language areas for each of the patients' languages (Paradis, 1987, 1995). Nonparallel recovery patterns, such as *selective, successive, antagonistic, mixed* and *differential recovery,* support such a dissociation between or among languages, lending clinical support to this hypothesis. For example, if, as in Silverberg and Gordon (1979), a patient with a single left-hemisphere lesion presents with nonfluent aphasia in her native language (Spanish), and fluent aphasia in her second language, L2 (Hebrew), with a more complete recovery of Hebrew, her more-used language, one can conclude that her first language, L1, (Spanish) was

---

[1] Because there is no substantial agreement yet that knowing more than two languages affects brain organization in markedly different ways from knowing only two, we use the term 'bilingualism' at most points in this paper to include multilinguals as well.

focally stored in the left hemisphere, while her more preserved L2 (Hebrew) was diffusely represented in the two cerebral hemispheres.

Paradis proposed both a third and a fourth model, the *Tripartite Systems Hypothesis* which we cover in section V. of this paper, and the *Subsystems Hypothesis* (Paradis, 2004) in which there is redundant representation of a bilingual's language: both a unified single language/cognitive system and subsystems representing each of the languages. This hypothesis Paradis describes as the most comprehensive as it is congruent with all the patterns of recovery in addition to the bilingual individual's ability to access the elements of both languages at each level of linguistic structure. Both parallel impairment in aphasia or differential impairment can be explained by this hypothesis.

Clearly, Paradis's categories do not yield mutually exclusive theories of which only one can hold. Rather, it would appear that different individuals manifest different patterns of recovery from aphasia, which may simply reflect micro-level differences in the brain-damage leading to aphasia, but, more likely, reflect differences in the way the two or more language were acquired and maintained, resulting in slightly differing brain systems underlying their pre-morbid processing. Before we turn to the factors that have been discussed with respect to such individual differences, let us consider the other topics that have arisen vis-à-vis localization of language in the bilingual: studies of lateralization, and studies of specific differences within the left hemisphere.

In the mid-20th century, when *lateral dominance* was of great interest to discussions of language localization in monolinguals, it became a question of interest concerning language localization in bilinguals as well. Gloning and Gloning (1965) and April and Tse (1977) thought they observed an unduly greater proportion of crossed aphasia—aphasia in a right-hander resulting from a right-hemisphere lesion— in bilingual speakers than had been reported for monolinguals. This would have suggested more right-hemisphere involvement in language processing among the bilinguals than among otherwise comparable monolinguals. Comparisons of consecutive cases (e.g., as in Charlton, 1964), however, suggest that, rather, such cases are more likely to get reported than they are to occur. Thus, on the basis of incidence of crossed aphasia, one would have to conclude that there is no more right-hemisphere involvement for language for bilinguals than for monolinguals.

In addition to studies of aphasia, techniques like dichotic listening and tachistoscopic presentation that were employed to study laterality in normal individuals were applied to various groups of bilinguals, with confusing results vis-à-vis the laterality issues. In a series of studies reviewed in Obler et al. in 1982, the methodological problems in the studies conducted to that time were deemed so great as to render the question unanswered. In a more recent review, Hull and Vaid (2005) conclude that there is greater right-hemisphere participation for earlier-learned second languages than for later ones. Albert and Obler (1978) had suggested, by contrast, that the right hemisphere could be particularly involved in early stages of second-language acquisition. In any event, while lateral dominance studies account for a lower proportion of studies of either monolingual or bilingual brain organization for language today than they once did, there may still be interesting subtleties to discover in the relative contributions of the two cerebral hemispheres to language organization and processing in the bilingual.

By the 1970 and 1980s, localizationist interest turned from lateral dominance to the question of what happens *within the left hemisphere* of the bilingual. Cortical stimulation techniques permitted Ojemann and Whitaker (1978) to suggest, based on two case studies, that the first-learned language was more narrowly distributed in the peri-Sylvian language region, while the second-learned language was more broadly distributed. While Whitaker pulled back from this position somewhat (personal communication), the focus on areas in and around the left-hemisphere cortical areas commonly associated with language has continued, as we shall see in section IV.

III. Individual-Differences Approaches

To address the issue of individual differences, we must step back chronologically to the beginnings of modern neurolinguistics with the early aphasiologists of the end of the 19th century. Localizationists were battling holists –those neurologists who eschewed localization, preferring to consider the brain a unified entity— at this time and researchers interested in bilingual patients began proposing *behavioral* explanations for how the bilingual brain is organized. The first of these was *order of acquisition* of the two or more languages. In his 1881 essay titled *Les maladies de la mémoire*, Ribot proposed that the language learned earliest in life would be the first to recover in a patient with bilingual aphasia. Later termed *Ribot's rule*, this position proposes that the native language would recover first because the first learned language is *overlearned* and thus less susceptible to loss following brain damage (Paradis, 1995). *Ribot's rule* was supported by Freud (1891), who added that a lesion in the brain would never affect a native language and spare a subsequently learned language. Freud asserted that a later learned language, as a "superimposed set of associations" (p. 61) would be impaired before the primary associations created by the learning of the mother tongue.

Ribot's rule was challenged by Pitres, a French physician and professor of anatomy, physiology and clinical medicine at the Faculty of Medicine in Bordeaux. Pitres (1895) argued that the rule of Ribot was inadequate to explain all cases of nonparallel recovery in bilingual aphasia. He described a series of clinical cases in the literature in which Ribot's rule did not hold.

In his 1895 article, Pitres proposed that the most *familiar* and most *used* language prior to the stroke would have the most stable cortical associations and would therefore be the first language to recover. In other words, the language that the patient was using most routinely and immediately prior to the onset of aphasia would be expected to recover first; this was because this "overused" language had the most solidly established cortical associations. This could be the patient's native language, or a language learned later in life. In several of the clinical cases highlighted in his 1895 paper, the language of the environment also seemed to have a decisive influence on the linguistic recovery and the order of restitution of languages.

As Albert and Obler (1978) pointed out, researchers such as Krapf (1957, in Paradis, 1983) and Swiss neurologist Minkowski (1963) reported on clinical cases that did not fit either *Ribot's rule* or *Pitres' rule*. They postulated that the *affect* and emotional valence associated with a language for a patient would influence which language would recover first. Krapf suggested that the patients' personal situation prior to lesion onset and the emotional significance of the various languages in patients' life history would influence how patients' languages recover from aphasia. In particular, if the native language returns first, he suggested that this would represent for that patient "the special need to communicate with the first guardian of their vital interests; in other words, with their mother" (Paradis, 1983, p.

571). If the patient had a poor relationship with the maternal figure in his or her life, then a non-native language that "provides a feeling of security" (Paradis, 1983, p. 571) would recover first.

By the middle of the 20th century, as the field of applied linguistics developed, certain psychologists took an interest in language, second-language teaching became a discipline of academic study, and a number of additional factors were nominated as related to second-language acquisition and its intended product, bilingualism. Additionally, those such as order of acquisition that had been mentioned in the 19th century were given new attention.

Age of Acquisition considerations, one might argue, hearken back to Ribot's19th-century beliefs about the importance of order of acquisition in brain-organization for bilinguals' language. However, for Ribot, order was the crucial issue, whereas for Penfield (1953) and for Lenneberg (1967) a *critical period* for second-language learning was available before puberty. Since they raised the issue, researchers have identified different critical periods past which native-like pronunciation and grammatical usage in the second language is unusual. Birdsong and Molis (2001) and Birdsong (2005) discuss these critical periods and neural plasticity in second language acquisition. Rather than identifying a specific limit, both articles emphasize age as a continuum that negatively correlates with linguistic attainment; thus for many, the term *sensitive period* has replaced that of *critical period.* Other factors that may constrain native-like fluency are the type of languages paired together and second language frequency and context of use. (See Hyltenstam and Abrahamsson (2003) for a detailed critical review of this topic)

In a return to studies of cognitive abilities and emotional contributions to second-language learning, Abu-Rabia and Kehat (2004) investigated the critical period hypothesis in ten cases of individuals with native-like pronunciation in Hebrew although they were later learners with a range of L2 acquisition from the ages of 7 to 40 years. The variables that seemed to impact language proficiency were the *amount and type of L2 use* (informal, formal), individual *motivation, awareness, ability to self-monitor,* and *learning style.*

Beyond the early notions of native-language status, language use and emotional significance of a language, and their respective influence on language localization and recovery from aphasia, language *automaticity* and *type of bilingualism* have also been proposed as factors that influence language localization and organization in bi- and multilingual speakers' brains. In a precise contradiction of Pitres, Kainz (1960, in Paradis, 1983) proposed that the language most vulnerable to aphasia in bi-and multilingual speakers was the language that was most automatic and used most unconsciously. He stated that we converse in the native language automatically, without conscious reflection, whereas a later learned language, which requires more volitional and conscious effort to use, "delivers a stronger stimulus to the impaired apparatus" (Paradis, 1983, p. 637).

Type of bilingualism, reflecting the manner of acquisition of the two or more languages, with particular focus on the coordinate vs. compound bilingual dichotomy, was investigated by Lambert and Fillenbaum (1959, available in Paradis, 1983). They hypothesized that coordinate bilinguals, who learned their languages at different times in life, would have their languages controlled by more "functionally separated neural structures" (Paradis, 1983, p. 626) than compound bilinguals, who learned two or more languages simultaneously. If this were the case, then coordinate bilinguals would always evidence nonparallel aphasia recovery profiles, while compound bilinguals would evidence parallel aphasia recovery profiles.

Paradis (1995) critiqued this hypothesis, claiming a lack of definitive clinical cases in support of this hypothesis, even from the authors' own research.

Particular *talent* or lack thereof in second language acquisition has been another individual-difference factor that has entered the discussion. Schneiderman and Desmarais (1988) fleshed out how Geschwind and Galaburda's (1985) theory of brain organization for talent might underlie exceptional adult second-language learners, and in the same book (Obler and Fein, 1988), Novoa et al. (1988) provided a cognitive-neuropsychological case study of a talented learner as evidence in support of the theory. Since that time, Sparks et al. (e.g., 1999) have elaborated on the particular difficulties adults with learning differences may have in learning a second language, and Ijalba (in preparation) demonstrates that even adults who have not been diagnosed as dyslexic but bear the symptoms of it may show particular difficulty acquiring a second language in adulthood. Indeed, consistent with Geschwind and Galaburda's hypothesis that neuronal-level differences underlie both dyslexia and talent, Lamm and Epstein (1989) demonstrated both gender-differences (in favor of girls) and handedness differences (in favor of right-handers) between normal and particularly poor English-learning Hebrew-speaking adolescents.

In her discussion of the neural architecture implicated in talented second-language learning, Kalbfleisch (2004) includes connections between the limbic system and the prefrontal cortex. Subcortical structures such as the basal ganglia, thalamus, and cerebellum show as much evidence of activation in demanding cognitive-specific tasks as do interhemispheric connections and higher-level corticocortical circuits. Strong working memory, processing speed and advanced visuo-spatial skills are all dependent on rich afferent and efferent neural networking.

Indeed, working memory has been linked to an unusual facility with language acquisition. A component of working memory crucial in language performance is what Baddley et al. (1998) describe as the phonological loop, an on-line storage mechanism to hold unfamiliar sound patterns in memory while more permanent sound-word connections are being made. Multilingual individuals provide us with an opportunity to examine the strength of phonological and other types of working memory in language performance, and how these cognitive skills are neuroanatomically mediated. In fact one of the criticisms of studies purporting to show differential mediation for various languages is that the differences seen in neuro-imaging research could be a reflection of memory skills or other extra-linguistic cognitive abilities. (Price, et al., 1999; Paradis, 2004).

Of course language expertise and working memory are particularly taxed in *simultaneous interpretation*, the job requiring professionals to listen to speech in one language and translate it, while listening, into another. Christoffels et al. (2005) compared trained Dutch-English interpreters, bilingual university students and bilingual teachers of English. Speed, accuracy and memory abilities distinguished the interpreters from the university students, however only on memory tasks did the interpreters outperform the English teachers. The authors concur with earlier studies that working memory is necessary for simultaneous translating but again pose the question of whether interpreters self-select for inherent talent or develop their talent during practice on their jobs. Indeed, Signorelli (in preparation) suggests that with advancing age, simultaneous interpreters may lose their working-memory advantage over comparable non-interpreter multilinguals. That they continue to function well in their profession suggests that practice enables them to develop skills that compensate for the diminishing of working memory associated with age.

Having discussed the issues covered in individual-differences work, we can turn to conclude our localizationist review with the literature of the 1990s and first years of the 21st century: the literature on brain imaging and what it appears to have taught us about organization of the bilingual brain. As the reader will see, practitioners of these techniques often incorporate certain of the individual-differences factors into their imaging designs.

IV. Imaging the Bilingual Brain

For the past two decades, brain-imaging techniques such as magnetic resonance imaging (MRI) and positron emission tomography (PET), have been acknowledged as useful tools for the study of neurologically intact brains. With respect to language, the primary focus has been to investigate brain activation as it relates to specific language tasks in monolinguals. Both PET and fMRI (functional MRI) techniques enable researchers to track brain activity when a healthy participant is engaged in specific language tasks, e.g. reading correct and anomalous sentences, in real time. These two techniques use regional cerebral blood flow (rCBF) to demonstrate both location and level of activity. In an area of the brain that is active, synaptic activity, which requires energy, will be present. As a result of the synaptic activity, an increase in blood flow will occur.

For a PET scan, a person ingests or is injected with a slightly radioactive substance that emits positrons (i.e. positive electrons), which can be tracked. When this radioactive substance is added to glucose, the fuel of our brains, PET scans show levels of brain activity as well. As the resolution of PET scans has improved, researchers have used this technique to discover which parts of the brain a person uses to perform specific tasks and the related level of activity of each part.

Functional, real time features of the MRI technique rest on the magnetic properties of hemoglobin, oxygen metabolism, and blood flow. By using the blood oxygenation level dependence (BOLD) contrast, deoxygenated (paramagnetic) blood and oxygenated (diamagnetic) blood distort a static magnetic field differently.

Both PET and fMRI techniques use a subtraction method to determine what part of the brain is engaged in a particular language task. For such imaging studies, two sets of images are compared, namely, brain activity during a control state and brain activity during the experimental language task. Fundamental to a strong imaging study are the carefully selected control state and the experimental language task. A drawback of the subtraction method is the fact that language tasks are inherently complex and activation patterns can not always reliably be related to specific language aspects or tasks. Even at the single-word level, imaging experiments result in extensive activation at both cortical and subcortical levels (Raichle, 1996). In studies of monolinguals, imaging work tends to reinforce that the traditional peri-Sylvian language area is involved in language production and comprehension, but, in addition, it often implicates subcortical areas whose contributions to language had been less often studied until the advent of imaging. Even the roles of the traditional left-hemisphere language areas have been expanded through the use of brain imaging; most notably, Broca's area seems to be involved not only in language production, but in syntactic and lexical processing for comprehension as well (Binder et al., 1997). A series of studies has returned to discussion of right-hemisphere contributions to language processing as well (e.g., Just et al., 1996).

Regarding bilingualism, fMRI and PET studies have focused on the questions the bilingual aphasia literature led researchers to, as we discussed above: the extent of overlap or differentiation between the language areas responsible for each of the bilingual's languages. As detailed below, many studies have reported that later acquired languages may involve broader activation locations than the first acquired language. As we said above, although these studies do not all reach precisely the same conclusions, the evidence from them generally suggests that largely overlapping but sometimes distinct cortical areas are involved in the comprehension and production of first and second languages. In designing imaging studies of bilinguals, moreover, the researchers often investigate not only the neural basis of second language processing and its relationship to first-language processing; they also incorporate the questions of how a number of the individual-differences factors we discussed above are reflected in inter-individual patterns of brain organization for language. Their findings with respect to age of L2 acquistion, degree of proficiency, exposure to the L2, different language tasks, and working memory are covered in sections IV.B,C,D,E and F respectively.

IV a. Cerebral Activation in First Versus Second Languages

A large number of studies have focused on the question of whether cortical representation for two languages is shared or separate. Whereas some studies have described differences in topographic activation between L1 and L2 processing (Perani et al., 1996; Dehaene et al., 1997; Kim et al., 1997; Pillai et al., 2003), a number of other studies have supported shared cortical activation areas (Klein et al., 1994, 1995, 1999; Perani et al., 1998; Chee et al., 1999). The most distinct cortical activation was reported in an fMRI study in which participants used widely different L1 and L2 pairs of languages, such as English-French, Korean-English and Spanish-English. While silently describing to themselves what they did during the morning, afternoon or evening of the previous day, late bilinguals showed different activation between L1 and L2, and these differences were only found in the left inferior frontal cortex, i.e. in Broca's area (Kim et al., 1997).

Another manifestation of differential activation is seen in the several studies that have reported that the native language showed fewer activation locations than did second languages (Yetkin et al., 1996; Chee et al., 2001; Luke et al., 2002). However, other studies reported greater activation in the first language (Perani, et al., 1996; Dehaene et al., 1997; Halsband et al., 2002)

Using PET, Perani et al. (1996) studied nine late bilinguals who acquired their second language after age seven. Participants were asked to listen to stories in L1, L2 and an unknown language. Partially different cerebral substrates were active for the L1 and L2. While the were listening in L1, the peri-Sylvian language areas; inferior frontal gyrus, the superior and middle temporal gyrus, the temporal pole and angular gyrus and homologous right hemisphere areas were activated,. On the contrary, during L2 listening, only the bilateral superior and middle temporal gyri remained active, whereas other previously active areas showed reduced activation (See Figure 1).

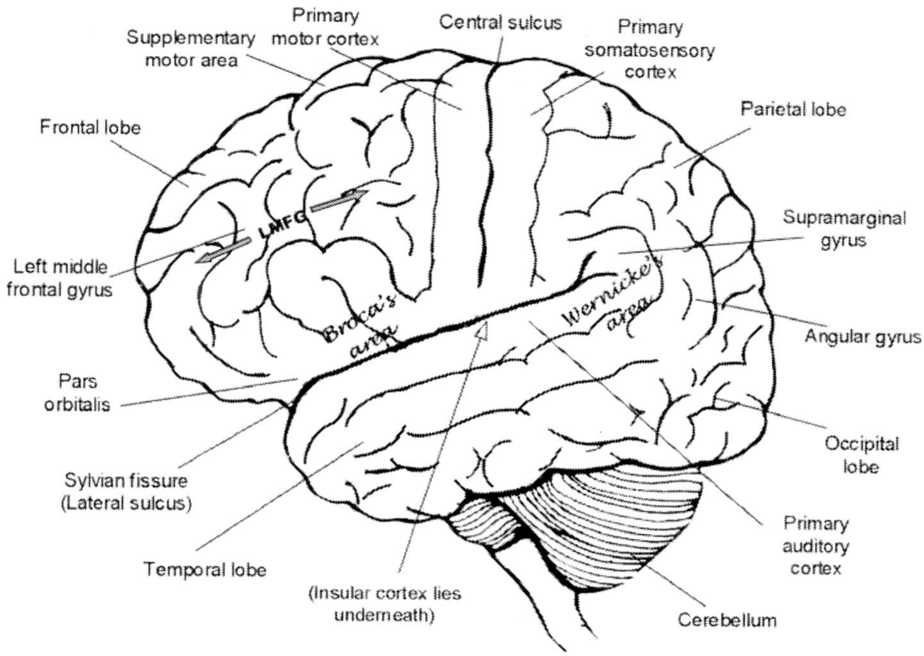

Figure 1. Left cerebral hemisphere, lateral view.

Usually, activation differences between L1 and L2 are reported in cases of late acquisition or low proficiency bilinguals. One infers that variables such as age of second language acquisition, degree of proficiency and effect of daily usage, seem to play a crucial role in activation-pattern differences. In addition, specific task and procedural variables impact results and, thus, the conclusions drawn from imaging and cortical stimulation research.

IV b. Cerebral Activation in Early Bilinguals Compared to Late Bilinguals

As mentioned above, a number of imaging studies have proposed that the pattern of representation for the native and second language may vary in bilinguals, depending upon the age of second language acquisition (Kim et al., 1997; Dehaene et al., 1997; Hernandez et al., 2001). The fMRI study of Dehaene et al. (1997), for example, emphasized the age of acquisition and inter-subject variability in the cortical representation of L2 processing. In this study, participants who had been exposed to L2 after age seven showed common activation areas in left hemisphere during listening to stories in L1. However, in L2 listening they showed very diverse patterns of activation ranging from left hemisphere lateralization to complete right hemisphere dominance.

Conversely, some bilingual-brain studies using PET reported overlapping left hemisphere activation across two languages in participants who learned the second language after age five and were considered highly proficient as adults (Klein et al., 1994, 1995). Similar activation is reported by bilinguals who speak two very different languages, e.g. Chinese and English.

Even though these two languages have markedly different phonological systems and use differing orthographic systems (ideographic and more 'phonemic'), brain activation within similar areas was observed among early and late (after age 12), highly fluent bilinguals (Chee, Tan and Thiel, 1999). Thus, one must consider the possibility that language proficiency plays a more important role than age of acquisition in determining bilingual brain processes..

IV c. Cerebral Activation in Proficient and Non-Proficient Bilinguals

Several authors have proposed that proficiency in each language is responsible for the different cerebral activation patterns that have been reported (Klein et al., 1994, 1995; Perani et al., 1998; Illes et al., 1999; Chee at al., 1999, 2001; De Bleser et al., 2003; Briellmann et al., 2004). An fMRI study by Perani et al.(1998) showed that degree of mastery of L2 is a more crucial determinant of brain activation than age of acquisition. Comparing highly proficient early bilingual and highly proficient late bilinguals who learned their L2 after age 10, Perani et al, reported no differences in the areas of activation on a listening task. Both groups showed overlapping activation patterns in the left superior and middle temporal gyri and in the bilateral temporal poles. A similar conclusion was drawn from many other studies, even in the case of bilinguals who had moderate proficiency in their L2 (e.g., Hasegawa et al., 2002) and these results suggest that despite the late age of second language acquisition, proficient bilinguals activate similar cortical areas for L1 and L2.

However, conflicting findings are also reported in some articles: namely, that late bilinguals who have high or moderate proficiency in L2 show different activation in L1 compared to L2 in some language tasks. (Perani et al., 1996; Dehaene et al., 1997; Kim et al., 1997; Hernandez, Martinez and Kohnert, 2000; De Bleser et al., 2003). To investigate the importance of proficiency, De Bleser et al. (2003) studied cognate and noncognate words in a lexical retrieval task in L1 and L2 using PET. Participants in this study were 11 late bilinguals who are not native-like but have good proficiency. Overlapping activation patterns for cognate naming in both L1 and L2 and for noncognate naming in L1 were evident. By contrast, for noncognate naming in L2, more extended brain activation was observed in the left prefrontal area.

One recent fMRI study, conducted by Watenburger et al. (2003), was designed to elucidate how age of acquisition and proficiency influence the cortical representation of grammatical and semantic judgments in L2. In this study, both late high-proficient and late low-proficient bilinguals who acquired L2 after age six evidenced differential activation in Broca's area and various subcortical structures for grammatical processing when L2 was compared to L1. However, during a semantic judgment task, only late low proficient bilinguals showed greater activation in the left frontal gyrus. Based on these results, the authors concluded that age of L2 acquisition has a more pronounced effect on the neural representation of grammatical processing and that degree of proficiency is more crucial for semantic processing.

IV d. The Role of Exposure and Usage of L2

Recently, it has been argued that not only age of acquisition or proficiency, but also the role of environmental exposure on cerebral language representation should be taken into consideration when studying brain activation in bilinguals. Using fMRI, Perani et al. (2003) addressed this issue in two groups of early-acquisition, high-proficiency bilinguals using lexical search and retrieval tasks. Their participants were six Spanish-speaking and five Catalan-speaking bilinguals who acquired their second language (Catalan and Spanish respectively) just after the age of three when children first attend school, and were living in Catalonia where Catalan was used in everyday social contexts. Thus, the two groups were only different in terms of amount of daily L2 usage; the exposure to L2 (Spanish) was less for the Catalan native speakers than it was, mutatis mutandi, for the native Spanish speakers. More extensive activation was seen in the left dorsolateral frontal area when the Catalan native-speakers produced words in Spanish. This finding may be an indication that language exposure and usage can influence the neural organization in early, high proficient bilinguals.

IV e. Cerebral Activation Patterns in Different Language Components and Tasks

Whether the tasks targeted lexical, semantic or syntactic performance, the majority of studies show that early bilinguals activate overlapping cortical areas when processing L1 and L2 (Kim et al., 1997; Chee et al., 1999, 2000; Hernandez et al., 2000; Urbanik et al, 2001). This similarity was found in orthographically and phonologically different languages as well. (Chee et al., 1999).

However, some studies have demonstrated that task difficulty contributes to brain activation patterns, and this has ramifications for studies of L2, since imperfect mastery of one's L2 will render performance of many tasks more difficult (Dewaele 2002; Hasegawa et al., 2002; Yokoyama et al., 2006; Klein et al., 2006). Yokoyama et al.(2006) investigated whether late bilinguals employ different cortical networks to process structurally complex sentences in L1 and L2. During a task requiring participants to judge active and passive sentences, differential activation patterns between L1 and L2 were found in the processing of passive sentences. A significant interaction between sentence type and language (L1, L2) in the left pars orbitalis was revealed. The results of this study indicate that late bilinguals use similar neural bases to comprehend both L1 and L2; however, for structurally complex sentences, activation showed differences between L1 and L2. In addition to age of L2 acquisition and proficiency, then, differences in grammatical structure affect cortical activity during the comprehension of L1 and L2.

Recently, using both PET and fMRI techniques with a semantic priming task, Crioion et al. (2006) reported that the left caudate plays an important role in monitoring and controlling lexical selection in bilinguals. In their experiment, highly proficient bilinguals showed greater activation in the head of the left caudate when the prime and target words were in different languages or had different meaning. The authors argued that this result was supported by neuropsychological studies of bilingual patients who had lesions in this area and showed involuntary switching from one language to another (Abutalebi, Miozzo, and Cappa, 2000).

Thus, it is assumed that bilinguals rely on cortical-subcortical circuits to selectively access lexical representation (Abutalebi, Cappa, and Perani, 2001) (See Figure 2).

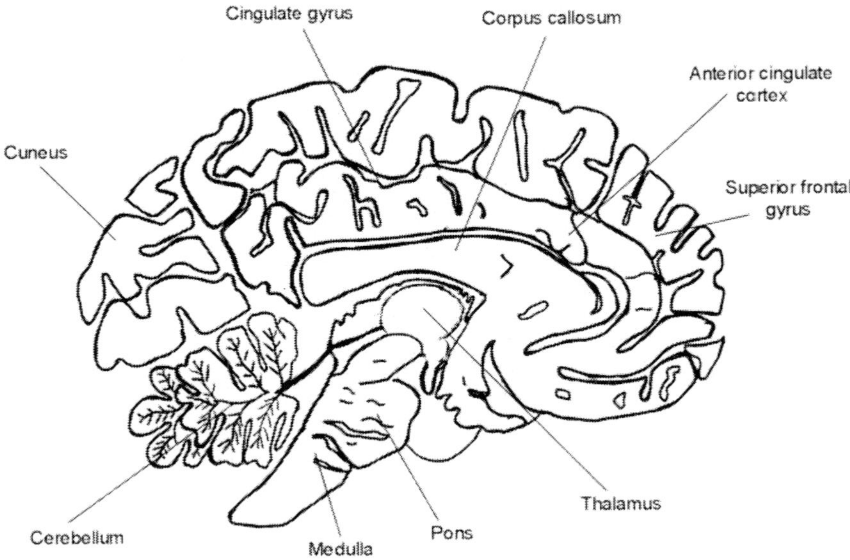

Figure 2. Midsagittal view of left cerebral hemisphere.

IV.f Working Memory

Strong phonological working memory (PWM) as an indicator for one language talent—that of achieving high proficiency—, has been discussed and investigated in several papers. In an fMRI study, Chee et al. (2004) compared two carefully matched groups of bilinguals, one with high proficiency and one with low proficiency in their L2, by giving them a PWM task. Significant differences were found between the groups, implying the use of different cognitive strategies. The less proficient L2 group demonstrated activation of the anterior cingulate and deactivation of the anterior medial frontal gyri, and right cuneus (Figure 3) . The anterior cingulate has been linked to the early stages of learning and is thought to be involved in adaptive regulation of behaviors such as evaluating the appropriateness of a response and the affective consequence. (Lu and Pederson, 2004). In contrast to the less proficient group, the highly proficient group showed greater activation in the left inferior frontal region within which the left inferior frontal gyrus corresponds to sublexical processing of phonology and the left anterior insula is implicated in subvocal rehearsal. Perani (2005) questioned whether the differences in the two proficiency groups in the Chee et al. study were the cause or the consequence of superior phonological working memory. This question can be addressed by looking at talented language users and translation.

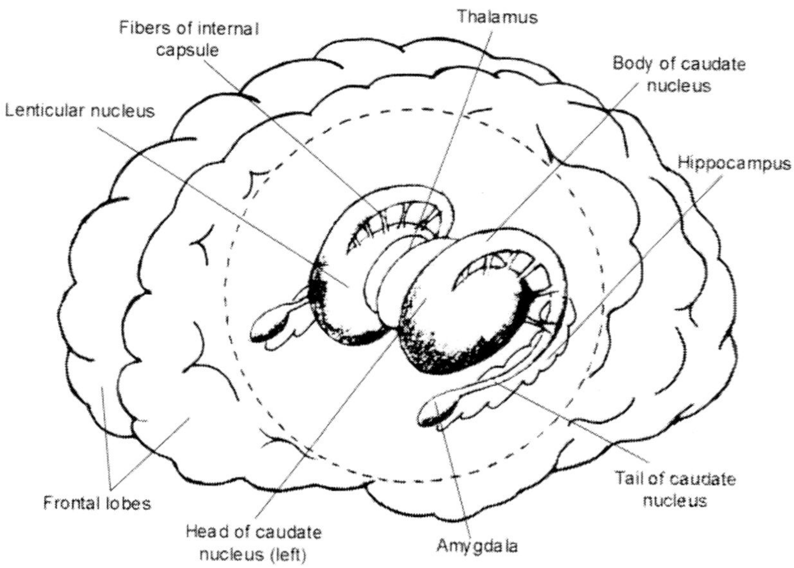

Figure 3. Left superior view of underlying subcortical areas.

Translation and simultaneous interpreting make substantial demands on working memory. Using a translation task, Price et al. (1999) noted the activation of the canonical language areas but also found areas external to the language region were activated such as the attention system that consists of the anterior cingulate and bilateral subcortical structures. They suggested that translation involves not only regulating activity in regions responsible for articulation (ie., supramarginal gyrus) but also in areas associated with articulation such as the cerebellum, the left anterior insula (as identified in Chee et al., 2004) and the supplementary motor area (SMA).

In sum, most of the findings from imaging studies support overlapping neural representation for L1 and L2 in early, proficient bilinguals. In addition, bilinguals who acquire their second language later but have become highly proficient in their second language, appear to involve shared brain areas in the processing of both languages. However, for late bilinguals whose proficiency remains low, separate activation may be observed, perhaps especially in the frontal cortex.

We have not dealt with critiques of fMRI and PET techniques in this paper as they are beyond the scope of this paper (the interested reader can find them in Bub 2000, and with reference to bilinguals in Abutalebi, et al. 2005), . Because of the numerous factors identified in the literature on bilingual brains, both prior to the imaging literature and within it, we recommend that readers approach each study with an organized set of questions in order to make comparisons across studies more interpretable. The most important issues to consider are:

1. What is the level of proficiency of the participants in each of their languages?
2. Are the participants early or late bilinguals, and what age demarcates the distinction employed?
3. What has been the extent of exposure of L2?

4. Has working memory (WM) been assessed in the participants?
5. What linguistic aspects are being investigated, e.g. phonological, semantic, syntactic?
6. What is the control task?
7. What linguistic level is being tested, e.g. word level, sentence level?
8. To what extent does task-complexity enter into the study?
9. Are the scans of the whole brain, or exclusively of the left hemisphere?
10. Are subcortical regions studied?

These issues all have been shown to significantly influence the activation patterns observed and reported during language tasks in bilinguals. As neuroimaging techniques become even more sophisticated, eventually the above-mentioned variables will be further disentangled and a clearer picture of brain organization for bilingualism will emerge.

V. Language Differences

The final language-related factor we draw attention to here is that of **similarity** or lack thereof between the bilingual's pair of languages. As has been proposed over the years, it is plausible that there are cortical sites common to both languages and cortical sites distinct to both languages in a bilingual speaker. That is, there are areas where the languages share overlapping neural networks, and areas where there are distinct neural networks for the two languages. Items that are identical in the languages of bi- and multilinguals would be stored together, and items that are different in each language would be separately represented in the brain. Therefore, cognate lexical items (e.g., *lemon* in English and *limón* in Spanish) would be subserved by the same or closely linked cortical sites. This hypothesis, which Paradis labeled *The Tripartite System Hypothesis* (Paradis, 1987, 1995) also postulates that less proficient languages use more cortical space at the periphery of the language zones than more proficient languages do (Paradis, 1995).

The Tripartite System Hypothesis is supported by treatment-efficacy studies of bilingual aphasia which show a "mass effect" of therapy benefits confined to the areas of overlap between the two languages. Case examples of this phenomenon are found in Sasanuma and Park (1995, in Paradis, 1995) and Watamori and Sasanuma (1978). Additional support comes from cortical stimulation studies of normal bilingual speakers, which revealed cortical sites where both languages were affected by electrical stimulation, while other cortical sites, when stimulated, only affected one language (Ojemann and Whitaker, 1978). Goral et al. (2006), moreover, suggest that even the non-cognate items in a pair of languages that share many cognates and structures may be differently linked to their translation equivalents than are pairs of translation equivalent lexical items in languages that are structurally more distant.

In addition to cognates, what other *language-specific* factors should be considered? We first address the insights we have gained from studies of brain-injured individuals and then discuss how differences between languages in typical populations may impact brain organization.

From the middle of the twentieth century there have been assertions that it is possible that structural differences between languages in the bilinguals' pairs can bring about differential organization in the bilingual brain. Even within one language, there may be two systems. This can be learned from discussions of bidialectal aphasia, which Jean Jones (2002) and Jones et al.(submitted) observe, reflect very similar patterns to those seen among bilingual aphasics as reported in Paradis (1977) and Albert and Obler (1978). It can be seen, as well, in studies of differential breakdown of reading (or writing) in readers of languages that can be written in more than one script, most notably Japanese, that can serve as interesting models for bilingualism per se. Japanese dyslexics and alexics provide further evidence of the existence of these two reading pathways as the language can be written in Kana, a phonologically-based system, or Kanji, a symbol system derived from Chinese characters and more lexically-based. Korean has a similar dual graphic representation for reading and writing: Hangul (a syllabic script) and Hanja (ideographic). In both Japanese and Korean, selective reading impairment has been described as a result of brain damage and disruption of one of the two routes for reading. (Ohno, et al. 2002; Kwon et al. 2002, 2005) In neuroimaging studies of brain-intact Korean speakers, differences in activation showed ideographic reading involved the right fusiform gyrus and right temporal-occipital region, whereas the phonographic script was more bilaterally represented in the inferior parietal lobes (Lee, 2004).

In bilinguals, Chinese and English provide an example of spoken and written language contrasts that may be differentially represented. The alphabetic system of English, like that of many Indo-European languages, maps letters and letter groups to sounds in a semblance of grapheme to phoneme correspondence. Chinese, by contrast, uses morphosyllabic characters, and its phonemes are reflected to some extent in its orthographic system. This logographic reading system uses approximately 5,000 to 6,000 characters to represent syllables or whole words that do not correspond to phonemes the way alphabetic systems like English do. Chinese characters contain a series of strokes within into a square shape and require complex visuo-spatial processing to read. Early studies in reading Chinese characters suggest greater right than left hemisphere involvement, however subsequent hemodynamic studies have not shown script-related differences in hemispheric activation. (e.g., Chee, et al., 1999; Tan et al., 2000).

A recent study suggests a revision whereby both shared and language-specific cortical areas for reading in English and Chinese are identified. In a neuroimaging study of bilingual readers of Mandarin Chinese and English, Tham et al. (2005) found common areas of activation but also several distinct regions for both languages, in both right and left hemispheres, on a homophone matching task. Shared activation was noted in the inferior frontal and occipital gyri of the left hemisphere. Evidence for distinct representation was also found in both languages. In Mandarin, however, the left hemisphere showed unique activation in the medial frontal gyrus (implicated in the auditory comprehension of single words) and unique activation in English in the supramarginal gyrus (involved in auditory-visual integration). Results from Tan and colleagues highlighted language-specific regions for reading Chinese and English.[2] In a series of studies they noted reading Chinese activated occipital and fusiform regions bilaterally, and the middle frontal gyrus of the left hemisphere (LMFG), areas involved in processing spatial information and working memory (Tan et al. 2001, 2003; Tan, 2005, see also Perfetti, et al., in press; Figures 1 and 4) English reading

[2] In Tan et al. (2003), although bilingual speakers whose first language was English or Chinese showed activation of different neural regions in reading, for both types of bilinguals the regions activated for reading in the second language were largely the same as those of the first language .

activated brain regions in the left superior temporal lobe, implicated in phonological processing and phoneme to grapheme correspondence. (Shaywitz, et al., 1998; Booth et al., 2003; Simos, et al., 2005). Some orthographic-specific disruptions were also observed in a bilingual Cantonese-English speaker who suffered a left temporal lobe contusion. Eng and Obler (2002) observed reading performance in Chinese was more vulnerable to semantic errors whereas reading in English showed more visual errors. In addition errors in lexical tone were noted in Chinese whereas errors in lexical stress in weres seen in English.

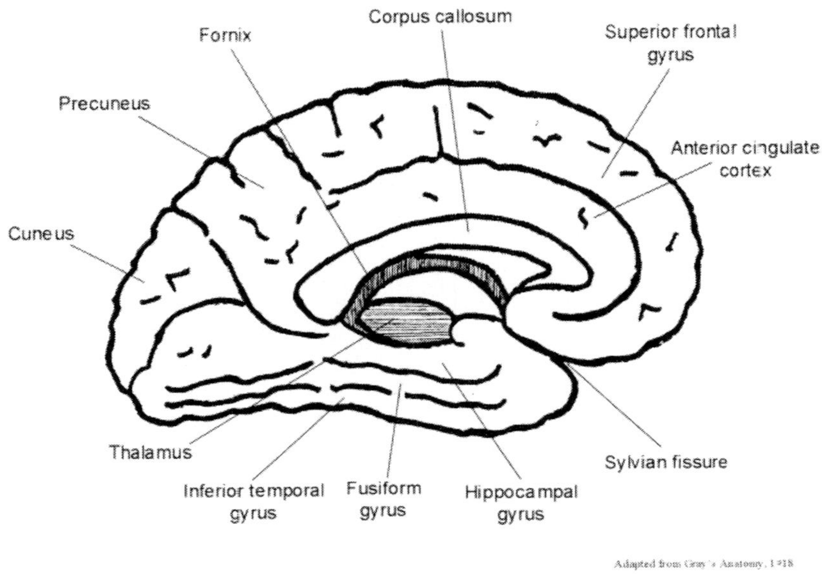

Figure 4. Medial surface of left cerebral hemisphere.

In a thorough review, Perfetti, Liu, and Fiez (in press) note multiple studies that demonstrate both overlapping and language specific activation. Several studies concurred with the involvement of the left superior temporal gyrus in alphabetic reading. Perfetti et al. distinguish this cortical mediation for phonological assembly, as in grapheme-phoneme correspondence in English, from the phonological retrieval needed to process syllables or whole words in Chinese. In their discussion they report the connection between phonological retrieval required by logographic Chinese reading to the dorsal left inferior parietal area and its probable syllable and word level mediation. They reviewed the evidence for more bilateral and visual processing when reading Chinese. Furthermore they suggested that Chinese learners of English may use more right hemisphere spatial processing including the fusiform region when they read English, than English readers learning Chinese. Although this language-specific activation in reading English and Chinese may result from the orthographic differences, it is unclear what impact the additional characteristic of lexical tone in Chinese could have on these results (Simos et al., 2005).

In addition to the *biscriptal* readers, speakers of a *signed language* and a spoken language (or, in principle, of two signed languages) provide supplementary insight into the factors that enter into brain organization for bilingualism.

If phonological/orthographic features can impact organization of languages in the brain, how is the bimodal sign-oral language represented cortically? A distinction should be made at the outset that degree of language proficiency is clearly impacted by hearing loss in deaf signers. As a double linguistic disadvantage, most deaf individuals from hearing families do not acquire sign language from their home environment in their early years, and hearing loss clearly impacts their acquisition of spoken language. This makes comparision of the cerebral processing of languages more problematic in different modalities than in a single spoken modality.

Studies that compare hearing and deaf signers provide a unique opportunity to expand our knowledge of the underlying linguistic representation when languages differ in sensory-motor constructs. Neville et al. (1998) compared typical hearing monolinguals, native congenitally deaf signers of ASL who learned English as a second language, and normal hearing bilingual signers of ASL who were also speakers of English via an fMRI study. On a reading and sign language processing task, all three groups demonstrated strong activation of the classical language areas in the left hemisphere. However when reading English, unlike their hearing participants, the deaf participants did not show activation of the canonical left hemisphere areas. In addition, when the normal hearing and deaf signers processed sign language, they did so bilaterally with extensive activation of concomitant areas of the right hemisphere.

The findings of this study by Neville and colleagues presented a challenge to earlier research that did not find language-modality specific neural substrates. In addition, the classical auditory-related structures appeared to be heavily involved in processing sign language, which seemed counterintuitive. Hickok et al. (1998) discussed these findings and referred to the differential activation of the superior-temporal lobe including the primary auditory cortex and the planum temporale (responsible for visual-auditory language processing) for hearing signers that was not activated when deaf signers watched ASL sentences. Hickok et al. remarked on the importance of these areas for speech perception as an explanation for these findings.[3] In addition they suggested the differences found could be modality dependent rather than linguistically dependent. In a subsequent study Hickok et al. (2002) compared signers with left and right hemisphere damage and discovered significantly greater language loss in the group with left-hemisphere damage. The greatest impairment in comprehension was observed in the signers with temporal lobe damage. The authors conclude that signed and spoken languages have a similar cerebral representation.

The results of other studies have demonstrated both shared and differential activation for spoken and sign languages. Braun, et al. (2001) found parallel activation of ASL and English in classic left hemisphere regions; however, the activation of structures on a PET study extended beyond these areas and included bilateral extrasylvian activation. In this study they evaluated language production in neurologically intact hearing signers and found a pattern of activation in the right hemisphere during both signing and speaking that varied during stages of discourse production. Using an ASL comprehension task, Newman, et al. (2001) also found strong left-hemisphere activation for both English and ASL but greater right hemisphere involvement for ASL. Buchsbaum, et al. (2005) studied brain-intact deaf signers and an aphasic signer. When compared to studies of hearing participants, areas in common included the posterior frontal cortex, the left temporal-parietal junction, and the bilateral

[3] See also Nakada, 2001

superior temporal sulcus. Neural areas specific to sign language included the dorsal posterior parietal regions, suggested by the authors to be important for working memory.

Certainly the idea is appealing that languages that differ markedly with regard to orthography (Chinese vs. English) or the mode of representation (ASL vs. English) could be differentially represented. However our review of the evidence of whether the majority of biscriptal or bimodal language users have shared or unique neural representation for their language pairs falls far short of definitive answers. Rather, these bilingual populations help us to continue to pose interesting questions about the complexities of brain functioning.

VI. Summary and Conclusion

The history of our field's study of the brain bases of bilingualism has oscillated between foci as broad as lateral dominance to the narrower ones permitted by current imaging technology. Individual differences in second-language proficiency, resulting from different histories of second-language acquisition and use, appear to be reflected somewhat differently in the brain of the adult bilingual. More right-hemisphere participation may be seen in earlier, less-proficient stages of acquiring the second language. And, within the left hemisphere, earlier acquisition of a second language and high proficiency appear linked to more overlap within the peri-Sylvian language area, than is later acquisition.

What the localizationist imaging techniques permit that earlier methods did not is a focus on subcortical areas involved in language processing. Indeed, inclusion of the limbic system in the subcortical regions permits a return to the emotional-links posited by aphasiologists with psychiatric bents such as Minkowski (1963) and Krapf (1957). Among second-language teaching professionals, emotional factors may be seen in the link between second-language learning success and motivation. Event Related Potential (ERP) studies will permit us to understand more about the relative timing of performance in a second language. Delays of even milliseconds, even in quite-proficient bilinguals, as Tom Walsten has pointed out (personal communication, 2006) can quickly accumulate under stressful conditions to result in less than fully native-like processing (see also Blumenthal et al., 2006, for discussion of the effects of stress on second-language performance).

Acknowledgements

Thanks to Mona Diane Conner for help with the figures, and to Yael Neumann for help with the neuroanatomy underlying them. Thanks to Mira Goral for discussing interpretations of some of the papers cited herein and helpful editorial suggestions on a penultimate draft.

References

Abu-Rabia, S., and Kehat, S. (2004). The critical period for second language pronunciation: Is there such a thing? Ten case studies of late starters who attained a native-like Hebrew accent. *Educational Psychology, 24*, 77-98.

Abutalebi, J., Cappa, S. F., and Perani, D. (2005). What can functional neuroimaging tell us about the bilingual brain? In Kroll, J. F. and De Groot, A. M. B. (Eds). *Handbook of Bilingualism: Psycholinguistic Approaches*. New York: Oxford University Press.

Abutalebi, J., Cappa, S. F., and Perani, D. (2001). The bilingual brain as revealed by functional neuroimaging. *Bilingualism: Language and Cognition. 4,* 179-190.

Abutalebi, J., Miozzo, A., and Cappa, S. F. (2000). Do subcortical structures control language selection in bilinguals? Evidence from pathological language mixing. *Neurocase, 6,* 101-106.

Albert, M. L., and Obler, L. K. (1978). *The bilingual brain: Neuropsychological and neurolinguisitic aspects of bilingualism* (pp. 95-158). New York: Academic Press.

April, R. S., and Tse, P. C. (1977). Crossed aphasia in a Chinese bilingual dextral. *Archives of Neurology, 34,* 766-770.

Baddeley, A., Gathercole, S., and Papagno, C. (1998). The phonological loop as a language learning device. *Psychological Review, 105*, 158-173.

Binder, J. R., Frost, J.A., Hammeke, T.A., Cox, R.W., Rao, S.M., and Prieto, T. (1997). Human brain language areas identified by functional magnetic resonance imaging. *Journal of Neuroscience 17,* 353-362.

Birdsong, D. (2005). Interpreting age effects in second language acquisition. In Kroll, J., and DeGroot, A. (Eds.). *Handbook of bilingualism: Psycholinguistic perspectives* (pp. 109-127). Oxford: Oxford University Press.

Birdsong, D., and Molis, M. (2001). On the evidence for maturational constraints in second-language acquisition. *Journal of Memory and Language, 44*, 235-249.

Blumenthal, P., Bradley, P., Britt, T., Cohen, J., Maxfield, N., McCubbin, J., Michael, E., Moore, P., Obler, L., Pilcher, J., Signorelli, T., Wallsten, T. (2006). Stress effects on bilingual language-professionals' performance. *International Journal of Bilingualism,10, 477-495.*

Booth, J. R., Burman, D. D., Meyer, J. R., Zhang, L., Gitelman, D. R., Parrish, T. R., et al. (2004). Development of brain mechanisms for processing orthographic and phonological representations. *Journal of Cognitive Neuroscience, 16*, 1234-1249.

Braun, A. R., Guillemin, A., Hosey, L., and Varga, M. (2001). The neural organization of discourse: An H215O-PET study of narrative production in English and American sign language. *Brain, 124*, 2028-2044.

Briellmann, R. S., Saling, M. M., Connell, A. B., Waites, A. B., Abbott, D. F., and Jackson, G. D. (2004). A high-field functional MRI study of quadri-lingual subjects. *Brain and Language, 89*, 531-542.

Bub, D. N. (2000). Methodological issues confronting PET and fMRI studies of cognitive function. *Cognitive Neuropsychology, 17*, 467-484.

Buchsbaum, B., Pickell, B., Love, T., Hatrak, M., Bellugi, U., and Hickok, G. (2005). Neural substrates for verbal working memory in deaf signers: fMRI study and lesion case report. *Brain and Language, 95*, 265-272.

Castles, A., and Coltheart, M. (1993). Varieties of developmental dyslexia. *Cognition, 47,* 149-180.

Charlton, M. H. (1964). Aphasia in bilingual and polyglot patients— A neurological and psychological study. *Journal of Speech and Hearing Disorders, 29,* 307-311.

Chee, M. W. L., Caplan, D., Soon, C. S., Sriram, N., Tan, E. W. L., Thiel, T., and Weekes, B. (1999). Processing of visually presented sentences in Mandarin and English studies with fMRI. *Neuron, 23,* 127-137.

Chee, M. W. L., Tan, E. W. L., and Thiel, T. (1999). Mandarin and English single word processing studied with functional Magnetic Resonance Imaging. *Journal of Neuroscience, 19,* 3050-3056.

Chee, M. W. L., Hon, N., Lee, H. L., and Soon, C. S. (2001). Relative language proficiency modulates BOLD signal change when bilinguals perform semantic judgments. *NeuroImage, 13,* 1155-1163.

Chee, M. W. L., Soon, C. S., Lee, H. L., and Pallier, C. (2004). Left insula activation: A marker for language attainment in bilinguals. *Proceedings of the National Academy of Sciences USA, 101,* 15265-15270.

Christoffels, I. K., De Groot, A. M. B., and Kroll, J. F. (2006). Memory and language skills in simultaneous interpreters: The role of expertise and language proficiency. *Journal of Memory and Language, 54,* 324-345.

Crinion, J., Turner, R., Grogan, A., Hanakawa, T., Noppeney, U., Devlin, J. T., et al. (2006). Language control in the bilingual brain. *Science, 312,* 1537-1540.

Coltheart, M., Curtis, B., Atkins, P. and Haller, M. (1993). Models of reading aloud: Dual-route and parallel-distributed-processing approaches. *Psychological Review,* 1089-608

De Bleser, R., Dupont, P., Postler, J., Bormans, G., Speelman, D., Mortelmans, L., et al. (2003). The organisation of the bilingual lexicon: a PET study. *Journal of Neurolinguistics, 16,* 439-456.

Dehaene, S. D., Dupoux, E., Mehler, J., Cohen, L, Paulesu, E., Perani, D., et al. (1997). Anatomical variability in the cortical representation of first and second languages. *NeuroReport, 8,* 3809-3815.

Dewaele, J.-M.. (2002). Individual differences in L2 Fluency: The effect of neurobiological correlates, in V. Cook, Ed., *Second language acquisition, 1: Portraits of the L2 user.* Clevedon: Great Britain: Multilingual Matters, 221-249.

Eng, N., and Obler, L. K. (2002). Acquired dyslexia in a biscript reader following traumatic brain injury: A scond case. *Topics in Language Disorders, 22,* 5.-19.

Fabbro, F. (2001a). The bilingual brain: Bilingual aphasia. *Brain and Language, 79,* 201-210.

Fabbro, F. (2001b). The bilingual brain: Cerebral representation of languages. *Brain and Language, 79,* 211-222.

Fletcher, J. M., Simos, P. G., Shaywitz, B. A., Shaywitz, S. E., Pugh, K. R., and Papanicolaou, A. C. (2000). *Neuroimaging, language, and reading: The interface of brain and environment.* In A Research Symposium on High Standards in Reading for Student from Diverse Language Groups: Research, Practice and Policy, Washington D.C.

Freud, S. (1891). *On aphasia: A critical study.* Translated by Stengel, E. (1953). New York: International Universities Press, Inc.

Ganschow, L. and Sparks, R. (1995). Effects of direct instruction in Spanish phonology on the native language skills and foreign language aptitude of at-risk foreign language learners. *Journal of Learning Disabilities,* 28, 107-120.

Geschwind, N., and Galaburda, A. M. (1985). Cerebral lateralization. Biological mechanisms, associations and pathology. *Archives of Neurology, 42,* 428-459.

Gloning, I. and Gloning, K. (1965). Aphasien bei polyglotten. Beitrag zur Dynamik des Sprachabbaus sowie zur Lokalisationsfrage dieser Storungen. *Wiener Zeitschrift fuer Nervenheilkunde, 22,* 362-397.

Goral, M., Levy, E. S., and Obler, L. K. (2002). Neurolinguistic aspects of bilingualism. *International Journal of Bilingualism,* 6, 411-440.

Goral, M., Levy, E. S., Obler, L. K., and Cohen, E. (2006). Cross-language lexical connections in the mental lexicon: Evidence from a case of trilingual aphasia *Brain and Language, 98,* 235-247..

Halsband, U., Krause, B. J., Sipila, H., Teras, M., and Laihinen, A. (2002). PET studies on the memory processing of word pairs in bilingual Finnish-English subjects. *Behavioural Brain Research,* 132, 47-57.

Hasegawa, M., Carpenter, P., and Just, M. (2002). An fMRI study of bilingual sentence comprehension and workload. *NeuroImage, 15,* 647-660.

Hernandez, A. E., Dapretto, M., Mazziotta, J., and Bookheimer, S. (2001). Language switching and language representation in Spanish-English bilinguals: an fMRI study. *NeuroImage, 14,* 510-520.

Hernandez, A. E., Martinez, A., and Kohnert, K. (2000). In search of the language switch; An fMRI study of picture naming in Spanish-English bilinguals. *Brain and Language, 73,* 421-431.

Hickok, G., Bellugi, U., and Klima, E. S. (1998). What's right about the neural organization of sign language? A perspective on recent neuroimaging results. *Trends in Cognitive Sciences 2*, 465-468.

Hickok, G., Love-Geffen, T., and Klima, E. S. (2002). Role of the left hemisphere in sign language comprehension. *Brain and Language, 82*, 167-178.

Horwitz, B., Amunts, K., Bhattacharyya, R., Patkin, D., Jeffries, K., Zilles, K., et al. (2003). Activation of Broca's area during the production of spoken and signed language: a combined cytoarchitectonic mapping and PET analysis. *Neuropsychologia, 41*, 1868-1876.

Horwitz, B., Rumsey, J. M., and Donohue, B. C. (1998). Functional connectivity of the angular gyrus in normal reading and dyslexia. *Proceedings of the National Academy of Sciences USA, 95*, 8939-8944.

Hull, R. (2003). *How does bilingualism matter: A meta-analytic tale of two hemispheres.*, Unpublished doctoral dissertation.Texas A and M University.

Hull, R. and J. Vaid. (2005). Clearing the cobwebs from the study of the bilingual brain: Converging evidence from laterality and electrophysiological research. In J. Kroll and A. DeGroot (Eds.), *Handbook of bilingualism: Psycholinguistic perspectives* (pp. 109-127). Oxford, Oxford University Press.

Hyltenstam, K., and Abrahamsson, N. (2003). Maturational constraints in SLA. In C. J. Doughty and M. H. Long (Eds.), *The handbook of second language acquisition* (pp. 539-588). Malden, MA: Blackwell.

Hyltenstam, K., and Abrahamsson, N. (2000). Who can become native-like in a second language? All, some, or none? On the maturational constraints controversy in second language acquisition. *Studia Linguistica, 54,* 250-166.

Ijalba, E. (in preparation). Dyslexia in Spanish-speaking English Learners, Doctoral Dissertation, City University of New York.

Illes, J., Francis, W. S., Desmond, J. E., Gabrieli, J., Glover, G., Poldrack, R., et al. (1999). Convergent cortical representation of semantic processing in bilinguals. *Brain and Language, 70,* 347-363.

Jones, J. E. (2002) The manifestation of agrammatism in a bidialectal speaker of African-American Vernacular English and Standard American English. Unpublished Doctoral Dissertation. City University of New York, NY.

Just, M. A., Carpenter, P.A., Keller, T.A., Eddy, W.F., and Thulborn, T.A. (1996). Brain activation modulated by sentence comprehension. *Science, 274,* 114-116.

Kainz, F. (1960). *Psychologie der Sprache*. Zweite, umgearbeitete Auflage (p. 330-334), vol. 2, Stuttgart: Enke.

Kalbfleisch, M.L. (2004). The functional neural anatomy of talent. *The Anatomical Record,* 277B (1), 21-36.

Kim, K., Rilkin, R., Lee, K., and Kirsch, J. (1997). Distinct cortical areas associated with native and second language. *Nature, 388,* 171-174.

Klein, D., Milner, B., Zatorre, R. J., Meyer, E., and Evans, A. (1995). The neural substrates underlying word generation: a bilingual functional-imaging study. *Proceedings of the National Academy of Sciences USA, 92,* 2899-2903.

Klein, D., Zatorre, R. J., Chen, J., Milner, B., Crane, J., Belin, P., and Bouffard, M. (2006). Bilingual brain organization; A functional magnetic resonance adaptation study. *NeuroImage, 31,* 366-375.

Klein, D., Zatorre, R.J, Milner, B., Meyer, E., and Evans, A. (1994). Left putaminal activation when speaking a second language: Evidence from PET. *NeuroReport, 17,* 2295-2297.

Krapf, E. (1957). A propos des aphasies chez les polyglottes. *Encéphale, 46,* 623-629.

Kwon, J. C., Lee, H. J., Chin, J., Lee, Y. M., Kim, H., and Na, D. L. (2002) Hanja alexia with agraphia after left posterior inferior temporal lobe infarction: A case study *Journal of Korean Medical Science, 17,* 91-95.

Kwon, M., Kim, J. S., Lee, J., Sim, H., Nam, K., and Park, H. (2005). Double dissociation of Hangul and Hanja reading in Korean patients with stroke**.** *European Neurology, 54*, 199-203.

Lambert, W., and Fillenbaum, S. (1959). A pilot study of aphasia among bilinguals. *Candadian Journal of Psychology, 13,* 28-34.

Lamm, O., and Epstein, R. (1999). Left-handedness and achievements in foreign language studies. *Brain and Language, 70*(3), 504-517.

Lee, K. M. (2004). Functional MRI comparison between reading ideographic and phonographic scripts of one language. *Brain and Language, 91*, 245-251.

Lenneberg, E. (1967). *Biological foundations of language*. New York: John Wiley.

Luke, K., Liu, H., Wai, Y., Wan, Y., Tan, L. H., (2002). Functional anatomy of syntactic and semantic processing in language comprehension. *Human Brain Mapping, 16,* 133-145.

Luu, P., and Pederson, S. M. (2004). The anterior cingulate cortex: regulating actions in context. In M. I. Posner (Ed.), *Cognitive neuroscience of attention*. New York: Guilford.

Marrero, M. Z., Golden, C. J., and Espe-Pfeifer, P. (2002). Bilingualism, brain injury, and recovery: Implications for understanding the bilingual and for therapy. *Clinical Psychology Review, 22*, 463-478.

Mazoyer, B. M., Tzourio, N., Frak, V., Syrota, A., Murayama, N., and Levrier, O. (1993). The cortical representation of speech. *Journal of Cognitive Neuroscience 5,* 467-479.

Minkowski, M. (1963). On aphasia in polyglots. In L. Halpern (Ed.), *Problems of dynamic neurology* (pp. 119-161). Jerusalem: Hebrew University,

Nakada, T., Fujii, Y., Yoneoka, Y., and Kwee, I. L. (2001). Planum temporale: Where spoken and written language meet. *European Neurology, 46*, 121-125.

Neville, H. J., Bavelier, D., Corina, D., Rauschecker, J., Karni, A., Lalwani, A., et al. (1998). Cerebral organization for language in deaf and hearing subjects: Biological constraints and effects of experience. *Proceedings of the National Academy of Science USA, 95*, 922-929.

Newman, A. J., Bavelier, D., Corina, D., Jezzard, P., and Neville, H. J. (2002). A critical period for right hemisphere recruitment in American Sign Language processing. *Neuroscience, 5*(1), 76-80.

Nichelli, P., Grafman, J., Pietrini, P., Clark, K. (1995). Where the brain appreciates the moral of a story. *NeuroReport, 6*, 2309-2313.

Novoa, L., Fein, D. and Obler, L. K. (1988). Talent in foreign languages: a case study. In L. Obler and D. Fein (Eds.), *The exceptional brain: Neuropsychology of talent and special abilities* (pp. 294-302), New York: Guilford.

Obler, L. K., Zatorre, R. J., Galloway, L., and Vaid, J. (1982). Cerebral lateralization in bilinguals: Methodological issues. *Brain and Language, 15*, 40-54.

Obler, L.K. and Fein, D. (1988). *The exceptional brain: Neuropsychology of talent and special abilities.* New York: Guilford.

Ojemann, G. A., and Whitaker, H. A. (1978). The bilingual brain. *Archives of Neurology, 35*, 409-412.

Ohno, T., Takeda, K., Kato, S., and Hirai, S. (2002). Pure alexia in a Japanese-English bilingual: dissociation between the two languages. *Journal of Neurology, 249*, 105-107.

Paradis, M. (1977). Bilingualism and aphasia. In H. Whitaker and H. Whitaker (Eds.), *Studies in neurolinguistics* (pp. 65-120), Vol. 3. New York: Academic Press.

Paradis, M. (1983). *Readings on aphasia in bilinguals and polyglots.* Canada: Marcel Didier, Inc.

Paradis, M. (1987). *The assessment of bilingual aphasia* (pp. 1-17) Hillsdale, NJ: Lawrence Erlbaum Associates.

Paradis, M. (1989). Bilingual and polyglot aphasia. In F. Boller and J. Grafman (Eds.), *Handbook of neuropsychology* (pp. 117-140), Vol. 2. Amsterdam: Elsevier.

Paradis, M. (1992). The Loch Ness Monster approach to bilingual language lateralization: A response to Berquier and Ashton. *Brain and Language, 43*, 534-537.

Paradis, M. (1995). *Aspects of bilingual aphasia.* Tarrytown, NY: Elsevier Science Inc.

Paradis, M. (1995). Bilingual aphasia 100 years later: consensus and controversies. In Paradis (Ed.), *Aspects of bilingual aphasia* (pp. 211-223). Oxford: Pergamon Press.

Paradis, M. (2004). *A neurolinguistic theory of bilingualism.* Amsterdam : John Benjamins.

Penfield, W. (1953). A consideration of the neurophysiological mechanisms of speech, and some educational consequences. *Proceedings of the American Academy of Arts and Science, 82*, 199-214.

Perani, D. (2005). The neural basis of language talent in bilinguals. *Trends in Cognitive Sciences, 9*, 211-213.

Perani, D., Dehaene, S., Grassi, F., Cohen, L., Cappa, S., Dupoux, E., Fazio, F., and Mehler, J. (1996). Brain processing of native and foreign language. *Neuroreport, 7*, 2439-2444.

Perani, D., Paulesu, E., Galles, N. S., Dupoux, E., Dehaene, S., Bettinardi, V., Cappa, S. F., Fazio, F., and Mehler, J. (1998). The bilingual brain. Proficiency and age of acquisition of the second language. *Brain, 121,* 1841-1852.

Perani, D., Abutalebi, J., Paulesu, E., Brambati, S., Scifo, P., Cappa, S. F., et al. (2003). The role of age of acquisition and language usage in early, high-proficient bilinguals; A fMRI study during verbal fluency. *Human Brain Mapping, 19,* 179-182.

Perani, D., Paulesu, E., Galles, N. S., Dupoux, E., Dehaene, S., Bettinardi, V., et al. (1998). The bilingual brain. Proficiency and age of acquisition of the second language. *Brain, 121*, 1841-1852.

Perfetti, C., Liu, Y., Fiez, J. and Tan, L. H. (in press) The neural bases of reading: The accommodation of the brain's reading network to writing systems In *The Neural Basis of Reading.* P. Cornelissen, M. Kringelbach, and P. Hansen, (Eds.), Oxford University Press.

Petersen, S. E., Fox, P. T., Snyder, A. Z., and Raichle, M. F. (1990). Activation of extrastriate and frontal cortical areas by visual words and word-like stimuli. *Science, 249,* 1041-1044.

Pillai, J. J., Araque, J. M., Allison, J. D., Sethuraman, S., Loring, D. W., Thiruvaiyaru, D., et al. (2003). Functional MRI study of semantic and phonological language processing in bilingual subjects; preliminary findings. *NeuroImage, 19,* 565-576.

Pitres, A. (1895). Etude sur l'aphasie des polyglottes. *Revue de Médecine*, 15, 873-899.

Poeppel, D. (1996). A critical review of PET-studies of phonological processing. *Brain and Language 55,* 317-351.

Price, C. J., and Mechelli, A. (2005). Reading and reading disturbance. *Current Opinion in Neurobiology, 15*, 231-238.

Price, C. J., Green, D. W., and von Studnitz, R. (1999). A functional imaging study of translation and language switching. *Brain, 122*(12), 2221-2235.

Price, C. J., Moore, C. J., and Frackowiak, R. S. (1996). The effect of varying stimulus rate and duration on brain activity during reading. *Neuroimage 3,* 40-52.

Pugh, K. R. (1996). Cerebral organization of component processes in reading. *Brain, 119,* 1221-1238.

Raichle, M. E. (1996). What words are telling us about the brain. *Cold Spring Harbor symposia on quantitative biology*, 61, 9-14.

Ribot, T. (1881). *Les maladies de la mémoire. Paris:*. Baillère.

Roux, F. E., Lubrano, V., Lauwers-Cances, V., Tremoulet, M., Mascott, C. R., and Demonet, J. F. (2004). Intra-operative mapping of cortical areas involved in reading in mono- and bilingual patients. *Brain, 127*, 1796-1810.

Sasanuma, S., and Park, H. S. (1995). Patterns of language deficits in two Korean-Japanese bilingual aphasic patients- A clinical report. In M. Paradis (Ed.), *Aspects of bilingual aphasia* (pp.111-123). Tarrytown, NY: Elsevier Science Ltd.

Schneiderman, E. I., and Desmarais, C. (1988). A neuropsychological substrate for talent in second-language acquisition. In L.K. Obler and D. Fein (Eds.), *The exceptional brain: Neuropsychology of talent and special abilities (pp.* 294-302). New York: Guilford.

Scoresby-Jackson, R. (1867). Case of aphasia with right hemiplegia. *Edinburgh Medical Journal, 12,* 696-706.

Signorelli, T. (in preparation). Working Memory in Simultaneous Interpreters. Doctoral dissertation, City Univesity of New York-Graduate Center.

Scott, S. K., and Wise, R. J. S. (2003). Functional imaging and language: A critical guide to methodology and analysis. *Speech Communication, 41,* 7-21.

Shaywitz, S. E., Shaywitz, B. A., Pugh, K. R., Fulbright, R.K., Constable, R.T., Mencl, W. E., et al. (1998). Functional disruption in the organization of the brain for reading in dyslexia. *Proceedings of the National Academy of Science USA, 95,* 2636-2641.

Silverberg, R., and Gordon, H. W. (1979). Differential aphasia in two bilingual individuals. *Neurology, 29,* 51-55.

Simos, P. G., Billingsley-Marshall, R. L., Sarkari, S., Pataraia, E., and Papanicolaou, A. C. (2005). Brain mechanisms supporting distinct languages. *Learning Disabilities Research and Practice, 20,* 31-38.

Sparks, R. L. Philips, L. Ganshow, L. and Javorsky, J (1999), Students classified as LD and the college foreign language requirement: A quantitative analysis, *Journal of Learning Disabilities*, 32, 566-580.

Stowe, L. A., Paans, A. M. J., Wijers, A. A., Zwarts, F., and Mulder, G. (1994). PET-studies of language: an assessment of the reliability of the technique. *Journal of Psycholinguistic Research, 23,* 499-527.

Stromswold, K., Caplan, D., Alpert, N., and Rauch, S. (1996). Localization of syntactic comprehension by positron emission tomography. *Brain and Language, 52,* 452–473.

Tan, L. H., Feng, C. M., Fox, P. T., and Gao, J. H. (2001). An fMRI study with written Chinese. *Neuroreport 12,* 83-88.

Tan, L. H., Spinks, J. A., Feng, C. M., Siok, W. T., Perfetti, C. A., Xiong, J., Fox, P. T., and Gao, J. H. (2003). Neural systems of second language reading are shaped by native language. *Human Brain Mapping, 18,* 158-166.

Tan, L. H., Spinks, J. A., Gao, J. H., Liu, H. L., Perfetti, C. A., Xiong, J., Stofer, K. A., Pu, Y., Liu, Y., and Fox, P. T. (2000). Brain activation in the processing of Chinese characters and words: a functional MRI study. *Human Brain Mapping, 10,* 16-27.

Tan, L.H., Laird, A., Li, K., and Fox, P. T. (2005). Neuroanatomical correlates of phonological processing of Chinese characters and alphabetic words: A meta-analysis. *Human Brain Mapping, 25,* 83-91.

Tham, W. W., Rickard Liow, S. J., Rajapakse, J. C., Choong Leong, T., Ng, S. E., Lim, W. E., et al. (2005). Phonological processing in Chinese-English bilingual biscriptals: An fMRI study. *NeuroImage, 28,* 579-587.

Vaid, J. and Hull, R. (2002). Re-envisioning the bilingual brain using functional neuroimaging: Methodological and interpretive issues. In F. Fabbro (Ed.), *The neurolinguistics of bilingualism: Essays in honor of Michel Paradis.* (pp. 315-355). Udine Forum: Udine University Press.

Veyrac, G. J. (1931). A study of aphasia in polyglot subjects. In M. Paradis (Ed.), *Readings on aphasia in bilinguals and polyglots* (pp. 320-338). Montreal: Didier.

Vingerhoets, G., Borsel, J. V., Tesink, C., van den Noort, M., Deblaere, K., Seurinck, R., (2003). Multilingualism: an fMRI study. *NeuroImage, 20,* 2181-2196.

Wartenburger, I., Heekeren, H., Abutalebi, J., Cappa, S., Villringer, A. and Perani, D. (2003). Early setting of grammatical processing in the bilingual brain. *Neuron, 37,* 159-170.

Watamori, T. S., and Sasanuma, S. (1978). The recovery processes of two English-Japanese bilingual aphasics. *Brain and Language, 6,* 127-140.

Yetkin, O., Yetkin, Z., Haughton, V., and Cox, R.W. (1996). Use of functional MR to map language in multilingual volunteers. *American Journal of Neuroradiology, 17,* 473-477.

Yokoyama, S., Okamoto, H., Miyamoto, T., Yoshimoto, K., Kim, J., Iwata, K., et al. (2006). Cortical activation in the processing of passive sentences in L1 and L2; An fMRI study. *NeuroImage, 30,* 570-579.

In: Speech and Language Disorders in Bilinguals
Editors: Alfredo Ardila and Eliane Ramos, pp. 47-67
ISBN 978-1-60021-560-5

Chapter 3

PSYCHOLINGUISTIC MODELS OF SPEECH PRODUCTION IN BILINGUALISM AND MULTILINGUALISM

Andrea Marini[1,2,3] ***and Franco Fabbro***[1,2]
1. University of Udine, Udine, Italy
2. IRCSS "E. Medea" "La Nostra Famiglia", San Vito al Tagliamento (UD), Italy
3. IRCCS "Santa Lucia", Roma, Italy

INTRODUCTION

Bilingualism is a complex psychological and socio-cultural phenomenon encompassing a number of individual and social dimensions (Butler and Hakuta, 2004). It constitutes a widespread phenomenon, as in the world approximately 7000 languages are spoken in just 160 countries. Therefore over 50% of the world population is bi- or even multilingual (Tucker, 1998; Grosjean, 1982, 1994). Moreover, in many countries the number of spoken languages is constantly growing due to massive immigration.

The issue of language representation and use in multilingual speakers and the related problem of multilingual competence can be approached at different levels of description. Indeed, they constitute a matter of interest not only for sociolinguistic models of language use and stratification, but also for psycholinguistic theories of language development and functioning, as well as neurolinguistic models of language representation in the brain.

In this chapter some of the most influential psycholinguistic models of language representation and speech production in multilingual speakers are introduced. The results from psycholinguistic and neurolinguistic investigations will be taken into account in order to discuss the assumptions of such models.

MODELS OF LANGUAGE REPRESENTATION IN MONOLINGUAL INDIVIDUALS

Psycholinguistics investigates the functional architecture of language and the processes involved in both oral and written language production and comprehension. Language is considered a complex cognitive function involving interaction of a number of different levels of processing: a word level for lexical processing; a sentence level for syntactic processing; a pragmatic level where words or sentences are contextualized and inferences are drawn; a text/discourse level where those sentences that constitute a written text or a spoken discourse are integrated in order to retrieve its general meaning or gist (Marini et al., 2005a, b; Marini and Nocentini, 2003; Caplan, 1992; Kintsch and van Dijk, 1978). Lexical and syntactic processing form the within-sentence or microlinguistic dimension of language responsible for intra-phrasal functions. Lexical processing organizes phonological or graphemical patterns into morphological strings and words, and determines the morphosyntactic context each word requires. All these aspects of lexical knowledge are assumed to be represented in a mental lexicon where phonetic, phonological, morphophonological, morphological, morphosyntactic and semantic information are stored for each word. Syntactic processing organizes the morphosyntactic contexts required by words in phrases and clauses in order to generate well-formed sentences. Pragmatic and discourse processing form the between-sentence or macrolinguistic dimension of language. They are responsible for inter-phrasal functions and utterance contextualization.

Each aspect of language processing is subserved by neurofunctionally distinct systems that can be separately compromised, inhibited or preserved following a brain lesion or after transient inhibition due to electrical stimulation, paroxystic charge or pharmacological inhibition (*e.g.* Ojemann, 1991). According to the Declarative/Procedural model (Paradis, 1994; 2004; Ullman, 2001; 2004), language learning and representation are assumed to be subserved by two anatomically and functionally distinct long-term memory systems (declarative and procedural, respectively). Procedural memory is a type of implicit memory subserved by frontal/basal ganglia circuits as well as portions of the parietal cortex, superior temporal cortex and the cerebellum (Fabbro, 1999; Ullman, 2001). Procedural memory underlies implicit linguistic competence. In the course of first language acquisition, it is involved in the process of learning and consequently executing sensori-motor and cognitive skills such as, for example, those involved in the articulation of the sounds of a language (*i.e.* phones) and in syntax. Declarative (or explicit) memory is subserved by bilateral medial and temporo-parietal structures, including the hippocampal region and the parahippocampal cortex (Fabbro, 1999; Ullman, 2001). It is implicated in conscious learning of facts and events and consists of two subtypes, semantic and episodic memory, respectively. *Semantic memory* is the system storing one's encyclopedic knowledge of the world (*e.g.* knowledge about the meaning of words, as well as knowledge about historical, geographical, social facts). *Episodic* (or *autobiographical*) *memory* refers to one's past experiences that can be consciously recalled. It is assumed that grammar (*i.e.* syntactic and morphosyntactic implicit competence) is acquired incidentally through procedural memory, whereas lexical-semantic explicit knowledge is overtly learned and stored in declarative memory (Paradis, 1994; Ullman, 2001; Fabbro, 1999; 2001). For example, procedural memory acquires and applies implicit syntactic rules such as principles of government and binding (Chomsky, 1988; 1995;

Pinker, 1999) or procedures of syntactic parsing (Frazier and Fodor, 1978), but it is declarative memory that deals with lexico-semantic aspects of the words the form the sentences. Furthermore, the procedural system "learns" and applies word formation rules to morphemes and lexical items stored in declarative memory. Moreover, once the access to a lexical item is granted, implicit memory procedures automatically generate the argument structure of that particular word and assign the thematic roles to the required arguments (morphosyntactic processing). As to phonetics, the articulatory programs necessary to produce the target phones of a language become automatized and are transferred to procedural memory, so that the speaker does not have to think about the articulatory movements while speaking.

According to Levelt (1989), the process of speech production is mediated by the central role of the mental lexicon and involves three subsystems: a pre-linguistic conceptual system (conceptualizer); a linguistic system (formulator); an output system (articulator) where production actually takes place. In the conceptualizer the speaker retrieves from long-term declarative memory all available data to formulate a mental model of the intended message. Indeed, declarative memory provides knowledge about what to say (message planning), what has previously been said (linguistic context) and the particular situation, place and time in which the communicative exchange takes place (Marini, 2001; Levinson, 1983; Johnson-Laird, 1980). During the phase of message planning, a supervisory attentional system (SAS: Green, 1998) is in charge of controlling the speakers' communicative intentions. Moreover, such system modulates the amount of information that the speaker intends to communicate and its relevance with respect to what has previously been said (Grice, 1975). This conceptual information is then sent to the formulator where the preverbal message is converted into a speech plan. At this stage, lexical processing matches the intended meaning formulated in the pre-linguistic phase with the corresponding lexical items stored in the mental lexicon. This match is performed through a multi-stage process which entails a phase of lexical selection and one of lexical access. The process of lexical selection, allows speakers to select the lexical items that correspond to the intended meaning (Levelt, 1989; Levelt, Roelofs and Meyer, 1999). How exactly this selection takes place is still debated, but it is likely achieved through an activation/inhibition mechanism (Green, 1986; 1998; Paradis, 1989; 1993). Each word is supposed to have its own specific activation thresholds as a function of its frequency of use and time elapsed since last activation (Luria, 1973; Paradis, 1989; 1993): The lower the threshold level, the easier the access; The higher the threshold level, the more difficult the access. In Green's theory, the activation of the target word is achieved through the co-occurring inhibition of its semantically-related competitors. Such inhibition would be obtained by raising the competitors' activation thresholds. For example, if the speaker's intention is to speak out the word "banana" (*e.g.* in a picture naming task), the activated concept corresponding to the idea of "banana" enters the lexicon where a selection mechanism is needed in order to select the target word ("banana") among all other semantically related lexical items ("pear", "orange", "apple", etc...). Consequently, the activation threshold of the competitors is raised while the target word ("banana") gets selected. At the end of the lexical selection process, the target word has been activated and the formulator gains access to its semantic, morphosyntactic and morphological features (lemma level of word representation) and then to its phonological form (lexeme level of word representation). In case of single word production (*e.g.* picture naming tasks) the lexical information is then transmitted to the output system where articulatory configurations corresponding to the phonemes to be uttered are programmed and then implemented. In case of sentence production, the process of lexical selection and the access to a word's lemma form the "functional level" of sentence processing, where the morphosyntactic structures requested by the selected lexical item (*i.e.* its argumental structure) guides the process of sentence generation by means of thematic roles assignment and phrase generation (noun phrase [NP], verbal phrase [VP], adjective phrase [AP], prepositional phrase [PP]). At the second level of sentence processing, the "positional level", the information contained in the lemmas of the selected lexical items is used to generate the grammatical relations among the phrases and to build up well-formed syntactic representations (Chomsky, 1988; 1995; Pinker, 1999; Caplan, 1992). It is now possible to access the syllabic and phonologic representations of the lexical items (their lexemes) and this information is sent to the output system where articulatory configurations corresponding to the phonemes to be uttered are programmed and then implemented.

What is Multilingualism?

There is no accepted definition of bilingualism and/or multilingualism among researchers as our intuitive knowledge of "bilingualism" falls short of a precise definition. According to Bloomfield (1933), bilinguals are those people who have a native-like control of two languages. We might therefore extend such interpretation to multilingual speakers, suggesting to consider multilinguals those people who have native-like control of more than two languages. However, such a rigid account of bilingualism and multilingualism introduces to the problem of the definition of quite abstract notions such as "balanced", "ideal" or even "perfect" bilingualism. Who is a perfect bilingual or multilingual? It is no doubt hard to find completely balanced or "perfect" bilinguals. When we turn to consider multilinguals, the issue becomes even more complex because we should be obliged to exclude from the count of multilingual speakers all those people who know three or more languages but simply not as much as they know their mother tongue (L1). Such a view of bilingualism (and consequently multilingualism) has been fiercely challenged by a number of studies. Rather, the focus has been shifted toward the degree of proficiency in two or more languages within the same individual. According to Weinreich (1953), a bilingual is a person who can use alternatively two languages to communicate, whereas Haugen (1953) introduced the notion of bilingualism as the simple ability to produce well-formed meaningful utterances in a second language (L2). According to Grosjean (1989; 1994; 1995; 1999), bilinguals are those people who use two or more languages in their every-day lives. However, not all multilingual speakers use their two languages all the time. Therefore an additional distinction must be introduced between multilinguals who use their languages daily and dormant multilinguals who know more than one language but use only one of them in their ordinary communicative interactions. Furthermore, Grosjean (1989) points out that bilinguals must not be considered as the sum of two complete or incomplete monolinguals, because the interaction of two or more linguistic competences in the same person produces a different but complete linguistic entity. It is an integrated whole with its own characteristics that cannot be simply reduced to the sum of the parts. Indeed, multilingual individuals can acquire their languages at different times and in different ways. Furthermore, they can use them with different people in different situations.

Therefore, bilinguals find themselves at various points of "a situational continuum which induce a particular speech mode. At one end of this continuum, bilinguals are in a totally monolingual speech mode … At the other end of the continuum, they are with bilinguals who share their two languages … and with whom they normally mix languages (code-switch and borrow): they are here in a bilingual speech mode … we should keep in mind that intermediary modes exist between the two" (Grosjean, 1989, 8).

Results from neuropsychological and neuroimaging investigations suggest that also at the neuroanatomical level the languages spoken by multilingual individuals have a complex neurofunctional organization (Fabbro, 2001). For example, several studies on bilingual or polyglot aphasic patients provide indirect arguments in favour of the hypothesis that in multilingual speakers the different languages are represented in distinct brain regions. Indeed, in some cases polyglot patients loose only one of the languages mastered before the insult (Albert and Obler, 1978; Paradis, 1995) and the different languages can be recovered at different degrees (Paradis, 1978). Neurosurgical studies provide further evidence for distributed cortical organization of the languages in multilingual speakers (Gomez-Tortosa et al., 1995). However, electrical stimulation and neuroimaging studies suggest that the cortical representation of the different languages in multilingual speakers may be complicated by several factors. For example, Ojemann and Whitaker (1978) and Rapport, Tan and Whitaker (1983) report the case of bilingual and polyglot epileptic patients who underwent language assessment while receiving cortico-electrical stimulation before neurosurgery. Interestingly, the authors detected centers *common* to all languages known by the patients along with centers showing *differential* inhibition effects. Furthermore, the L2 tended to have a more diffuse representation in the left hemisphere as opposed to the mother tongue. More recently, several studies have shown that the cortical representation of languages in multilingual speakers varies in function of two major factors: age of L2 acquisition and proficiency in the second language (*e.g.* Perani et al., 1998; Perani et al., 1996; Dehaene et al., 1997, Kim et al., 1997) (see below). Overall, results from neuroimaging investigations support the hypothesis that bilinguals are not simply two monolinguals in one person suggesting that even the multilingual brain is not the sum of two or more monolingual language systems "but is rather a unique and complex neural system which may differ in individual cases" (Abutalebi, Cappa and Perani, 2001, 188).

In what follows, a pragmatic definition of multilingualism will be privileged. Namely, multilingualism (or multilingual competence) will be intended as the command and use of two or more linguistic systems, whatever the level of proficiency and the age of acquisition of those languages. Bilingualism (or bilingual competence) will be considered a type of multilingualism, that is the command and use of two linguistic systems whatever the level of proficiency and the age of acquisition of both languages.

FACTORS AFFECTING THE ACQUISITION OF LANGUAGES IN MULTILINGUAL SPEAKERS

Several classifications have been proposed to distinguish among different types of bilingualism (Butler and Hakuta, 2004; Edwards, 2004). When the focus is on the proficiency in the two languages, a distinction has been introduced between balanced and dominant bilinguals (Peal and Lambert, 1962): a *balanced bilingual* masters the two languages to the same extent, whereas a *dominant bilingual* is more fluent in one language than in the other. As to when a second language has been acquired, it has been proposed to distinguish between early and late bilingualism: the expression *early bilingualism* refers to the early acquisition (in infancy) of both languages, whereas *late bilingualism* designates that the L2 has been acquired much later than the mother tongue. As to the effect that a second language exerts on the mother tongue, Lambert (1974) proposed to distinguish between additive and subtractive bilingualism, where *additive bilinguals* are those who improve their L2 without loosing L1 proficiency, and *subtractive bilinguals* those who lower the proficiency in their L1 while achieving a second language.

Some of these distinctions have proved empirically useful to distinguish among groups of bilingual participants for psycholinguistic and neurolinguistic experiments (Hamers and Blanc, 1990; Vaid, 1986). Indeed, several investigations have demonstrated that factors such as context and modalities of L2 acquisition (*e.g.* acquiring a second language in a Country where that language is currently spoken by means of its continuous use in real-life contexts, rather than learning it at school by means of conscious and effortful assimilation of rules and words) or the age when it has been learnt are particularly critical to determine good levels of proficiency in that language (Neville, Mills and Lawson, 1992; Neville, Coffey, Lawson, et al., 1997; Weber-Fox and Neville, 1996; Kim et al., 1997; for a review see Fabbro, 2001). One of the challenges for second language learners is the difficulty (in most cases impossibility) to acquire a native-like pronunciation of the L2. As to this respect, second language learners are faced with three main problems: an articulatory problem, consisting in the difficulty to acquire the correct articulatory configurations that allow them to produce the target phones; a word-level prosody problem, that is the production of words with correct intonation; a sentence-level prosody problem, consisting in the difficulty to learn how to correctly produce the intonation pattern of sentences during a conversation. Results from a number of investigations suggest that only those children who have been adequately exposed to the second language before the age of 8 will acquire native-like control of articulatory and prosodic aspects of speech production in L2 (Fabbro, 2004). For example, two groups of children who migrated to the USA and to The Netherlands when they were younger than 8 are reported to have acquired native-like phonetic/phonological competence in English and Dutch, respectively (Asher and Garcia, 1969; Snow, 1987; Flege and Fletcher, 1992) Interestingly, the accuracy in L2 pronunciation gets gradually lower for those people who moved to other Countries when they were older than 8 and lower than 21 years of age and remains low for those who have migrated after the age of 22. Therefore, it is possible to postulate three critical periods for the acquisition of native-like pronunciation in a second language: 1) Multilingual speakers acquiring two or more languages between 1 and 8 years of age will have a native-like pronunciation in all those languages; 2) Multilingual speakers learning a second, a third (or even more) languages between 9 and 21 years of age will develop a relatively good pronunciation in all of them; 3) Multilingual speakers learning two or more languages after the age of 22 will probably have a marked foreign accent. The existence of a "critical period" for language learning has been reported also for what regards grammatical development. For example, results from a series of experiments, where bilingual participants were tested with L2 grammaticality judgment tasks, showed a significant reduction in accuracy for those who had learnt the second language after the age of 8 (Johnson and Newport, 1989; Long, 1990). Further evidence for age-related effects on bilingual acquisition comes from electrophysiological studies where the cortical organization of the mother tongue and a second language was assessed using event-related potentials (ERPs) in a group of early bilingual participants compared to a group of late bilingual volunteers who had acquired the L2 after 7 years of age (Neville et al., 1992; 1997; Weber-Fox and Neville, 1996). In the early bilingual group the authors found that for both languages closed-class words were represented in the left frontal lobe, whereas open-class words usually involved post-rolandic cortical structures. Conversely, in late bilinguals L2 closed-class words were represented together with open-class words in post-rolandic areas and not in left frontal areas. Moreover, in an fMRI study, Kim et al. (1997) compared twelve proficient bilingual participants with diverse first and second languages in covert production tasks. The volunteers were divided in two groups: an early acquisition group, formed by six participants who had been exposed to both L1 and L2 during early infancy, and a late acquisition group, formed by six subjects who had learnt the second language after puberty. In the early bilingual group the authors found similar activation of Broca's and Wernicke's areas for both languages. In the late bilingual group, L1 and L2 shared similar activations of Wernicke's area but different activations (separated by approximately 8 mms) within Broca's area. These results suggested that the age of acquisition is a major factor affecting the cortical organization of a second language. It is noteworthy, however, that the authors did not specify in detail the levels of L2 proficiency for the participants involved in the experiment. This is a significant omission because the differences registered in Broca's activation in the late acquisition group may reflect differences at the morphosyntactic (functional and/or positional) and phonetic (articulatory) levels of sentence processing (see also Abutalebi et al., 2001; Fabbro, 2001). In a subsequent fMRI study, Chee, Tan and Thiel (1999) investigated the cerebral activation in two groups of Chinese (Mandarin) – English highly proficient bilinguals during word-stem completion tasks. The first group included fifteen participants who learned English before the age of 6 (early bilingual group). The second group included nine bilinguals who learned English after age 12 (late bilingual group). In this experiment, the authors found no group-related difference in the activation of frontal areas (left prefrontal region including the inferior frontal gyrus, left supplementary motor area and bilateral occipital and parietal regions). The divergent results obtained by Kim et al. (1997) and Chee et al. (1999) may depend not on the age of L2 acquisition (early vs. late acquisition), but on the levels of proficiency in the two languages and on the time spent speaking them. Therefore, the differential activation of left frontal areas reported by Kim et al. (1997) may reflect different levels of L2 proficiency between the two groups rather than the age of L2 acquisition. A possible solution to this problem can be found in the results of a recent fMRI experiment where three groups of Italian-German bilingual participants were compared in a series of grammatical and semantic judgment tasks (Wartenburger et al., 2003). The first group (Early Acquisition High Proficiency group [EAHP]) was formed by 11 bilingual participants who learned the two languages together since birth and showed high proficiency in both of them. The second group (Late Acquisition High Proficiency group [LAHP]) included 12 bilingual participants who learned German (L2) before 6 years of age but with high proficiency in both languages. The third group (Late Acquisition Low Proficiency group [LALP]) consisted of 9 bilingual volunteers who learned German (L2) after the age of 6 and had were low proficient in that language. The EAHP and LAHP groups had a perfect phonetic and morphosyntactic competence in the L2, whereas the participants included in the LALP group made a number of morphosyntactic errors coupled with a strong foreign accent. On the grammatical judgement task, the LAHP group showed greater activation in language-related areas than the EAHP group. At the same time, with respect to the LALP group, greater activation was found in the left temporo-parietal junction, the right lingual gyrus and right inferior parietal lobule in the LAHP group. These results suggest that age of acquisition and, to a lesser degree, proficiency level affect the cortical representation of grammatical processes in L2.

Models of Language Representation in Bilingual and Multilingual Individuals

The first systematic investigations of bilingualism began approximately 100 years ago as diary studies by researchers reporting on the linguistic development of their own children. Ronjat (1913) described the linguistic development of his son in a bilingual German-French environment. Leopold (1939; 1949) provided a detailed report of his daughter Hildegard's simultaneous acquisition of English and German. These studies represent a rich source of observations. However, the analyses of bilingual language development performed by the authors lacked of a systematic linguistic approach and were based on subjective impressions rather than rigorous scientific methodology.

One of the first attempts to formulate a model of lexical representation in bilinguals is the "compound-coordinate model" of bilingualism initially proposed by Weinreich (1953) and then revised by Ervin and Osgood (1954). In its original configuration, this model assumes that in bilingual individuals the phonological ("signifier") and semantic ("signified") aspects of the words in the two languages are represented in three possible configurations: coordinate, compound and subordinate, respectively. In a coordinate system the phonological representation of translation equivalents (*i.e.* words of different languages sharing the same meaning) matches two different meaning representations. In such a system, the bilingual individual would have two separate conceptual representations and two separate word forms for the Italian word "casa" and the corresponding English word "house" (Figure 1). In a compound representation, the two phonological forms are identified with a common meaning representation. Therefore, the two word forms "casa" and "house" are represented in the same conceptual system (Figure 2). A subordinate system is a word association model where the meaning representation of an L2 word (*e.g.* "house") is accessed through the meaning representation of the word of the mother tongue (*e.g.* "casa") (Figure 3).

Erving and Osgood (1954) suggested that coordinate or compound representation of two languages depends on the modalities of L2 acquisition. An individual learning two languages in separate cultural environments will develop a coordinate representation. This is for example the case of an English child who learns English as his mother tongue in an English-speaking Country and then Italian as L2 in an Italian-speaking environment. In contrast, a child learning two languages together in the same context will develop a compound structure. An individual learning a second language after a certain age in formal contexts will develop a subordinate representation. While speaking, subordinate bilinguals formulate what they want to say in their L1 and then translate it into L2. Therefore, in a subordinate representation the meanings of the L2 words are accessed only through a translation process.

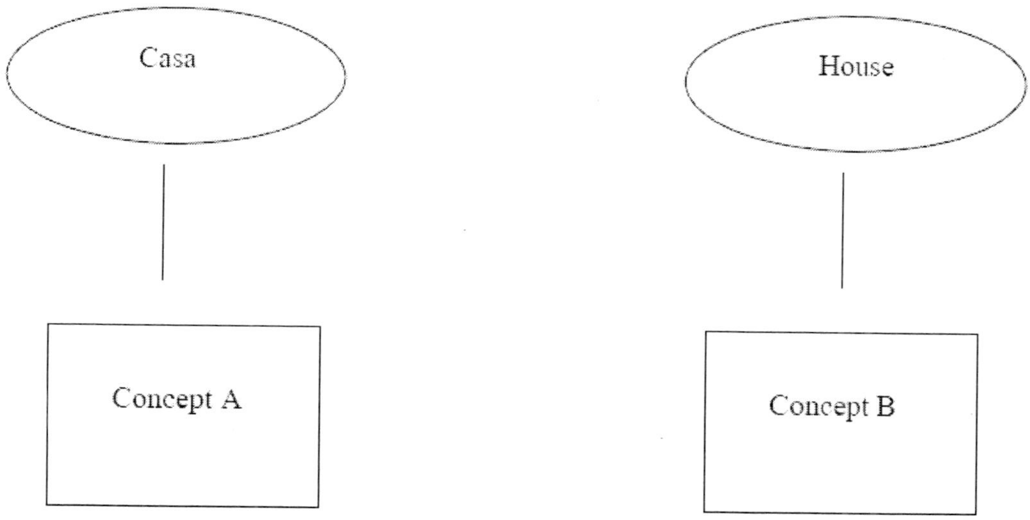

Figure 1. Representation of a coordinate system (adapted from Woutersen, Cox, Weltens, and De Bot, 1994).

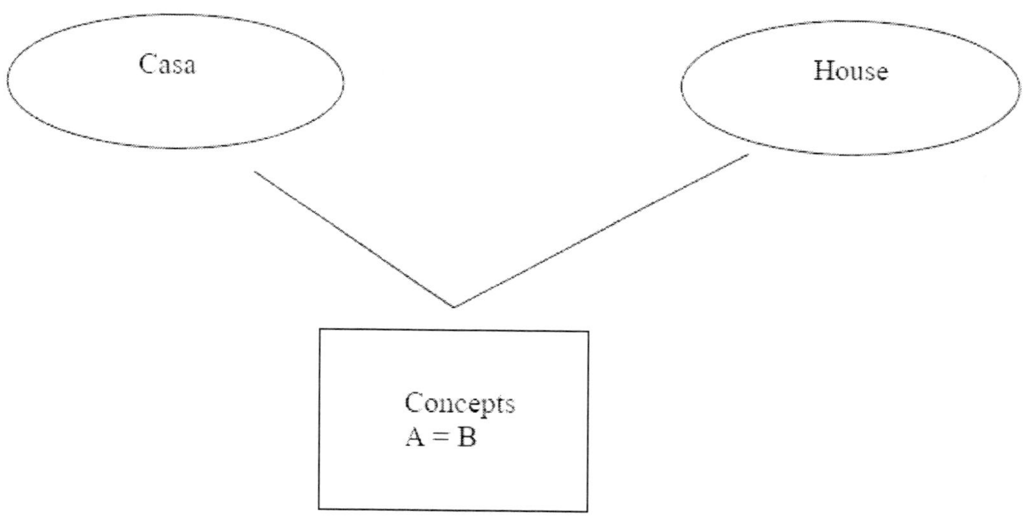

Figure 2. Representation of a compound system (adapted from Woutersen, Cox, Weltens, and De Bot, 1994).

The coordinate-compound model introduced important theoretical issues on the debate about language representation in bilingual individuals such as the hypothesis of a distinction between conceptual and lexical representation of words, and the problem of language storage in bilingual speakers.

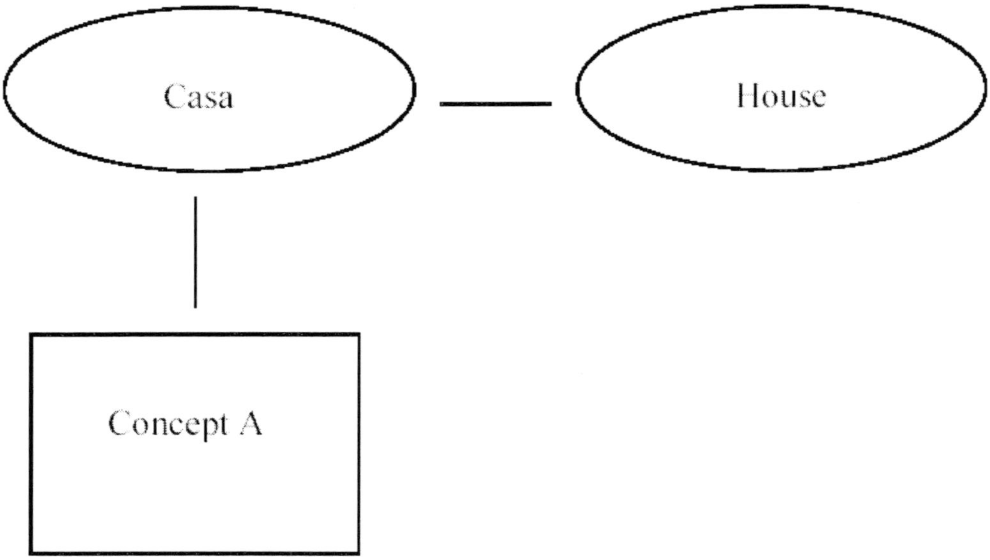

Figure 3. Representation of a subordinate system (adapted from Woutersen, Cox, Weltens, and De Bot, 1994).

As to the first problem, results from psycholinguistic and neurolinguistic studies support the hypothesis that the two languages of a bilingual individual access a common semantic system (*e.g.* Illes et al., 1999; Costa, Miozzo and Caramazza, 1999; Hermans, Bongaerts, de Bot and Schreuder, 1998; Potter, So, von Eckardt, and Feldman, 1984). For example, in an fMRI study aimed at investigating the brain activation patterns during semantic judgement tasks (concrete/abstract judgements) in a group of 8 late Spanish-English bilingual speakers who had learned their L2 after the age of 10, Illes et al. (1999) identified a shared frontal lobe system for semantic processing for both languages (left inferior frontal gyrus; in six of the participants the activation included also the right inferior frontal gyrus).

As to the problem of whether lexical knowledge of bilinguals' two languages is merged into one large lexical system or is kept separate in two distinct lexicons (*i.e.* a lexicon for L1 and a lexicon for L2), there is much less agreement, as two opposite hypotheses have been put forward and are currently debated (Grosjean, 1995): a two-lexicons view opposed to a one-lexicon view. Proponents of the two-lexicons hypothesis (Potter et al., 1984; De Groot, 1993; Kroll and Stewart, 1994) claim that the lexical representations in bilingual speakers are stored in two different lexicons and that information acquired in one language is available in the other only through a translation process. In contrast, according to the one-lexicon view (*e.g.* De Bot and Schreuder, 1993; De Bot, 1992; Paradis, 1987), the two languages of a bilingual speaker are stored in different subsystems of the same lexicon which can be activated to different extents, depending on which language is currently being used.

Within the theoretical framework of the two-lexicons view, the coordinated-compound model proposed by Weinreich has been extended and reformulated. Such models are usually defined "hierarchical" as they postulate that a word's conceptual representation (its "meaning" in the broadest sense) is separated from its lexical representation and that the words of the two languages of a bilingual individual are stored in two separate lexicons, one for the words of the L1, the other for those of the L2. Potter et al. (1984) proposed a Word

Association Model and a Concept Mediation Model based on Weinreich's subordinate system and compound system, respectively. According to the Word Association Model, L2 words do not have a direct access to the corresponding concepts but must first be translated in the corresponding L1 lexical representations that, in turn, have direct access to the conceptual system. This model is assumed to represent the organization of the two languages in non-fluent low proficient bilinguals such as for example second language learners in the early stages of L2 acquisition. In the Concept Mediation Model the lexical items of both lexicons (L1 and L2) are supposed to have direct access to the conceptual system by means of direct conceptual-lexical links. This system is hypothesized to reflect the competence of bilinguals who have reached high levels of proficiency in their L2. Taken together, the Word Association Model and the Concept Association Model entail a developmental hypothesis of language representation in bilinguals, as the shift from lexical to conceptual mapping is assumed to reflect growing levels of proficiency in the L2. Such hypothesis has been tested in a number of studies (see Kroll and de Groot [1997] for an extensive review on this issue). For example, Chen and Leung (1989) and Kroll and Curley, (1988) compared the reaction times (RTs) of more and less fluent bilinguals in a picture naming task and a word translation task. Under the assumption that picture naming is achieved through concept mediation, it was hypothesized that similar RTs in both tasks would imply the recourse to a concept mediation strategy, whereas shorter RTs at the word translation task would imply the recourse to a lexical translation strategy. Indeed, less proficient bilingual individuals at earlier stages of L2 acquisition were faster in the word translation task than in the picture naming task (use of the lexical translation strategy), whereas in the more proficient bilinguals the RTs were comparable across the two tasks (recourse to the concept mediation strategy). Therefore, experimental results seem to support the proficiency-related shift from a Word Association to a Concept Association representation of the bilinguals' two languages. However, neither of the two models could account for the translation asymmetry effect (Kroll and Dussas, 2004; Kroll and Sholl, 1992) reported in both early and advanced bilinguals in a number of empirical observations, that is the fact that bilinguals usually translate faster and more accurately in the L2 to L1 rather than in the L1 to L2 direction. In order to explain the translation asymmetry effect, Kroll and Stewart (1994) proposed a Revised Hierarchical Model where both the Word Association and the Concept Association Model were incorporated (figure 4).

The Revised Hierarchical Model maintains the idea of independent lexical representations for the two languages known by the bilingual and of a shared conceptual system for both languages. However, it also introduces some important innovations to the previously presented models. We will briefly consider some of the main assumptions of the model. It is assumed that the extension of the lexicon of the L1 is larger than that of the L2, as even highly proficient bilinguals usually know more words in the native language than in their subsequently learned languages. In order to account for the translation asymmetry effect, the connections between the two languages (L1 and L2) and the concept-system are supposed to be asymmetrical and to reflect the modalities of L2 acquisition. It is postulated that translating from L2 to L1 entails a direct access to the L1 lexical form, whereas translating from L1 to L2 is supposed to activate not only the corresponding translation equivalent in L2, but also the conceptual representation of the L1 word thus engaging a semantic route as well. The forward translation direction (from L1 to L2) is assumed to be particularly challenging for less proficient bilinguals, because in these individuals the link between the second language and the conceptual store is still weak. Indeed, experiments on translation generally support these predictions (e.g. Kroll, Michael, Tokovicz, and Dufour, 2002).

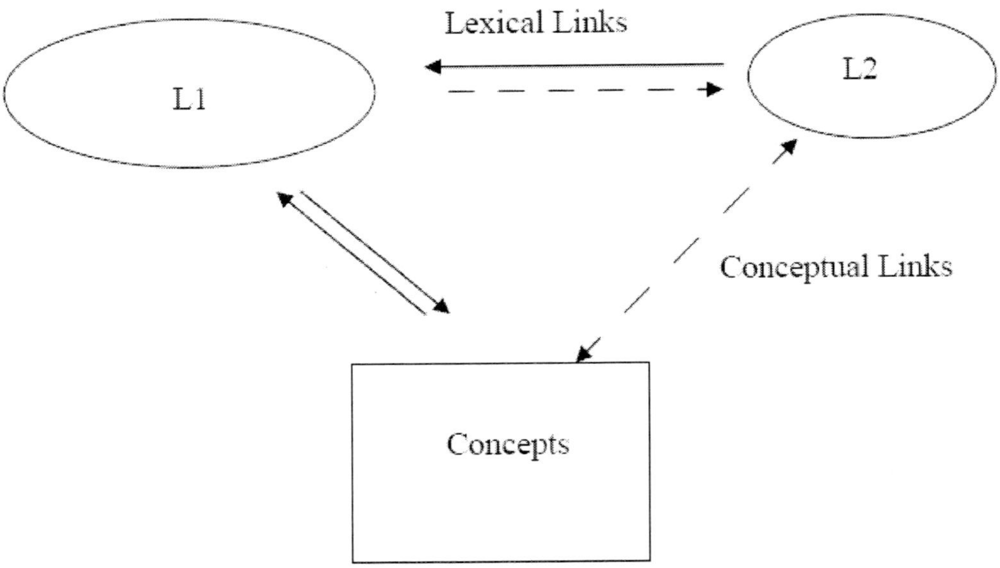

Figure 4. The Revised Hierarchical Model (adapted from Kroll and Stewart, 1994).

Even if appealing, the two-lexicons view has been challenged by a number of neurophysiologic and neuroimaging studies that, at least at the macroscopical level, evidenced a similar cerebral representation for L1 and L2 lexicons in both early and late bilinguals (Klein et al., 1999; Chee et al., 1999; Illes et al., 1999; Hernandez et al., 2000). For example, in a Positron Emission Tomography (PET) study Klein et al. (1999) found that Chinese (L1) – English (L2) bilinguals showed similar cerebral activation patterns for both languages when involved in verb generation tasks (left inferior frontal, dorso-lateral frontal cortex, temporo-parietal cortices, and right cerebellum). Furthermore, results from the afore mentioned study by Chee, Than and Thiel (1999) provide additional evidence in favour of the hypothesis that the cortical representation of words even in typologically different languages such as English and Mandarin may involve the same cortical areas. Overall, as it will be shown in the next paragraph, results from both experimental and clinical studies suggest that age and modalities of acquisition, as well as language use probably affect the neuroanatomical and functional organization of the lexicon.

The Functional Architecture of the Bilingual Speech Production System

Several hypotheses have been put forward to account for the functional architecture of the bilingual speech production system. In most cases these are the reformulation of models originally proposed for monolingual speakers. Indeed, psycholinguistic theorizing has usually held monolingualism as the canonical form of language use (Vaid, 2002), implicitly assuming that monolingual acquisition and processing are the norm. Such monolingual prejudice has proved to be misguiding in cognitive research on multilingualism and has conditioned the modelling of bilingual and multilingual competence. In fact, quite no one can be considered purely monolingual as even monolingual children usually grow up in a social environment where more than one variety of the same language is spoken (*e.g.* the so-called "dialects"). Therefore, they learn to use a certain variety of the language they are exposed to in specific linguistic and/or extra-linguistic contexts, and other varieties in different contexts. In other words, even those children who are generally regarded as monolingual will develop a multilingual competence, based on lexical, grammatical and pragmatic/discursive knowledge relative to each of the varieties of the language to which they are exposed. Let's consider the case of a Canadian born in Quebec. He may acquire Quebecois as his mother tongue (L1) and use it in familiar contexts, standard French as a second language (L2) used as language of education and in formal contexts, and eventually English as a third language (L3), used not in daily/life interactions but, for example, to write scientific articles or to give lectures at international congresses.

The issue of language production in polyglots raises several problems. A major question concerns the functional architecture of the multilingual lexicon, that is how words are represented, selected and accessed in multilingual speakers. One of the most influential models of language production is the "bilingual production model" (de Bot, 1992; de Bot and Schreuder, 1993), based on Levelt's "speaking model" (1989). In what follows we will attempt to integrate the model proposed by de Bot (1992) with data from recent psycholinguistic, neurophysiologic and neuroimaging investigations.

De Bot's bilingual production model hypothesizes the existence of three subsystems for language production (a conceptualizer, a formulator and an articulator, respectively), a subsystem for comprehension (speech-comprehension system), and a lexicon involved in both production and comprehension.

In multilingual speakers, the conceptualizer is assumed to be language independent. It elaborates the conversational conventions and the contextual information in order to signal "which language to choose". It is at the level of the formulator that the language to be used in the interaction will be chosen. The formulator is considered a procedural system working on a system of declarative knowledge: the lexicon. Adopting Paradis' (1987) subset hypothesis, De Bot (1992) proposed that L1 and L2 words form different subsets within one and the same lexicon. Experimental and clinical studies suggest that age and modalities of acquisition, as well as language use probably affect the organization of both formulator and lexicon. In multilingual individuals who have acquired two or more languages from birth, the formulator is probably represented in common cortico-subcortical cerebral structures. In this case the different languages would be maintained separate merely by neurofunctional mechanisms. When a second language is learned after the age of 8, however, the neurofunctional systems accounting for grammar and phonology are most likely to be separate also at the neuroanatomical level (Fabbro, 1996; Kim, Relkin, Lee and Hirsch, 1997). Furthermore, in fluent bilinguals the lexicon is probably represented in common neural structures (parieto-temporal areas) and the neurofunctional separation between languages might depend on word use relationships.

In the formulator the preverbal message is converted into a speech plan by means of two processes: lexical selection and lexical access, respectively. When considering multilingual competence, it becomes important to explain how a multilingual speaker selects the correct lexical node in the target language preventing cross-language interference. As to this respect, two major hypotheses have been proposed. The first states that the intended meaning in the preverbal message selectively activates the lexical items only of the selected language and not those of the other language(s) (Soares and Grosjean, 1984; Macnamara and Kushnir, 1971). Such view has been generally abandoned in favour of an alternative hypothesis claiming that the intended meaning activates the subsets of words belonging to the languages mastered by the speaker and that the target word is selected by creating an imbalance in their activation levels (De Bot, 1992; Green, 1986, 1998). It is postulated that each subset has its own specific activation thresholds[1] (Luria, 1973; Green, 1986, 1998; Paradis, 1989; 1993) and can be selected by means of activation and inhibition processes[2] (Inhibitory Control Model, Green, 1998). Inhibition is generally automatic and avoids interferences among the languages that form the multilingual competence. The selection of the target lexical node is obtained by creating a differential level of activation in the two or more lexicons of the multilingual speaker by means of both activation of the target words and reactive inhibition of its competitors. In other terms, the selection of a word in one language automatically triggers an inhibition process of the competitors in the other language(s). Consider the case of a trilingual individual who knows Italian (L1), English (L2) and Dutch (L3). In this case, the activation of the word 'bike' (L2) will inhibit the corresponding lexical items in L1 (*i.e.* Italian "bicicletta") and L3 (*i.e.* Dutch "fiets") as well as semantically and phonologically similar words in the three languages. The multilingual speaker's languages can receive three states of activation (Green, 1986). They can be selected, active or dormant depending on the communicative situation. A language is selected when it has been chosen for the interaction. The selected language controls the speech output. A language is active when it has not been chosen as the main code for the communicative exchange but is kept active during the whole interaction. It works in parallel to the selected language but has no direct access to the outgoing speech processing. A dormant language does not receive any activation and consequently does not play a role in ongoing processing. In the multilingual competence, one language is always selected while the other(s) language(s) can be either active or dormant. In this framework it is possible to explain the code-switching phenomenon. Language switching occurs quite commonly for instance in bilingual communities where both languages have the same social status (see Grosjean, 1998). The habit of bilingual individuals to alternate between languages within one coherent discourse may determine low thresholds of activation of switching phenomena and a reduction in both languages' mutual inhibition. In such bilingual communities, it is quite normal for individuals to switch from one language to the other while speaking informally. In other communities, however, such behavior is intentionally avoided for sociolinguistic reasons. For example, in Brussels, where both French and Flemish are official languages, a public official or a bank employee would never switch between the two languages and would stick to his/her interlocutor's language, even though

[1] A cerebral lesion can lower the activation threshold of a language, which is thus not lost, but simply inaccessible through the usual activation threshold. Generally, such activation threshold is lower for comprehension than for expression. For this reason, there are cases of bilingual aphasic patients with preserved comprehension of a language associated to impaired production in it (Paradis, 1996).

[2] It is likely that inhibitory relations among languages are organized differently in simultaneous interpreters in which both languages are concurrently activated for many hours a day. In this particular profession, the activation thresholds of the two languages are thus quantitatively different as opposed to those of the other polyglots.

most natives understand and speak both languages. In Belgium each linguistic community has a strong identity which is fiercely defended also through language use. This switching mechanism is not peculiar only to polyglot speakers, but also to monolingual individuals who use it to select among different linguistic registers according to the communicative context. For example, an individual may ask his/her interlocutor to close the door by using a courtesy form ("Will you please close the door?") or a direct form ("Close the door"). In Paradis' (1993) opinion, the system accounting for the selection of one of the two registers is similar to that accounting for the selection of one language rather than another. Many neurologists and neurolinguists have discussed the possible neurological organization of the switch mechanisms. Some of them, generally defined as *localizationists*, claim that the activation of a specific language (for example L1) and the concurrent inhibition of the other languages (*e.g.* L2, L3, and the like) is subserved by specific brain areas. For example, Leischner (1943) claimed that this center is localized in the left supramarginal gyrus, whereas, according to Stengel and Zelmanovicz (1933) and Zatorre (1989), it is localized in anterior structures of the left hemisphere. In Lebrun's opinion (1971), the switching mechanism is localized in the right hemisphere. Other authors have criticized the idea of an anatomical center governing language switching. Goldstein (1948), for example, suggested that any cerebral lesion impairs switching between mental processes, and that the faculty of switching is only an example of the more general faculty of abstraction. Paradis (1993) claims that switching mechanisms are only one aspect of a more general system involved in decision-taking processes. In Paradis' opinion, the switch function is part of a general system responsible for the selection of behaviors such as standing up or sitting down, speaking Italian or English, etc. Recent evidence suggests that the language switching mechanism involves the dorsolateral prefrontal cortex (Fabbro, Skrap, and Aglioti, 2000; Hernandez, Dapretto, Mazziotta, and Bookheimer, 2001; Holtzeimer, Fawatz, Wilson, and Avery, 2005). Indeed, Fabbro et al. (2000) report the case of a bilingual patient with a lesion to the left anterior cingulated and to the frontal lobe (marginally involving also the right anterior cingulate area). After that lesion, the patient presented pathological switching between languages in the absence of any other linguistic impairment.

Once the target lexical node has been selected, the formulator gains access to its semantic, morphosyntactic and morphological features (lemma level) and then to its phonological form (lexeme level). In case of single word production the lexical information is directly transmitted to the articulator. In case of sentence production, however, the information stored in the lemma level of word representation is used to generate the argumental structure and hence the syntactic organization of the sentence. At this point, the articulator converts the speech plan into actual speech. During speech production in bilinguals both selected and active languages are simultaneously activated at all levels with the exception of the articulatory subsystem, which remains inactive for the non-selected language (de Bot, 1992). The articulator transforms the strings of syllables of the selected language in articulatory patterns. It is assumed that syllable articulatory programs are automatized and that the level of automatism correlates with the level of proficiency which, in turn, is a function of age of L2 acquisition. In other words, a multilingual speaker can pronounce as a native speaker words and sentences in two or more languages only if he/she has correctly automatized the syllable articulatory programs before the age of 8. Advanced bilinguals, usually early bilinguals, may have only one large articulatory system containing all syllable articulatory programs for all the languages they master, whereas less proficient bilinguals, usually late bilinguals, may have independent stores for each language (*e.g.* Flege and Fletcher, 1992).

References

Abutalebi J, Cappa SF and Perani D (2001). The bilingual brain as revealed by functional neuroimaging. *Bilingualism Lang. Cogn.*, 4: 179-190

Albert, M.L., and Obler, L.K. (1978). *The bilingual brain*. New York: Academic Press.

Asher J, and Garcia R (1969). The optimal age to learn a foreign language. *Modern Language Journal*, 28: 334-341

Bloomfield L (1933). *Language*. New York: Holt, Rinehart and Winston

Butler YG and Hakuta K (2004). Bilingualism and Second Language Acquisition. In T K Bhatia and W C Ritchie (eds.) *The Handbook of Bilingualism*. (pp. 114-144). Blakwell Publishing. Malden , MA

Caplan D (1992). *Language. Structure, processing and disorders*. Cambridge, Massachusetts: MIT Press

Chee, M. W. L., Tan, E. W. L., and Thiel, T. (1999). Mandarian and English single word processing studied with functional magnetic resonance imaging. *The Journal of Neuroscience,* **19,** 3050–3056.

Chen H-C. and Leung Y.S. (1989). Patterns of lexical processing in a nonnative language. *J. Exp. Psychol. Learn. Mem. Cogn.*, 15, 316-325.

Chomsky N (1988). Language and problems of knowledge: the Managua Lectures, MIT Press, Cambridge, Massachusetts

Chomsky, N. (1995). *The minimalist program*. Cambridge, MA: MIT Press.

Costa, A., Miozzo, M., and Caramazza, A. (1999). Lexical selection in bilinguals: Do words in the bilingual's two lexicons compete for selection? *Journal of Memory and Language, 41*, 365–397.

Costa A, and Caramazza A (1999). Is lexical selection in bilingual speech production language-speciWc? Further evidence from Spanish–English and English–Spanish bilinguals. *Bilingualism: Language and Cognition, 2*, 231–244.

Costa A, and Santesteban M (2004a). Bilingual word perception and production: Two sides of the same coin? *Trends in Cognitive Sciences, 8*(6), 253.

Costa A, and Santesteban M (2004b). Lexical access in bilingual speech production: Evidence from language switching in highly proWcient bilinguals and L2 learners. *Journal of Memory and Language, 50*, 491–511.

de Bot K (1992). A bilingual production model: Levelt's speaking model adapted. *Applied Linguistics, 13*, 1–24.

de Bot, K., and Schreuder, R. (1993). Word production and the bilingual lexicon. In R. Schreuder and B. Weltens (eds.), *The bilingual lexicon* (pp. 191-214). Amsterdam: John Benjamins.

de Groot A.M.B. (1993). Word-type effects in bilingual processing tasks: Support for a mixed-representational system. In R. Schreuder and B. Weltens (eds.) *The bilingual lexicon* (pp. 27-51). Amsterdam: John Benjamins

Dehaene, S., Dupoux, E., Mehler, J., Cohen, L., Paulesu, E., Perani, D., van de Moortele, P.F., Lehéricy, S., and Le Bihan, D. (1997). Anatomical variability in the cortical representation of first and second language. *Neuroreport*, 8(17):3809-15

Edwards, J.V. (2004). Foundations of bilingualism. In T.K.Bhatia and W.C. Ritchie (eds.), *The handbook of bilingualism* (pp. 7-31). Blakwell Publishing. Malden , MA

Erwin, S., and Osgood, C. (1954). Second language learning and bilingualism. *Journal of abnormal and social psychology. Supplement*. 49, 139-146

Fabbro, F. (1996) . Neurofunctional aspects of bilingual aphasia. *Journal of the Israeli Speech Hearing and Language Association, 19*: 13-15.

Fabbro F (1999). *The neurolinguistics of bilingualism: An introduction*. Hove, UK: Psychology Press.

Fabbro F (2001). The bilingual brain, cerebral representation of languages. *Brain and Language, 79*, 211–222.

Fabbro F (2004). *Neuropedagogia delle lingue*. Astrolabio, Roma, Italy

Fabbro F, Skrap M, and Aglioti S (2000). Pathological switching between languages after frontal lesions in a bilingual patient. *Journal of Neurology, Neurosurgery, and Psychiatry, 68*, 650–652.

Flege, J.E. and Fletcher, K.L. (1992). Talker and listener effects on degree of perceived foreing accent. *Journal of the Acoustical Society of America*, 91: 370-389.

Frazier L, and Fodor JD (1978). The sausage machine: a new two-stage parsing model. Cognition, 6, 291–325.

Goldstein, K. (1948). Disturbances of language in polyglot individuals with aphasia. In *Language and language disturbances* (pp. 138-146). New York: Grune and Stratton.

Green DW (1986). Control, activation and resource. *Brain and Language, 27*, 210–223.

Green DW (1998). Mental control of the bilingual lexico-semantic system. *Bilingualism: Language and Cognition, 1*, 67–81.

Grice HP (1975). Logic and conversation. In Cole P, Morgan JL (eds.) *Syntax and semantics: Vol. 3: Speech acts*, Academic Press, New York , 41-58

Grosjean F (1982). *Life with Two Languages. An Introduction to Bilingualism*. Cambridge: Harvard University Press

Grosjean F (1989). Neurolinguists beware! The bilingual is not two monolinguals in one person. *Brain and Language*, 36, 3-15

Grosjean F (1994). Individual bilingualism. In: Asher R E (ed.) *The Encyclopaedia of Language and Linguistics*. Pergamon Press, Oxford: 1656-60

Grosjean F (1995). A psycholinguistic approach to code-switching: The recognition of guest words by bilinguals. In L. Milry and P. Muysken (eds.), *One speaker, two languages* (259-275). Cambridge: Cambridge University Press.

Grosjean, F. (1998). Studying bilinguals: Methodological and conceptual issues. *Bilingualism: Language and Cognition*, 1: 131-149.

Grosjean F (1999) Individual bilingualism. In B. Spolsky (ed.) *Concise Encyclopaedia of Educational Linguistics*, pp. 284-90. London: Elsevier

Hakuta K (1986) *Mirror of language: The debate on bilingualism*. New York: Basic Books

Hamers JF, and Blanc MHA (1990). *Bilinguality and Bilingualism*. Cambridge: Cambridge University Press.

Haugen, E. (1953). Bilingualism in the Americas. Montgomery, AL: University of Alabama Press.

Hermans, D., Bongaerts, T., de Bot, K., and Schreuder, R. (1998). Producing words in a foreign language: Can speakers prevent interference from their first language? *Bilingualism: Language and Cognition*, 1: 213-229.

Hernandez A.E., Martinez, A., and Kohnert, K. (2000). In search of the language switch: An fMRI study of picture naming in Spanish-English bilinguals. *Brain and Language*, 73: 421-431.

Hernandez, A.E, Dapretto, M., Mazziotta, J., and Bookheimer, S. (2001). Language switching and language representation in Spanish-English bilinguals: An fMRI study. *Neuroimage*, 14: 510-520.

Holtzeimer, P., Fawatz, W., Wilson, C., and Avery, D. (2005). Repetetive transcranial magnetic stimulation may induce language switching in bilingual patients. *Brain and Language*, 94, 274-277.

Illes, J., Francis, W., Desmond, J., Gabrieli, J., Glover, G., et al. (1999). Convergent cortical representation of semantic processing in bilinguals. *Brain and Language*, 70: 347-363.

Johnson, J.S.and Newport, E.L. (1989). Critical period effects in second language learning: The influence of maturational state on the acquisition of English as a second language. *Cognitive Psychology*, 21: 60-99.

Johnson-Laird PN (1980). Mental models in cognitive science. *Cognitive Science*, 4, 71-115.

Kim, K.H.S., Relkin, N.R., Lee, K.-M. and Hirsch J. (1997). Distinct cortical areas associated with native and second languages: *Nature*, *388*: 171-174.

Kintsch W, and Van Dijk T (1978). Toward a model of text comprehension and production. *Psychological Review*. *85*, 363-394

Klein, D., Milner, B., Zatorre, R., Zhao, V., and Nikelski, J. (1999). Cerebral organization in bilinguals: A PET study of Chinese-English verb generation. *NeuroReport*, 10: 2841-2846.

Kroll J.F. and Curley J. (1988). Lexical memory in novice bilinguals: the role of concepts in retrieving second language words. In P.M. Gruneberg and R. Sykes (eds.) *Practical Aspects of Memory* (Vol. 2): John Wiley and Sons. London, UK

Kroll J.F. and Dussas P.E. (2004). The comprehension of words and sentences in two languages. In T.K. Bhatia and W.C. Ritchie (eds.) *The handbook of bilingualism* (pp. 169-200). Blackwell Publishing. Malden, MA

Kroll, J.F., and de Groot, A.M.B. (1997). Lexical and conceptual memory in the bilingual: Mapping form to meaning in two languages. In A. de Groot and J. Kroll (eds.), *Tutorials in bilingualism: Psycholinguistic perspectives* (pp. 169-199). Mahwah, NJ: Lawrence Erlbaum Associates.

Kroll J.F., Michael E., Tokovicz N. and Dufour R. (2002). The development of lexical fluency in a second language. *Second Language Research*, 18, 137-171

Kroll J.F. and Sholl A. (1992). Lexical and conceptual memory in fluent and nonfluent bilinguals. In R.J. Harris (ed.) *Cognitive processes in bilinguals* (pp. 191-206). Amsterdam: Elsevier Science.

Kroll JF, and Stewart E (1994). Category interference in translation and picture naming: Evidence for asymmetric connections between bilingual memory representations. *Journal of Memory and Language, 33*, 149–174.

Lambert WE (1974). Culture and language as factors in learning and education. In F F Aboud and R D Meade (eds.) *Cultural Factors inLearning and Education*. Bellingham, W A: Western Washinghton State University.

Lebrun, Y. (1971) The neurology of bilingualism. Word, 27 (1-3), 179-186

Leischner, A. (1943). Aphasia of deaf-mutes. In Paradis, M. (Ed.), *Readings on Aphasia in Bilinguals and Polyglots*. Montreal: Didier, 1983, pp.423-444.

Leopold W. (1939-1949). *Speech development of a Bilingual Child* (4 vols.) Evanston, IL: North-western University Press

Levelt WJM (1989). *Speaking: From intention to articulation*. Cambridge, MA: MIT Press.

Levelt WJM, Roelofs A, and Meyer AS (1999). A theory of lexical access in speech production. *Behavioral and Brain Sciences, 22*, 1–37.

Levinson S (1983). *Pragmatics*. Cambridge University Press, Cambridge

Long MH (1990). Maturational constraints on language development. *Studies in second language acquisition*, 12: 251.285

Luria, A.R. (1973). *The working brain: An introduction to neuropsychology*. New York: Penguin Education.

Macnamara, J., and Kushnir, S.L. (1971). Linguistic independence of bilinguals: The input switch. *Journal of Verbal Learning and Verbal Behavior,* 10: 480-487.

Marini, A. (2001). *Elementi di psicolinguistica generale*, Springer Verlag, Milano, Italy

Marini A., Carlomagno S., Caltagirone C., and Nocentini U. (2005a). The role played by the right hemisphere in the organization of complex textual structures. *Brain and Language.* 93/1, 46-54

Marini A., Boewe A. and Carlomagno S. (2005b). Assessment of age-related differences in the processing of textual descriptions. *Journal of Psycholinguistic Research*. 34/5, 439-463

Marini, A., and Nocentini, U. (2003). *Comunicazione verbale e emisfero destro*. Springer Verlag, Milano, Italy

Martin R C, Newsome M R and Vu H (2002). Language and lexical processing. In V S Ramachandran (Ed.) *Encyclopaedia of the Human Brain*. Vol. 2 (pp. 631-643). Academic Press. San Diego.

Meisel J M (2004). The Bilingual Child,. In T K Bhatia and W C Ritchie (eds.) *Handbook of Bilingualism*. pp. 91-113. Blakwell Publishing. Malden , MA

Neville, H.J., Mills, D.L. and Lawson, D.S. (1992). Fractionating language: different neural subsystems with different sensitive periods. *Cerebral Cortex*, *2*: 244-258.

Neville, H.J., Coffey, S.A., Lawson, D.S., Fischer, A., Emmorey, K. and Bellugi, U. (1997). Neural systems mediating American Sign Language: Effects of sensory experiences and age of acquisition. *Brain and Language*, *57*: 285-308.

Ojemann, G.A. (1991). Cortical organization of language. *The Journal of Neuroscience*, 11: 2281-2287

Ojemann, G.A., and Whitaker, H.A. (1978). The bilingual brain. *Archives of Neurology,* 35: 409-412.

Paradis, M. (1978). Bilingual linguistic memory: Neurolinguistic considerations. Paper presented at the Annual Meeting of the Linguistic Society of America, Boston, 28 December.

Paradis, M. (1987). Neurolinguistic perspectives on bilingualism. In M. Paradis and G. Libben, *The assessment of bilingual aphasia* (pp.1-17). Hillsdale, NJ: Lawrence Erlbaum.

Paradis, M. (1989). Bilingual and polyglot aphasia. In F. Boller and J. Grafman (eds.), *Handbook of Neuropsychology*. Vol. 2, 117-140. Amsterdam: Elsevier.

Paradis, M. (1993). Linguistic, psycholinguistic, and neurolinguistic aspects of 'interference' in bilingual speakers: The activation threshold hypothesis. *International Journal of Psycholinguistics*, *9*: 133-145.

Paradis, M. (1994). Neurolinguistic aspects of implicit and explicit memory: implications for bilingualism and second language acquisition. In N. Ellis (Ed.), *Implicit and Explicit Language Learning*. London: Academic Press, 393-419

Paradis, M. (1995). The need for distinctions. In M. Paradis (ed.), *Aspects of bilingual aphasia* (pp. 1-9). Oxford: Pergamon Press.

Paradis, M. (1996). The cognitive neuropsychology of bilingualism. In: A. De Groot and J. Kroll (Eds.), *Tutorials in Bilingualism: Psycholinguistic Perspectives*.. Hillsdale, NJ: Erlbaum.

Paradis M (2004). *A neurolinguistic theory of bilingualism*. Amsterdam: John Benjamins.

Peal E and Lambert WE (1962). The relation of bilingualism to intelligence. *Psychological Monographs*, 76, 1-23

Perani, D., Paulesu, E., Sebastian-Gallés, N., Dupoux, E., Dehaene, D., Bettinardi, V., Cappa, S., Fazio, F., and Mehler, J. (1998). The bilingual brain: Proficiency and age of acquisition of the second language. *Brain*, 121: 1841-1852.

Perani, D., Dehaene, S., Grassi, F., Cohen, L., Cappa, S., Paulesu, E., Dupoux, E., Fazio, F., and Mehler, J. (1996). Brain processing of native and foreign languages. *NeuroReport*, 7: 2439-2444.

Pinker S (1999). Words and rules: the ingredients of language. New York: Basic Books.

Potter M.C., So K., Eckardt V. and Feldman L. (1984). Lexical and conceptual representation in beginning and proficient bilinguals. *Journal of Verbal Learning and Verbal Behavior*, 23, 23-38

Rapport, R.L., Tan, C.T., and Whitaker, H.A. (1983). Language function and dysfunction among Chinese- and English-speaking polyglots: Cortical stimulation, Wada testing, and clinical studies. *Brain and Language*, 18: 342-366.

Ronjat J. (1913). *Le développement du langage observé chez un enfant bilingue*. Paris : Champion.

Snow C (1987). Relevance of the notion of a critical period to language acquisition. In Bornstein MH (ed.) *Sensitive Periods in Development: Interdisciplinary Perspectives*, Erlbaum, Hillsdale, NJ

Soares, C. and Grosjean, F. (1984). Bilinguals in a monolingual and a bilingual speech mode: The effect of lexical access. *Memory and Cognition*, 12: 380-386.

Stengel, E. and Zelmanowicz, J. (1933). Über polyglotte motorische Aphasie. *Zeitschrift für die gesamte Neurologie und Psychiatrie*, *149*: 292-311.

Tucker GR (1998). A global perspective on multilingualism and multilingual education. In J Cenoz and F Genesee (eds.) *Beyond bilingualism: Multilingualism and multilingual education*. Clevedon, England: Multilingual Matters. 3–15

Ullman MT (2001). The declarative/procedural model of lexicon and grammar. Journal of Psycholinguistic Research, 30(1), 37–69.

Ullman MT (2004). Contributions of memory circuits to language: the declarative/procedural model. Cognition, 92, 231-270

Vaid J (Ed.) (1986). *Language Processing in Bilinguals: Psycholinguistic and Neuropsychological Perspectives*. Hillsdale, NJ.: Erlbaum.

Vaid J (2002). Bilingualism. In V S Ramachandran (ed.) *Encyclopaedia of the Human Brain*. Academic Press, Elsevier. Vol. 1, 417-434

Wartenburger I, Heekeren HR, Abutalebi J, Cappa SF, Villringer A, and Perani D (2003) Eatly settings of grammatical processing in the bilingual brain. *Neuron*, 37:159-170

Weber-Fox, C.M. and Neville, H.J. (1996). Maturational constraints on functional specializations for language processing: ERP and behavioral evidence in bilingual speakers. *Journal of Cognitive Neuroscience*, *8*: 231-256.

Weinreich U (1953). *Languages in contact*. New York: The Linguistic Circle of New York

Woutersen M., Cox A., Weltens B. and De Bot K. (1994). Lexical aspects of standard dialect bilingualism. *Applied Psycholingusitics*, 15, 447-473.

Zatorre, R.J. (1989). On the representation of multliple languages in the brain: Old problems and new directions. *Brain and Language*, *36*: 127-147.

In: Speech and Language Disorders in Bilinguals
Editors: Alfredo Ardila and Eliane Ramos, pp. 69-89
ISBN 978-1-60021-560-5

Chapter 4

CODE-SWITCHING AND CODE-MIXING IN BILINGUALS: COGNITIVE, DEVELOPMENTAL, AND EMPIRICAL APPROACHES

Dana M. Basnight-Brown and Jeanette Altarriba
Department of Psychology
University at Albany, State University of New York
Albany, New York 12222, USA

The study of how individuals use and process two or more languages is an extremely important area of research, especially as the world's bilingual population continues to increase. It has been reported that currently, a majority of people worldwide are bilingual (Bhatia and Ritchie, 2004; Edwards, 2004; Tabouret-Keller, 2004). Although much of the research conducted in the domain of cognitive psychology has focused on the interesting question of how a bilingual represents or stores both of their languages in memory, there is a growing body of literature designed to explore how bilinguals process and switch in and out of languages. This usually occurs in speech production when an individual is speaking one language (i.e., referred to as the *matrix* or *base language*) and then rapidly replaces a word or phrase in that language with a word in the other language (i.e., *guest language*) (Li, 1996). For example, Heredia and Altarriba (2001, p. 164) introduced an example of code-switching that could be observed in the informal speech of a Spanish-English bilingual: "Dame una hamburguesa sin *lettuce* por favor?" ("Give me a hamburger without *lettuce* please?"), where in this statement the English word *lettuce* is used in place of its Spanish translation.

Although the terms *code (language)-mixing* and *code-switching* are used interchangeably in current discussions (Heredia and Altarriba, 2001), differences between the two phenomena have been pointed out in previous work. *Code-mixing* was originally described as using words and phrases from one language in place of those in the other language *within* a single sentence (i.e., the previous example where switching languages occurs within one sentence) (Sridhar and Sridhar, 1980, p. 408). On the other hand, *code-switching* has been described as switching between languages based on changes in the speech situation, where the topic or members of the conversation change (see e.g., Altarriba and Santiago-Rivera, 1994, for further discussion). This implies that code-switching does not occur within a sentence, whereas code-mixing is intra-sentential and does not rely on situational changes in the conversation (Sridhar and Sridhar, 1980). Since more recent work has not focused on differences between these two terms, the current chapter will refer to the switching between languages (i.e., whether it be within topics, paragraphs, sentences, etc.) as code-switching, the terminology most frequently used within the domain of cognitive psychology.

Several different reasons as to why bilinguals code-switch have been proposed (Heredia and Altarriba, 2001). One of the most common reasons is that bilinguals use words from the other language because they do not know the proper word in the language they are currently using. Therefore, they go in and out of languages because they do not have all the necessary vocabulary in both languages (Grosjean, 1982). However, Heredia and Altarriba (2001) have suggested that the absence of lexical knowledge may not be responsible, but rather the ease/difficulty of retrieval is responsible. A bilingual may know the needed word in both languages, but they may use the needed word more frequently in one language as compared to the other, and therefore, they are able to retrieve the word faster from memory in that language. Secondly, bilinguals may code-switch because the expression or feeling that they are trying to communicate has a better translation in one language or because no identical translation in the other language exists (Heredia and Altarriba, 2001; Wei, 2002). Altarriba (2003) explains this situation by providing the example of the Spanish word *cariño,* described as a combination of the English words liking and affection, although neither English word in and of itself is capable of fulfilling the true definition and meaning of the Spanish word. Research has also revealed that code-switching may be used as a defense mechanism in clinical settings where individuals may speak in their second or less dominant language in order to remove themselves from a painful or hurtful emotional experience (Altarriba and Santiago-Rivera, 1994). Lastly, code-switching also appears to have advantages in the marketplace (Luna and Peracchio, 2005), where it has been shown that persuasive advertising for products and services increases when advertisements or slogans that are normally presented in the second language (L2) include code-switches to the first language (L1) (e.g., "Twenty million *hijas* are covered by AFLAC, is yours?, where the word *hija* replaces the English word *daughter;* Luna and Peracchio, 2005, p. 760).

The aim of the current chapter is to discuss general code-switching patterns that have been observed in bilinguals, with a focus on the cognitive processes that underlie the switch between languages. Several theories and models of bilingual processing are briefly discussed in terms of the processes responsible for controlling the switch. The current chapter will explore if there is a cognitive cost (i.e., time consuming process) involved in code switching and if so, how it is affected as level of proficiency and developmental stages evolve over time. Lastly, code-switching patterns will also be discussed in terms of how they are influenced by various contextual constraints, stimulus manipulations, and differing task responses.

THEORIES AND MODELS BEHIND THE PROCESSES INVOLVED IN CODE-SWITCHING

The Revised Hierarchical Model (RHM)

One of the main questions that arises in bilingual research, and code-switching more specifically, is how bilinguals access or select the appropriate response when they have competing or alternative choices. As Green (1998a) suggests, this issue appears to be linked to the question of how a bilingual's two languages are represented in memory, but there are some differences as these models and accounts are not always designed to address issues in processing and selecting between the two languages. One of the most recent and widely cited models of bilingual language representation is the Revised Hierarchical Model (RHM) introduced by Kroll and Stewart (1994). This developmental model is able to account for a portion of the bilingual data that has been reported (however, see Altarriba, 2000, and Altarriba and Mathis, 1997, for further discussions). Figure 1 depicts this model, which shows a distinction between the conceptual and lexical levels of language representation.

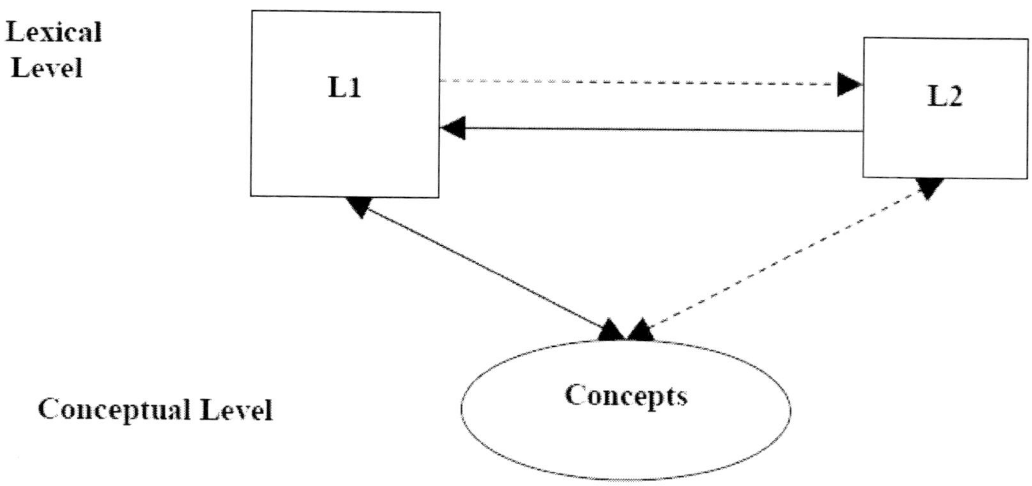

Figure 1. The Revised Hierarchical Model (Kroll & Stewart, 1994).

Each language is depicted as containing a separate and independent lexicon (i.e., mental dictionary), where the lexicon of the first (or dominant) language is pictured as being larger since vocabulary knowledge for this language is expected to be greater. The link between the L1 lexicon and concepts appears to be bi-directional and very strong, since a child acquiring their first language would form the strongest link between that language's lexicon and the corresponding concepts. However, as a person acquires a second language, especially if it occurs later in life, L2 words would be integrated into memory by developing a pathway that is attached to the lexicon of the first language. The solid directional line connecting the L2 lexicon to the L1 lexicon explains this process. The opposing directional arrow between the L1 and L2 lexicon is described as a weaker link since this is not the direction in which a bilingual first acquires the translations of the new language. Finally, the connection between the L2 and concepts is illustrated as being weaker as well. However, it has been suggested that this link may increase in strength as the bilingual becomes more proficient or fluent in their second language (Kroll and Stewart, 1994). Although this model is advantageous in that it can account for changes in a bilingual's proficiency level over time, it is not able to address how one language is selected over another. For example, the model does not provide an explanation as to how "a person translating from one language to another avoids naming the word to be translated" (Green, 1998a, p. 68).

The Idea of a Dual Switch Mechanism

The process of selecting between languages and of switching in and out of two languages has introduced several questions. How active are both languages when switching is occurring? Does one language have to be inhibited in order to achieve a correct response? Are there rules to code-switching or certain circumstances dictating when it can occur? Is there a cognitive cost to code-switching behavior?

It has been shown empirically that switching between languages is a time consuming process, a finding that can be traced back to many decades ago when research on bilingualism was just beginning to emerge (Kolers, 1966; Macnamara and Kushir, 1971). Kolers (1966) reported that bilinguals were slower to read passages of text containing mixed languages (French and English) as compared to monolingual text (text that was only in French or only in English). This finding led Macnamara and Kushnir (1971) to propose that switching between languages was a time consuming process because the bilingual linguistic system required that each language be either "on" or "off." Their idea was based on the assumption that a switch mechanism determined which lexicon could be used and which one could not. Because both lexicons or linguistic systems could not be activated at the same time, processing material that contained mixed languages would be slowed down. This theory seemed plausible; however, it was later refuted by research that showed that both languages could be activated at the same time (Dijkstra and van Heuven, 1998; Grosjean, 1997). Grosjean (1997) suggested that both languages could be active, but if a bilingual selects one language to use, the activation of that language must be greater than the activation of the other (second) language. Furthermore, a current model of bilingual processing, the Bilingual Interactive Activation (BIA and BIA+) Model, is a computer-simulated model that provides support for the dual activation of a bilingual's two languages (Dijkstra and van Heuven, 1998). Although this model is not specifically designed to predict code-switching behavior, it is a model that stresses that bilingual language processing in word recognition is nonselective and many of its processes can be applied to various aspects of bilingualism (Grainger and Dijkstra, 1992; see also Dijkstra and van Heuven, 1998, for a review of this model).

Other data in the bilingual research literature also seem to support the idea that both languages may be engaged simultaneously during the course of language processing. Those data stem from the use of the Stroop color-word task, within and between languages (Brauer, 1998; Dyer, 1971; Kiyak, 1982; Preston and Lambert, 1969; Tzelgov, Henik, and Leiser, 1990). In the typical monolingual version of this task, words that label colors are presented either in a congruent condition (e.g., the word *red* printed in the color red) or an incongruent condition (e.g., the word *red* printed in the color blue). The participant's task is to name the color the word is printed in and not the word itself. This is a timed task, and it is generally found that color naming suffers from significantly more interference in the incongruent condition, as compared to the congruent condition. It is often thought that this interference results from the competition involved between reading the word (an automatic process) and naming the color. This competition then produces interference. This task has been used in the bilingual literature to explore the activation and processing of words across a bilingual's two lexicons. Across languages, if one sees a word in one language but is asked to respond in a second, known language, interference is often observed. Typically, the bilingual Stroop effect is studied in two language conditions:

- Congruency between the language in which words are written (e.g., English) and the language in which answers are requested (e.g., English)
- Incongruency between the language in which words are written (e.g., English) and the language in which answers are requested (e.g., Spanish)

Within-language interference is typically larger than between-language interference, in most studies. However, the important point for the current discussion is the idea that the inability to suppress or inhibit naming a word that appears in a language different from that required to perform a naming response indicates that indeed both mental lexicons of a bilingual speaker may be activated at the same time. Thus, it is conceivable that this "fluidity" in the activation of multiple languages can contribute to circumstances in which code-switching and language-mixing can occur. At the very least, these conditions can be viewed within the context of an experimental laboratory situation and more than likely, can translate to the natural, speaking environment.

In summary, recent research as a whole appears to show that bilinguals are capable of simultaneously activating both of their languages; however, this finding implies that one language is either activated more than the other and/or that the language not in use must be inhibited to some degree.

The Inhibitory Control Model (ICM)

In an effort to extend some of the ideas introduced by the Revised Hierarchical Model and to explain some of the processing shortcomings not accounted for by this and other models, Green (1998a) proposed the Inhibitory Control Model (ICM) that was designed to explain issues such as how a bilingual translating a word from the L2-L1 avoids naming the word in the L2, and vice versa. This model is depicted in Figure 2. In this model, there is a language independent *conceptualizer*, similar to the conceptual store of the RHM, which is involved in constructing the conceptual information during a linguistic task. The conceptualizer is motivated by the linguistic *goal* (G) that the bilingual hopes to fulfill (e.g., such as translating from L2-L1, speech production in L2, etc.). The lexical-semantic system is similar to the lexicons of the RHM in that it contains the words from the bilingual's two languages, but it differs because the lexical items from both languages are depicted in the same store. However, each word or lexical entry has a *lemma* associated with it, which is language specific. Lemmas are best described as entries in the lexicon that contain information on the morphology, syntax, and phonology for each lexical item (Levelt, 1989).

Wei (2002) describes each lemma as being "tagged for a specific language," a property of the lexical system that is vital to understanding how processing occurs in the ICM.

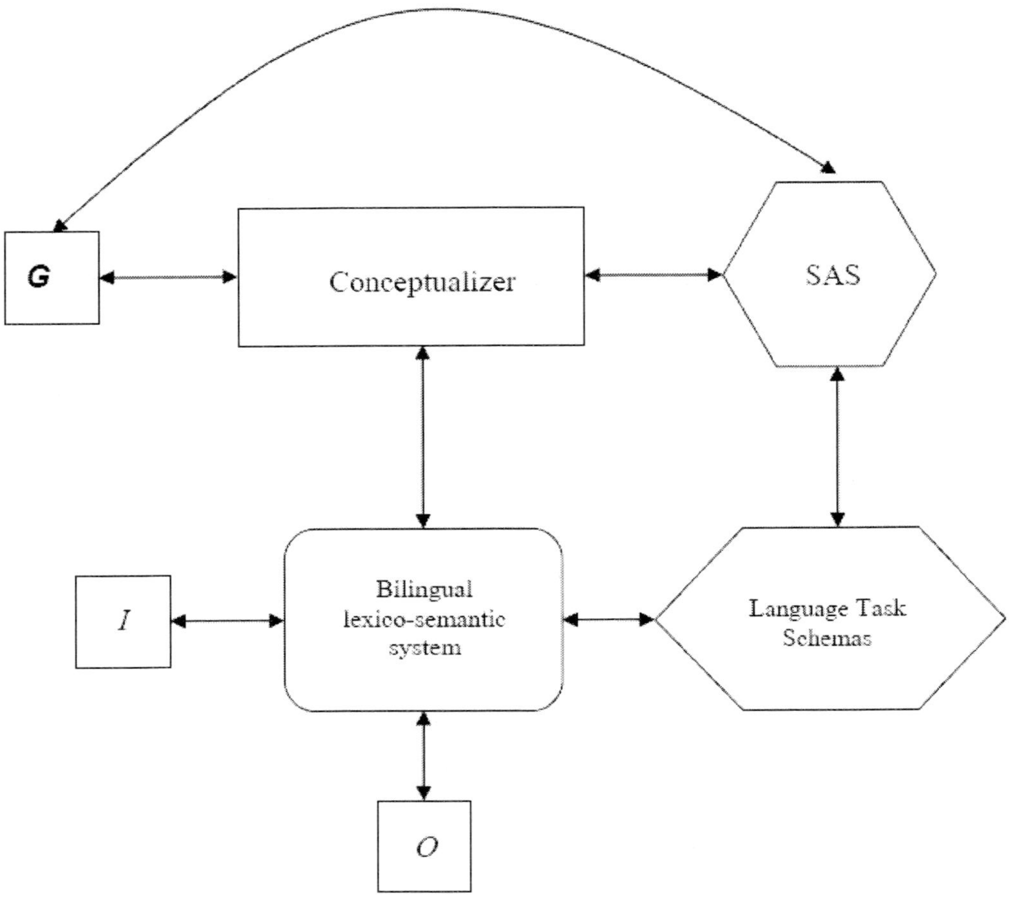

Figure 2. The Inhibitory Control Model (Green, 1998a).

The *language task schemas* are "mental devices or networks that individuals may construct or adapt on the spot in order to achieve a specific task and not simply to structures in long term memory" (Green, 1998a, p. 69). These schemas are task specific in that if a bilingual needs to translate from L2-L1, they must access a "L2-L1 translation schema" to complete this task. If the bilingual needs to produce a certain word in the L1 they will be required to activate a "L1 word production" schema. Therefore, each language has a task schema that works with the lexicon, and competition arises between the schemas for each language (see de Groot, 1998 and Green, 1998b for a more in depth discussion on the use of the term *schema* in this model).

If the required task has been performed before, the task specific schema just needs to be retrieved from memory; however, if the task is new and cannot be performed automatically, the *supervisory attentional system* (SAS) will assist. The SAS also acts as a mediator between the task required and the goal that one is trying to achieve. The task schema in turn works together with the lexico-semantic system to determine which words are produced, as shown by the output (O). The task schema is very influential in that it can manipulate the amount of activation of the different lexical entries in the lexical system. It can control the language output by inhibiting or activating different representations.

With regards to code-switching, when the matrix language changes, the language schema must change to accompany the new (guest) language. The language schema of the matrix language must then become inhibited. However, after the code-switch, when the bilingual returns to using the matrix language, inhibition of the guest language must occur. The switch cost observed in bilingual code-switching is most simply due to the amount of time it takes for a task schema to recover from inhibition (Thomas and Allport, 2000). It is important to point out that inhibitory processes can occur in two different locations in the model. Inhibition can occur at the schema task level, as suggested above, but it can also occur at the lexical level where specific language tags may be suppressed. When this occurs, the task schema remains the same. For example, participants performing a lexical decision task (i.e., a task in which a string of letters is presented and a participant presses one key if it is a real word or a different key if it is a nonword) can continue using a "*lexical decision schema,*" they just need to wait until the appropriate language tag is activated so that they can respond (Green, 1998a, p. 74). Switch costs of this nature are generally smaller and reflect a cost that occurs within the lexical system, as compared to the larger costs that have been reported outside the lexical system when task schema switches occur (von Studnitz and Green, 1997). The magnitude of switching costs that have been reported in the literature will be discussed more in depth in a later section.

Thus, the ICM implies that language activation is nonselective, the conceptual/semantic component activates lexical entries in both languages (a similar assumption proposed by the BIA and BIA+ models (Dijkstra and van Heuven, 1998)). Once this activation takes place, the lexical entries of the language that is not going to be used are inhibited. Lastly, there is a relationship between the cost involved and the inhibitory process, such that the cost or amount of time needed to switch is predicted to increase as the level of inhibition increases. The more activation there is of lexical entries in both languages, the greater the inhibition will be for the language that is not going to be used. Therefore, the competition between two languages is expected to be greater for proficient bilinguals, who will in turn show more inhibition than less proficient bilinguals (Green, 1998b). In addition, less proficient bilinguals will take a longer amount of time to switch back to their L1 or dominant language, since it is assumed that this language (L1) will have experienced more inhibition. In contrast, when switching to the L2, this less dominant language would not be inhibited to as large a degree resulting in an easier, faster switch (Green, 1998a). Overall, the extant data appear to indicate that factors outside of the properties of the lexicon itself can mediate the extent to which differential costs occur as bilinguals switch between lexicons (see e.g., Thomas and Allport, 2000). More will be said about this conclusion, as it relates to the ICM model, in a later section of this chapter.

Rules that Appear to Govern Code-Switching Behavior

While some research has focused on the cognitive aspects of code-switching—the cost involved and the processing mechanisms that underlie a language switch, other theories take a more linguistic perspective that is based on empirical research conducted on naturalistic speech behavior and the structures that appear to accompany language switches. For example, do bilinguals follow the syntactic structure of only one language when code-switching or do they use the syntactic rules of both languages, if indeed the two languages follow different rules? For example, in the Spanish language, adjectives describing a noun usually appear after the noun (e.g., la casa *verde),* whereas in English they usually precede the noun (e.g., the *green* house). An additional possibility has been introduced by Mahootian (1993), who suggests that bilinguals use a combination of the two language structures, resulting in code-switching patterns that are determined by a "third grammar."

Some of the earliest constraints reported in code-switching grammar implied that code-switching could not occur at a bound-morpheme boundary (Sankoff and Poplack, 1981), prepositions and other linguistic units like quantifiers and determiners (e.g., *some, all, those, many*) could not be switched, and the language in which a verb is used should dictate where the object will appear in the sentence (Mahootian, 1993). Some of these constraints are supported by Wei (2002), where code-switching patterns in Chinese-English bilinguals have been examined. His research has suggested that sentences containing code-switches only include content morphemes (i.e., nouns, verbs) from the guest language, while system morphemes (i.e., determiners) in the sentence are always presented in the matrix language. However, MacSwan (2000) argues that several of the original constraints do not always hold true. He introduces the very simple idea (i.e., Minimalist Program) that "all grammatical relations and operations which are relevant to monolingual language are relevant to bilingual language, and only these" (p. 43). According to this viewpoint, code-switching structure is not contingent on any principles of grammar; however, the phonology of each language remains separate and is language specific (see MacSwan, 2000 for an in depth review of this theory).

The idea of a divided phonological system has been supported by research conducted on bilingual speech production (Grosjean and Miller, 1994). In this study, voice onset times of French-English bilinguals were recorded as they read stories presented in either a monolingual or mixed language context. The results indicated that when a switch occurred, the phonology of the matrix language did not continue to influence the guest language, but rather the bilinguals were capable of shifting phonology very quickly. This finding proves to be very interesting because it suggests that language switches "involve a total change, not only at the lexical level but also at the phonetic level" (Grosjean and Miller, 1994, p. 205).

Although the study of when and where code-switches occur is useful in the study of bilingualism, Sankoff (1998) points out that one fundamental component of code-switching is that it is unpredictable, meaning that even if one knows the places and situations in which a code-switch can occur, one cannot predict that a code-switch will occur at that specific time and place. Further, "if a switch occurs at some point in a sentence, this does not constrain any potential site(s) later in the sentence either to contain another switch or not to—there are no *forced switches*" (Sankoff, 1998, p. 39).

Thus far, switching has been examined in terms of the models or theories that might predict certain outcomes and the ways in which code-switching and language-mixing may be governed by various rules that seem to be pervasive in the extant data. The following section, however, turns to the more developmental aspects of language switching behavior and attempts to draw certain conclusions related to maturational differences that occur from a lifespan perspective. To that end, this section will examine how the grammatical structure of code-switching is learned in bilingual children, as well as how low and high levels of proficiency influence code-switching patterns.

DEVELOPMENTAL ASPECTS OF CODE-SWITCHING

Code-Switching in Children and Adults

Those interested in the development of childhood bilingualism have studied code-switching patterns in the natural speech of children, usually by way of case study, where the speech of one child is examined in depth (Lanza, 1992; Meisel, 1989). One question that has been highly debated in this domain of research is the age at which a child can begin to code-switch. It has been suggested that code-switching observed in infants is not the result of linguistic awareness and the mixing of the two languages, but rather the behavior is the result of the infant confusing the two languages as they begin to differentiate between them (Lanza, 1992). The absence of linguistic awareness at a very young age has been referred to as "the unitary language system hypothesis" (Genesee, 1989). However, there have been studies suggesting that children's code switching patterns really do not differ that much from what has been observed in adults.

An examination of code-switching in a two-year-old Norwegian-English bilingual (Lanza, 1992) revealed that the child's code switching patterns did not differ much from adults, but rather the individuals who were involved in the conversation with the child determined the pattern of code-switching used. This finding has been supported by research conducted on children three years old and older who revealed that the main factor influencing code-switching patterns was who was participating, while setting and topic were less influential variables (Fantini, 1985; McClure, 1981). However, according to the present authors, it is possible that as bilinguals get older, the influence of topic on code-switching may become a more important factor because the bilingual will have more life experiences stored in memory and they may tend to change how they code-switch (i.e., altering which language is the matrix language and which is the guest language) based on what experiences they are talking about (e.g., childhood stories versus politics or work-specific jargon) (see Bentahila and Davies, 1992, for further elaboration on these latter examples). In addition, Heredia and Altarriba (2001) suggested that individuals might code switch depending on certain specialized knowledge they have regarding specific topics. These "specialized topics" might moderate the frequency and nature of code switching within particular domains of knowledge.

The most obvious and interesting finding in Lanza's (1992) study was that the child tended to make *grammatical* code-switches in Norwegian when speaking to her English dominant mother, but when speaking to her Norwegian dominant father, she only appeared to make *lexical* switches in English. Based on this observation, it was suggested that the child in this study was Norwegian dominant, which implies that those examining code-switching in children (and adults too) need to take into account dominance issues and context (Lanza, 1992), two points that will be discussed more in the following section. More importantly, this finding indicates that young children are able to develop some sort of linguistic awareness for their two languages.

Studies that have investigated code-switching behavior in groups of child bilinguals, as opposed to longitudinal case studies, are able to provide more insight into the underlying processes that dictate how bilingual children use their two languages. In an interesting study conducted by Lederberg and Morales (1985), code-switching in children and adults, as well as code switching experience, was examined. In this study, Mexican-American bilinguals who were born in the U.S. were placed into one of four groups: 1) 8-10 years old, 2) 10-11.5 years old, 3) 12-13 years old, and 4) adults (18-43 years old). In addition, a second group of adult bilinguals (28-35 years old) who were born in a Spanish speaking country, but who moved to the U.S. as adults participated. Based on research by Poplack (1980), it was hypothesized that this second group of bilinguals would not have as much experience code-switching as the individuals who grew up in the U.S.

In the experiment, participants had to determine whether sentences containing code-switches were grammatical and if not, they had to correct them so that they fit the rules of how they would naturally code-switch. Data from the two groups of adult bilinguals revealed that the bilinguals who emigrated to the U.S. late in life did not perform as well as American born bilinguals. However, a more in-depth analysis of the different types of sentences revealed that both groups used similar response patterns and appeared to make judgments using the same rules, suggesting that "the rules governing code-switching are not based on extensive exposure to code-switching" (p. 134).

Across the age groups, the results indicated that the two youngest groups of bilinguals accepted more sentences than the older groups, especially on the mixed verb sentences (e.g., the boy was *aprending* how to read; note the combination of the English word learning and its Spanish translation *aprendiendo*). This implies that there may be some type of developmental change in one's code-switching behavior. The authors suggest that children growing up in bilingual environments may create more general or flexible rules of grammar as compared to monolinguals or to adult bilinguals, such that they think it is appropriate to incorporate inflections or derivations from one language into the other language. However, Lederberg and Morales (1985) point out that other issues, an increase in general language knowledge and sentence structure or an increased ability to make grammatical judgments, could also be responsible for the developmental change they observed in code-switching, a finding that has been supported by Paradis, Nicoladis, and Genesee (2000). It is possible that children of this age have not fully conceptualized how words, sentences, and phrases interact, and therefore they believe that they can break up these linguistic forms in whatever manner they choose.

Paradis et al. (2000) examined code-switching behavior in two-year-old French-English bilinguals every six months over an eighteen-month time frame. They examined several of the constraints proposed in code-switching behavior and discovered that over time, the children violated one of the constraints less frequently, pointing to a developmental change in code-switching. However, like Lederberg and Morales (1985), the authors propose that since a change was observed for only one of the constraints when several were examined, it is possible that a developmental change in code-switching was not responsible, but that the child's general syntactic and linguistic knowledge matured. Overall, their results suggested that the children exhibited code-switching behavior that resembled that found in adults, which contradicts the idea of a developmental shift in code-switching.

In conclusion, it appears that code-switching in children is really not that different from what has been observed in adults, but that changes in children's overall linguistic knowledge and experience are responsible for developmental changes that have been reported. However, research conducted on aging bilinguals has revealed that changes do occur in code-switching behavior when one gets older (Hernandez and Kohnert, 1999). As one ages, code-switching appears to become a more difficult and slower process, with more errors being reported in experimental tasks. This is most likely due to increased task demands placed on the executive processing system of older adults. In the next section, the influence of age of acquisition and language dominance will be explored in order to see if those variables are capable of influencing how bilinguals code-switch.

The Influence of Age of Acquisition, Dominance, and Language Type on Code-Switching

The issue of proficiency and language dominance is obviously a very important one for those conducting research on bilingualism. Originally, it was assumed that a person's L1 was their more dominant language. However, more recent suggestions and empirical research have suggested that this is not the case for all bilinguals (Altarriba, 1992; Altarriba and Basnight-Brown, 2007; Heredia, 1997). Often, Spanish-English bilinguals in the United States who have grown up in Spanish speaking homes and communities, but who have attended school in predominantly English speaking environments, appear to show a shift in language dominance, such that their L2 (English) tends to become their more dominant language. This is an important issue to consider and one that can greatly influence how one interprets code-switching behavior, because the first language learned cannot always be assumed to be the more dominant language.

As expected, research has shown that individuals who are less proficient in their second language have more difficulty code-switching (Rakowsky, 1989; Toribio, Roebuck, Lantolf, and Perrone, 1993; cited in Toribio, 2001). McClure (1981) reported that Spanish-English bilingual children with low proficiency in their L2, tend to code-switch "at the word level," usually by substituting L2 nouns into sentences, while code-switching of more balanced Spanish-English bilingual children exhibits switches in more advanced parts of speech. Bentahila and Davies (1992) found a similar effect of proficiency in adult bilinguals, when they examined code-switching occurrences in the natural speech of balanced and unbalanced Arabic-French bilinguals. As compared to the more balanced bilinguals, the less proficient bilinguals (i.e., native Arabic speakers with lower French proficiency) appeared to use Arabic for grammatical aspects of sentences (e.g., prepositions, pronouns, etc.) and French primarily for nouns and verbs. In addition, the less proficient group also made switches within single words, a pattern not observed by the balanced group. The authors also point to the influence of the L2 learning environment as an influential factor, a suggestion that proves to be an important one. Because the age of acquisition of French was later for the less-proficient as compared to the balanced bilinguals, this group learned French in a formal school setting where vocabulary and grammatical rules were often taught by rote memorization. Therefore, it is not surprising that this group of bilinguals revealed a tendency to use memorized French lexical entries "within a clearly Arabic background structure," especially when talking about specific or technical topics that where learned within the context of French (Bentahila and Davies, 1992, p. 453).

In a recent study designed to examine the automatic processing that underlies code-switching by using a naming task (i.e., participants name aloud the word presented on the computer screen and the response latency is recorded in milliseconds (ms)), an effect of proficiency also proved to be salient (Costa and Santesteban, 2004). Spanish-Catalan and Korean-Spanish bilinguals who were less proficient in their second language appeared to have a more difficult time switching from the less proficient (L2) language into their native language (L1). This cost in task-switching diminished when bilinguals who were highly proficient in both Spanish and Catalan performed the same task, suggesting that different processing mechanisms are responsible for how switches occur in balanced and unbalanced bilinguals (Costa and Santesteban, 2004).

However, a less dominant or weaker language does not always influence code-switching in a negative way. Chan, Chau and Hoosain (1983) reported that their Chinese-English bilingual participants code-switched to English (L2) words when the words were harder to retrieve in Chinese. They suggested that code-switching in "natural and spontaneous" environments occurs due to greater cognitive and emotional availability of the words in the L2, a finding supported more recently in the research literature (Altarriba, 2003; Altarriba and Santiago-Rivera, 1994; Bentahila and Davies, 1992; Heredia and Altarriba, 2001).

Thus, it appears that a bilingual's proficiency level is capable of influencing the mechanisms that underlie the code-switching process, but that there are several instances where a less proficient (L2) language can be advantageous for code-switching. In the following section, the influence of environmental cues and task situations on code-switching will be discussed, as well as a more in-depth explanation of the costs involved when switching between languages.

Cognitive Studies of Task Switching and the Cost Involved

Contextual and Task Determinants of Code-switching

Although there has been a plethora of research conducted on code-switching in linguistic and socio-linguistic domains, it is only more recently that research studies on the cognitive aspects of code-switching, where cognitive experimental paradigms are used, have begun to increase in number. These studies are particularly interesting because they attempt to examine the automatic processing that underlies code-switching.

It has been reported that code-switching behavior can change depending on the level of stress in the environment (Javier and Marcos, 1989), the individuals participating in the conversation (e.g., acquaintance vs. spouse) (Yoon, 1992), the type of task (e.g., brainstorming) (Blot, Zárate, and Paulus, 2003), sentence context (Li, 1996), and the constraints placed on the word stimuli used in the task (Grainger and Beauvillian, 1987; Orfanidou and Sumner, 2005; Thomas and Allport, 2000). All of these studies suggest that the environmental or linguistic context that a bilingual is performing in can influence their code-switching behavior.

Whereas most of the studies discussed so far have been concerned with language production in code-switching, Li (1996) conducted a very interesting study aimed at determining how listeners of code-switched speech recognize and process mixed languages.

In his first experiment, Chinese-English bilinguals were presented with auditory sentences that were in Chinese, but which contained a code-switched word in English. A gating procedure was used—a task which involves presenting code-switched words at increasing intervals and requiring participants to determine the target word (i.e., the code-switched word). For example, the first gate would begin at the onset of the word and last for 30-50 ms; the second gate would include an additional 30-50 ms of the word, and so forth until the entire word has been heard. Li (1996) explains that the motivation behind this task is that it allows one to examine how much phonetic information about a word is needed in order for someone to identify what word is being said.

An additional manipulation included in this experiment was context (short vs. long) in which the code-switched word appeared. A short prior context sentence appeared as "his/her *flight* is delayed" and a long prior context sentence as "he/she boarded a delayed *flight,*" where *flight* was the code-switched word and the rest of the sentence appeared in Chinese. The results revealed that context definitely played a role in how the code-switched words were processed. In the long context, where participants were given more contextual information, it was observed that on average, only 59% of the word was needed in order for the bilingual to determine the correct word, whereas 72% of the word needed to be presented in order for participants to identify it in the short context. A similar pattern of results was replicated in a second experiment where Li (1996) used a word-shadowing task with the goal of tapping into even more automatic processes. In this type of task, participants heard the same sentences and were asked to name aloud the word that appeared after a predesignated point. Overall, this study provided insight into the way in which context can influence code-switching by showing that "context operates from early on to help bilingual listeners select the appropriate word" (Li, 1996, p. 772).

Additional studies have attempted to determine how code-switching behavior and the costs involved are influenced by manipulations of the type of word stimuli included in experiments (Grainger and Beauvillian, 1987; Orfanidou and Sumner, 2005; Thomas and Allport, 2000). Thus far, within the current chapter, the cost of switching has been generally defined by the extra time it takes a bilingual person to process a word in one language after hearing or reading a word or text in the other language. In the following experiments where participants are presented with hundreds of experimental trials where the words presented alternate languages at fixed or random points, the cost of language switching is defined as the difference in the mean reaction time (usually measured in milliseconds) between switch and nonswitch trials. For example, the amount of time needed to recognize an L1 word when it was preceded by an L2 (switch) trial would be compared to the time needed to recognize this same L1 word when preceded by an L1 (nonswitch) trial. A language switch could therefore be measured from the less dominant (L2) language to the more dominant (L1) language, or vice versa (L1-L2).

In a study conducted by Grainger and Beauvillian (1987), French-English bilinguals were presented with word lists that were mixed (i.e., lists that included a combination of words in both French and English) and with those that were not (i.e., lists containing only French or only English words). One word was presented at a time and participants performed a lexical decision task, where they pressed one key if the target word presented was in English or French and a second key if the word presented was a nonword in either language. The results indicated that the bilinguals were slower to recognize words in the mixed lists as compared to those that were not. Whereas French words in Experiment 1 were pronounceable using

English phonology (e.g., *trop*), French words in Experiment 2 were not (e.g., *oiseau*), and vice versa for English words (e.g., *cough*). An additional set of nonwords containing orthographies that were language specific was also created. The results from this experiment revealed that the cost of switching languages was greatly decreased when the words were orthographically specific to their respective languages. Participants could recognize those words faster because their orthographic form made them unique to one of the bilingual's two languages, which resulted in the lemmas of only one language being activated. This finding suggests that the cost of language switching occurs within the lexical system.

In an effort to further examine the locus of control responsible for code-switching costs, Thomas and Allport (2000) extended the experimental ideas put forth by Grainger and Beauvillian (1987). These authors pointed out that the participants in Grainger and Beauvillian's study might have been using a strategic process when performing the lexical decision task, which might be responsible for the results reported. Because of the types of nonwords used by Grainger and Beauvillian, it is suggested that participants may have hit the "yes" key whenever they saw words that were orthographically specific to only one language. This type of strategic processing is problematic because the bilinguals would not need to retrieve any lexical information in order to perform the task.

Thomas and Allport (2000) corrected this potential confound and discovered that orthographic specificity did not influence the cost of switching, but rather the magnitude of the cost was similar for words with both language-specific and non-specific orthographic forms. The finding is of particular interest because it suggests that "switch costs are a feature of the response mechanism rather than the lexicon and that the task schemas for the bilingual's two languages compete to control the response" (p. 51), which implies that the processes underlying language switching in bilinguals can be viewed as being similar to the cognitive control that dominates switching between any two simple tasks (Rogers and Monsell, 1995). The finding of a locus of control that is outside of the lexicon supports the theories posited by the ICM that was discussed in the first section of the present chapter, where Green's (1998a) model implied that word recognition was non-selective and that switch costs could be the result of response behavior.

Further support for the ICM comes from a recent study where the influence of language specific and non-specific orthography on code-switching was examined in Greek-English bilinguals (Orfanidou and Sumner, 2005). It was suggested that bilinguals of this nature, those who knew two languages that did not share the same alphabet, should be able to provide better insight into the mechanisms responsible for code-switching because words with language specific orthographies could be designed so that they were truly specific to each individual language. Two lexical decision experiments (i.e., word-nonword discrimination tasks) that included language specific and non-specific orthographic words in Greek and English were conducted in blocked, in terms of wordtype, (Exp.1) and unblocked (mixed) (Exp. 2) designs (Thomas and Allport used a mixed design only). The results from Experiment 1 revealed that there was an overall cost of switching (830 ms for switch trials vs. 788 ms on nonswitch trials = cost of 42 ms), but more importantly, the cost of switching was larger for the language non-specific words as compared to the language specific words, a finding that appears to contradict that reported by Thomas and Allport (2000). The results from Experiment 2 also indicated a significant switch cost (mean reaction time of 845 ms for switch trials vs. 800 ms for nonswitch = cost of 45 ms), but the difference between the non-specific and specific orthographic words reported previously was no longer reliable.

One of the main implications of Orfanidou and Sumner's (2005) study is that both experiments revealed an interaction between the magnitude of the switching cost and the type of response (response repetition), indicating that the locus of code-switching costs occurs at the response level. However, the fact that the language switching cost was influenced by the type of stimuli in Experiment 1, does suggest that in a blocked design, costs may be influenced to some degree by mechanisms within the lexical system. In conclusion, Orfanidou and Sumner (2005) were able to determine that "switching between language schemas causes costs from at least two independent sources, one at the level of the response initiation and one at an earlier level that is sensitive to stimulus properties and context via their implications for strategic control" (p. 36).

Switch Costs Obtained in Experimental Tasks Requiring Different Types of Responses

Whereas many of the studies just discussed used a lexical decision task to examine language switching, several other studies have used tasks that required the participant to make different types of decisions regarding the code-switched language stimuli that are presented (Meuter and Allport, 1999; von Studnitz and Green, 2002). In a study conducted by Meuter and Allport (1999), bilinguals were presented with single digits (from 1-9) on the computer screen and were instructed to name aloud the number in either their L1 or L2. Each number appeared in the center of either a blue or yellow rectangle, where the color of the shape was used to indicate which language (L1 or L2) the response should be in. The results revealed that as expected, response times were slower on switch trials as compared to nonswitch trials. Of greater interest was the finding of an asymmetry in the switch cost, such that costs in the L2-L1 direction (143 ms) were larger than those observed in the L1-L2 direction (85 ms). This finding also supports the ICM, where it was hypothesized that there was a positive correlation between the level of activation and inhibition. Because the dominant (L1) language is expected to be activated to a larger degree, this language also experiences greater inhibition. Therefore, L2-L1 switch costs are predicted to be larger because switching from a less dominant to a more dominant language requires one to overcome the large amount of inhibition associated with the L1 word.

A second study that used a different experimental task to examine code-switching in bilinguals required the participants to determine whether the English and German presented words were animate or inanimate (von Studnitz and Green, 2002). The results revealed that analogous to previous studies, participants were slower when responding to switch trials as compared to language nonswitch trials. In addition, the authors manipulated whether the correct response was repeated across two trials (e.g., animate-animate) or whether it was not (e.g., animate-inanimate). The data from this manipulation revealed that when the bilinguals were presented with switch trials that required the same response, response latencies were longer. The fact that the magnitude of the switch cost was found to interact with the type of response is interpreted as meaning that the cost of switching is not the direct result of processes occurring at the lexical level, but rather that it is due to "costs that arise in the course of mapping decisions onto responses" (p. 248).

In summary, studies that have used cognitive methodology and experimental tasks to explore code-switching suggest that there is a true cost involved when switching between two languages. This finding supports those reported in many of the linguistic and socio-linguistic fields that have shown that moving in and out of languages takes more time as compared to operating in a monolingual mode. However, many of the studies discussed in the current section are particularly useful because they are able to provide numerical estimates of the cost involved in switching and the cognitive capacity that is needed to perform a switch. Taken together, they also indicate that the result of this cost appears to be controlled by processing mechanisms that reflect the different and competing response schemas that the bilinguals are alternating between during code-switching. Furthermore, the costs observed under these experimental paradigms can most likely be applied to language processing in a more natural setting or environment. It has even been suggested that this concept could be extended to include monolinguals, in that those speaking in one language may use similar mechanisms to task switch between a "polite schema and a slang schema" (Orfanidou and Sumner, 2005).

Conclusions and Future Research Directions

The idea that bilingual speakers can at once, keep their languages apart when necessary, but switch between them as if they were both "available" poses an interesting conundrum that researchers have investigated from several perspectives. Is it that one language is suppressed or inhibited while the other one "takes the floor"? Or are both languages activated to some degree, simultaneously, when a bilingual is thinking about or producing utterances? The current chapter examined various aspects of code-switching from developmental perspectives to the extant models that purport to explain how switching between languages takes place. Through time, various "switching mechanisms" have been proposed. Switching behavior is seen to be moderated by a variety of influences, and the idea is often that one language is essentially "switched off" while another language is "switched on" (see e.g., Macnamara and Kushnir, 1971). However, empirical evidence (e.g., bilingual Stroop data) seems to indicate that one cannot always simply switch one language off in favor of another. Rather, the issue is one of suppressing or inhibiting the irrelevant language to some extent while performing a task in the relevant language (see e.g., Preston and Lambert, 1969 and Tzelgov et al., 1990). This argument seems plausible given that there is an apparent cost to switching between languages, as there might be in switching between other types of cognitive tasks (Meuter and Allport, 1999). It is likely that the model that stands to account for the bulk of the data related to language switching is that proposed by Green—The Inhibitory Control Model (ICM) (see Green, 1998 a and b). The idea that a language schema—not merely a word—is activated when an alternate language is to be engaged allows for a host of other relevant information pertinent to the language mode to also be engaged. Thus, in a more holistic sense, this model allows for the fact that one does not merely activate a single lexical representation, but likely through a process of spreading activation (Collins and Loftus, 1975), more information can be activated and accessed through the activation of a schema. Different devices also act to inhibit, activate, or otherwise control output in ways that one might predict given the extant literature.

The current chapter also explored the grammatical constraints that exist in the process of switching between languages. From a listener's perspective, it appears as though code switching does not occur in a haphazard manner. Rather a listener perceives the concepts or semantics involved in mixed-language speech as fitting together nicely—making sense—despite the language changes that are involved. Though some would argue that there is no specific "grammar" for language switching (see e.g., MacSwan, 2000), it is the case that the motivation a speaker has to forge a switch is usually such that it assists in the communicative process. Ultimately, a speaker wants to be understood. Thus, logic would dictate that switches are somehow "programmed" such that they occur in instances that lead to a clear understanding of the concepts being described and communicated. Further research should examine the ways in which this kind of pragmatic nuance to language switching occurs across various languages as well as various linguistic situations.

It is quite clear, just from the point of view of a casual observer, that children code switch, too, particularly in cases in which they are being raised in a bilingual environment. Whether the bilingual environment is the home/family environment or a school or educationally-based program outside of the home, children who are exposed to more than one language tend to blend those languages in some way (Lanza, 1992). Children ultimately develop linguistic awareness of their two languages and of certain relationships between them allowing them to switch between the two languages in patterned ways. The development of code-switching behavior seems to be moderated not so much by experience doing so, as by an increase in general knowledge, linguistic or otherwise (Lederberg and Morales, 1985). Thus, could this ability be somehow governed by innate processes? Could a variant of Chomsky's Language Acquisition Device (Chomsky, 1968) guide the development of code switching as it is touted to do for other language abilities? Future research should examine more closely the relationship between age and mode of acquisition and the frequency and nature of code-switching behavior across the lifespan.

Finally, the current chapter examined the ways in which empirical approaches have been designed to formalize the cost involved in switching between languages. The work of Allport and colleagues (e.g., Meuter and Allport, 1999; Thomas and Allport, 2000), for example, demonstrates the fact that "cost" in switching can be quantified in terms of milliseconds involved in responding. That cost in response is comprised of a host of processes that occur in terms of the access of language entries, the activation of those entries and suppression or inhibition of others, and the actual production of a response. Researchers have been able to capture those processes in terms of time and have developed clever paradigms to examine just what features of language representation moderate those costs. Clearly, switching takes time, and the nature and direction of those switches influences the amount of time involved in measurable ways.

While neurological approaches to code-switching represent an area that is out of the scope of the present chapter, many fine works are emerging that attempt to explore the ways in which the brain and patterns of activation within the brain change as different languages are accessed (see e.g., Ijalba, Obler, and Chengappa, 2004; Jackson et al., 2004; Muñoz, Marquandt, and Copeland, 1999; and Proverbio, Leoni, and Zani, 1999). Shanon (1991), for example, points to the issue of multilingualism and the representation of language in the case of polyglots. Thus, future research on code-switching and language-mixing should examine cases in which more than two languages are involved. How are costs distributed across switches that occur across different languages within an individual—languages that might represent different levels of proficiency or fluency? Though these questions appear complex, it is certainly the case that increasing globalization will provide for more and more instances in which individuals do maneuver across several languages and do so successfully. How is this accomplished? Note as well that the case of interpreters and professional translators also poses an interesting population for further study (see de Groot and Christoffels, 2006). Clearly, any cognitive model that purports to explain how switching takes place and the variables that moderate those switches must not exclude the ability to switch across more than one language. Further, as with the more basic bilingual research in memory and general cognitive processing, it is important to investigate language switching across a variety of languages—those that share a similar etymology as well as those that arose from very different origins. How do different language origins play a role in moderating how easily switching can take place in a fluent speaker? These are some of the many interesting questions that can be pursued in this area of investigation. The current chapter, therefore, should serve as a starting point for many of these topics of inquiry.

References

Altarriba, J. (1992). The representation of translation equivalents in bilingual memory. In R.J. Harris (Ed.), *Cognitive processing in bilinguals* (pp. 157-174). Amsterdam: Elsevier.

Altarriba, J. (2000). Language processing and memory retrieval in Spanish-English bilinguals. *Spanish Applied Linguistics, 4*, 215-245.

Altarriba, J. (2003). Does *cariño* equal "liking"? A theoretical approach to conceptual nonequivalence between languages. *International Journal of Bilingualism, 7,* 305-322.

Altarriba, J., and Basnight-Brown, D.M. (in press, 2007). Methodological considerations in performing semantic and translation priming experiments across languages. *Behavior Research Methods, Instruments, and Computers.*

Altarriba, J., and Mathis, K.M. (1997). Conceptual and lexical development in second language acquisition. *Journal of Memory and Language, 36*, 550-568.

Altarriba, J., and Santiago-Rivera, A.L. (1994). Current perspectives on using linguistic and cultural factors in counseling the Hispanic client. *Professional Psychology: Research and Practice, 25,* 388-397.

Bentahila, A. and Davies, E.E. (1992). Code-switching and language dominance. In R.J. Harris (Ed.), *Cognitive processing in bilinguals* (pp. 443-458). Amsterdam: Elsevier.

Bhatia, T.K., and Ritchie, W.C. (2004). Bilingualism in South Asia. In T.K. Bhatia and W.C. Ritchie (Eds.), *The handbook of bilingualism* (pp. 780-807). Malden, MA: Blackwell Publishing.

Blot, K.J., Zárate, M.A., and Paulus, P.B. (2003). Code-switching across brainstorming sessions: Implications for the revised hierarchical model of bilingual language processing. *Experimental Psychology, 50* (3), 171-183.

Brauer, M. (1998). Stroop interference in bilinguals: The role of similarity between the two languages. In A.F. Healy and L.E. Bourne (Eds.), *Foreign language learning: Psycholinguistic studies on training and retention* (pp. 317-337). Mahwah, NJ: Lawrence Erlbaum Associates.

Chan, M.C., Chau, H.L.H., and Hoosain, R. (1983). Input/output switch in bilingual code switching. *Journal of Psycholinguistic Research, 12* (4), 407-416.

Chomsky, N. (1968). *The acquisition of syntax in children from 5 to 10.* Cambridge: MIT Press.

Collins, A.M., and Loftus, E.F. (1975). A spreading activation theory of semantic processing. *Psychological Review, 82*, 407-428.

Costa, A., and Santesteban, M. (2004). Lexical access in bilingual speech production: Evidence from language switching in highly proficient bilinguals and L2 learners. *Journal of Memory and Language, 50,* 491-511.

de Groot, A.M.B. (1998). Retroactive of proactive control of the bilingual system. *Bilingualsism: Language and Cognition, 1,* 86-87.

de Groot, A.M.B., and Christoffels, I.K. (2006). Language control in bilinguals: Monolingual tasks and simultaneous interpreting. *Bilingualism: Language and Cognition, 9,* 189-201.

Dijkstra, T., and van Heuven, W.J.B. (1998). The BIA-model and bilingual word recognition. In J. Grainger and A. Jacobs (Eds.), *Localist connectionist approaches to human cognition* (pp. 189-225). Hove: LEA.

Dyer, F. N. (1971). Color-naming interference in monolinguals and bilinguals. *Journal of Verbal Learning and Verbal Behavior, 10,* 297-302.

Edwards, J.V. (2004). Foundations of bilingualism. In T.K. Bhatia and W.C. Ritchie (Eds.), *The handbook of bilingualism* (pp. 7-31). Malden, MA: Blackwell Publishing.

Fantini, A. (1985). *Language acquisition of a bilingual child: A sociolinguistic perspective.* Clevedon: Multilingual Matters.

Genesee, F. (1989). Early bilingual development: One language or two? *Journal of Child Language, 6,* 161-179.

Grainger, J., and Beauvillian, C. (1987). Language blocking and lexical access in bilinguals. *Quarterly Journal of Experimental Psychology, 39A,* 295-319.

Grainger, J., and Dijkstra, T. (1992). On the representation and use of language information in bilinguals. In R.J. Harris (Ed.), *Cognitive processing in bilinguals* (pp. 207-220). Amsterdam: Elsevier.

Green, D.W. (1998a). Mental control of the bilingual lexico-semantic system. *Bilingualism: Language and Cognition, 1,* 67-81.

Green, D.W. (1998b). Schemas, tags, and inhibition. *Bilingualism: Language and Cognition, 1,* 100-104.

Grosjean, F. (1982). *Life with two languages: An introduction to bilingualism.* Cambridge, MA: Harvard University Press.

Grosjean, F. (1997). Processing mixed languages: Issues, findings and models. In A.M.B. de Groot and J.F. Kroll (Eds,), *Tutorials in bilingualism: Psycholinguistic perspectives* (pp. 225-254). Mahwah, NJ: LEA.

Grosjean, F., and Miller, J.L. (1994). Going in and out of languages. *Psychological Science, 5* (4), 201-206.

Heredia, R.R. (1997). Bilingual memory and hierarchical models: A case for language dominance. *Current Directions in Psychological Science, 6,* 34-39.

Heredia, R.R., and Altarriba, J. (2001). Bilinguals language mixing: Why do bilinguals code switch? *Current Directions in Psychological Science, 10,* 164-168.

Hernandez, A.E., and Kohnert, K.J. (1999). Aging and language switching in bilinguals. *Aging, Neuropsychology, and Cognition, 6* (2), 69-83.

Ijalba, E., Obler, L., and Chengappa, S. (2004). Bilingual aphasia. In T.K. Bhatia and W.C. Ritchie (Eds.), *The handbook of bilingualism* (pp. 71-89). Malden, MA: Blackwell Publishing.

Jackson, G.M., Swainson, R., Mullin, A., Cunnington, R., and Jackson, S.R. (2004). ERP correlates of a receptive language-switching task. *The Quarterly Journal of Experimental Psychology, 57A* (2), 223-240.

Javier, R.A., and Marcos, L.R. (1989). The role of stress on the language-independence and code-switching phenomena. *Journal of Psycholinguistic Research, 18*, 449-472.

Kiyak, H.A. (1982). Interlingual interference in naming color words. *Journal of Cross-Cultural Psychology, 13,* 125-135.

Kolers, P. (1966). Reading and talking bilingually. *American Journal of Psychology, 3,* 357-376.

Kroll, J.F., and Stewart, E. (1994). Category interference in translation and picture naming: Evidence for asymmetric connections between bilingual memory representations. *Journal of Memory and Language, 33*, 149-174.

Lanza, E. (1992). Can bilingual two-year-olds code-switch? *Journal of Child Language, 19,* 633-658.

Lederberg, A.R., and Morales, C. (1985). Code switching by bilinguals: Evidence against a third grammar. *Journal of Psycholinguistic Research, 14* (2), 113-136.

Levelt, W.J.M. (1989). *Speaking from intention to articulation*. Cambridge, MA: MIT Press.

Li, P. (1996). Spoken word recognition of code-switched words by Chinese-English bilinguals. *Journal of Memory and Language, 35,* 757-774.

Luna, D., and Peracchio, L.A. (2005). Advertising to bilingual consumers: The impact of code-switching on persuasion. *Journal of Commercial Research, 33,* 760-765.

McClure, E. (1981). Formal and functional aspects of the code-switched discourse of bilingual children. In R. Duran (Ed.), *Latino language and communicative behavior* (pp. 69-94). Norwood, NJ: ABLEX.

Macnamara, J. and Kushnir, S. (1971). Linguistic independence of bilinguals: The input switch. *Journal of Verbal Learning and Verbal Behavior, 10,* 480-487.

MacSwan, J. (2000). The architecture of the bilingual language faculty: Evidence from intrasentential code switching. *Bilinugualism: Language and Cognition, 3* (1), 37-54.

Mahootian, S. (1993). *A null theory of code-switching*. Unpublished doctoral dissertation, Northwestern University, Evanston, IL.

Meisel, J. (1989). Early differentiation of languages in bilingual children. In K. Hyltenstam and L. Obler (Eds.), *Bilingualism across the lifespan: Aspects of acquisition, maturity, and loss* (pp. 13-40). Cambridge: Cambridge University Press.

Meuter, R.F., and Allport, A. (1999). Bilingual language switching in naming: Asymmetrical costs of language selection. *Journal of Memory and Language, 40,* 25-40.

Muñoz, M.L., Marquardt, T.P., and Copeland, G. (1999). A comparison of the codeswitching patterns of aphasic and neurologically normal bilingual speakers of English and Spanish. *Brain and Language, 66,* 249-274.

Orfanidou, E., and Sumner, P. (2005). Language switching and the effects of orthographic specificity and response repetition. *Memory and Cognition, 33* (2), 355-369.

Paradis, J., Nicoladis, E., and Genesee, F. (2000). Early emergence of structural constraints on code-mixing: Evidence from French-English bilingual children. *Bilingualism: Language and Cognition, 3* (3), 245-261.

Poplack, S. (1980). Sometimes I'll start a sentence in English y termino en español: Toward a typology of code-switching. In J. Amastae and L. Elias-Olivares (Eds.), *Spanish in the United States: Sociolinguistic aspects* (pp. 230-263). Cambridge: Cambridge University Press.

Preston, M.S., and Lambert, W.E. (1969). Interlingual interference in a bilingual version of the Stroop color-word task. *Journal of Verbal Learning and Verbal Behavior, 8,* 295-301.

Proverbio, A.M., Leoni, G., and Zani, A. (2004). Language switching mechanisms in simultaneous interpreters: an ERP study. *Neuropsychologica, 42,* 1636-1656.

Rakowsky, A. (1989). *A study of intra-sentential code-switching in Spanish-English bilinguals and second language learners.* Unpublished doctoral dissertation, Brown University, Providence, RI.

Rogers, R.D., and Monsell, S. (1995). Costs of a predictable switch between simple cognitive tasks. *Journal of Experimental Psychology: General, 124,* 207-231.

Sankoff, D. (1998). A formal production-based explanation of the facts of code-switching. *Bilingualism: Language and Cognition, 1,* 39-50.

Sankoff, D., and Poplack, S. (1981). A formal grammar for code-switching. *Papers in Linguistics, 14,* 3-46.

Shanon, B. (1991). Faulty language selection in polyglots. *Language and Cognitive Processes, 6* (4), 339-350.

Sridhar, S.N., and Sridhar, K.K. (1980). The syntax and psycholinguistics of bilingual code mixing. *Canadian Journal of Psychology, 34,* 407-416.

Tabouret-Keller, A. (2004). Bilingualism in Europe. In T.K. Bhatia and W.C. Ritchie (Eds.), *The handbook of bilingualism* (pp. 662-688). Malden, MA: Blackwell Publishing.

Thomas, M.S.C., and Allport, A. (2000). Language switching costs in bilingual visual word recognition. *Journal of Memory and Language, 43,* 44-66.

Toribio, A.J. (2001). On the emergence of bilingual code-switching competence. *Bilingualism: Language and Cognition, 4* (3), 203-231.

Toribio, A.J., Roebuck, R., Lantolf, J., and Perrone, A. (1993). *Syntactic constraints on code-switching: Evidence of abstract knowledge in a second language acquisition.* Unpublished manuscript, Cornell University, Ithaca, NY.

Tzelgov, J., Henik, A., and Leiser, D. (1990). Controlling Stroop interference: Evidence from a bilingual task. *Journal of Experimental Psychology: Learning, Memory, and Cognition, 16,* 760-771.

von Studnitz, R.E., and Green, D.W. (1997). Lexical decision and language switching. *International Journal of Bilingualism, 1,* 3-24.

von Studnitz, R.E., and Green, D.W. (2002). The cost of switching language in a semantic categorization task. *Bilingualism: Language and Cognition, 5* (3), 241-251.

Wei, L. (2002). The bilingual mental lexicon and speech production process. *Brain and Language, 81,* 691-707.

Yoon, K.K. (1992). New perspective on intrasentential code-switching: A study of Korean-English switching. *Applied Psycholinguistics, 13,* 433-449.

In: Speech and Language Disorders in Bilinguals ISBN 978-1-60021-560-5
Editors: Alfredo Ardila and Eliane Ramos, pp. 91-108

Chapter 5

Lexical and Semantic Organization and Retrieval

Maria L. Muñoz
Department of Communication Sciences and Disorders
TCU Box 297450,Texas Christian University
Fort Worth, TX 76129 USA

Words allow speakers and listeners to share meaning, even for things not present in the immediate context. If I tell you that I like to take my dogs for a walk. You, as the reader, can see me as a two legged human (I) having fun (like) moving forward at a moderate pace (walk) beside two or more barking, furry four-legged animals (dog/s). Our cultural, social, and academic experiences have created a shared corpus of English referents that allow us to convey meaning, in part, via the semantic and syntactic structures of our written and verbal communication. As a bilingual, I can also convey a shared experience with speakers of Spanish if I chose instead to linguistically represent my meaning as "Me gusta salir a caminar con mis perros."

Word production and comprehension are fundamental to communication between speakers of a given language. The linguistic process involved in manipulating even single words is complex. The brain of the speaker must formulate a thought, select a word form that best represents that thought, attach a phonological form to that thought, and instruct the muscles to produce that form. The brain of the listener must interpret the acoustic signal, recognize the phonemes the signal represents, construct the word form those phonemes represent, and attach meaning to the form. The bilingual brain has the additional requirement to choose and/or recognize the appropriate language for the interaction.

The process by which single word comprehension and production is accomplished has received significant attention in both the unilingual and bilingual literature. One approach to articulating the linguistic process has been the development of cognitive psychological models of single word comprehension and production (Caramazza, 1997). Historically, cognitive models have taken the form of connectionist models (Dell, Chang, and Griffin, 1999). The models attempt to capture the process of single word production or comprehension as a series of discrete, sequential steps that reflect the relatively independent stages of the process. The stages have been determined through a variety of methods, including examining patterns of normal speech errors (e.g. saying "Remember to bling blankets" instead of "Remember to bring blankets") and errors made by individuals with aphasia (One patient sees a picture of table and says "chair" while another says "dadle"). Bilingual models must additionally account for how and when a speaker focuses the recognition or production process to the single language of interest.

In this chapter, I will present an overview of models of the linguistic processing mechanisms that underlie semantic comprehension and lexical retrieval in unilinguals and bilinguals. First, I will provide a brief overview of a cognitive psychological model of word comprehension and production in a single language. Then, I review the processes underlying single word comprehension and production in speakers of multiple languages. Finally, I will address language processing issues unique to bilinguals (specifically proficiency, code-switching, and translation) within the context of the cognitive psychological model.

Unilingual Semantic Organization and Lexical Retrieval

Cognitive psychological models of semantic organization and lexical retrieval are particularly concerned with the way that knowledge about the world is represented with words and the process by which words are accessed (Hillis, 2001). While the process of word comprehension is often modeled independent from word production (Roelofs, 2003), they have much in common. For the sake of brevity, I will use one model to explain organization of the semantic system in the context of lexical comprehension and retrieval for a single language (Figure 1). Minimally, the linguistic process underlying lexical retrieval consists of three distinct components: modality specific output lexicon, semantic/conceptual system, and modality specific output lexicon (Hillis, 2001). For ease of comparison to the bilingual model, I have incorporated a fourth stage present in some but not all models, lexical selection (Foygel and Dell, 2000).

Phonological Input Lexicon

The process of comprehension is initiated by a stimulus entering into the sensory system, be it auditory or visual (e.g. "sensory input"). The sensory input in turn activates the first component in the linguistic process, the phonological input lexicon, or our mental dictionary of word forms. Simply put, the input lexicon refers to the point at which a stimulus becomes uniquely distinguishable and familiar (Raymer and Gonzalez Rothi, 2001). While this chapter is concerned primarily with the phonological input lexicon (e.g. word forms) it is important to note that speakers have modality specific input lexicons, e.g. separate dictionaries for visual, auditory, gestural, and written input (Caramazza and Miceli, 1990). The phonological input lexicon does not contain meaning, simply activation and selection of the mental representation that corresponds to the form of the auditory input.

Word comprehension first requires the activation of the phonological input lexicon, or the mental dictionary of word forms (Caramazza, 1997). However, introduction of the acoustic signal, i.e. word, activates the matching form and similar forms. Roelfs (2003) indicates that all words that are compatible in form with the target are activated in parallel. In particular, words with the same initial phoneme are activated while words with a different initial phoneme are suppressed (McClelland and Elman, 1986; Norris, 1994). Of those word forms activated, the target receives the strongest activation which leads to activation of the word meaning. As shown in Figure 1, hearing "dog" would most strongly activate the form *dog*, but weaker activation would be evident for phonologically related words (*doll, door, log, fog*).

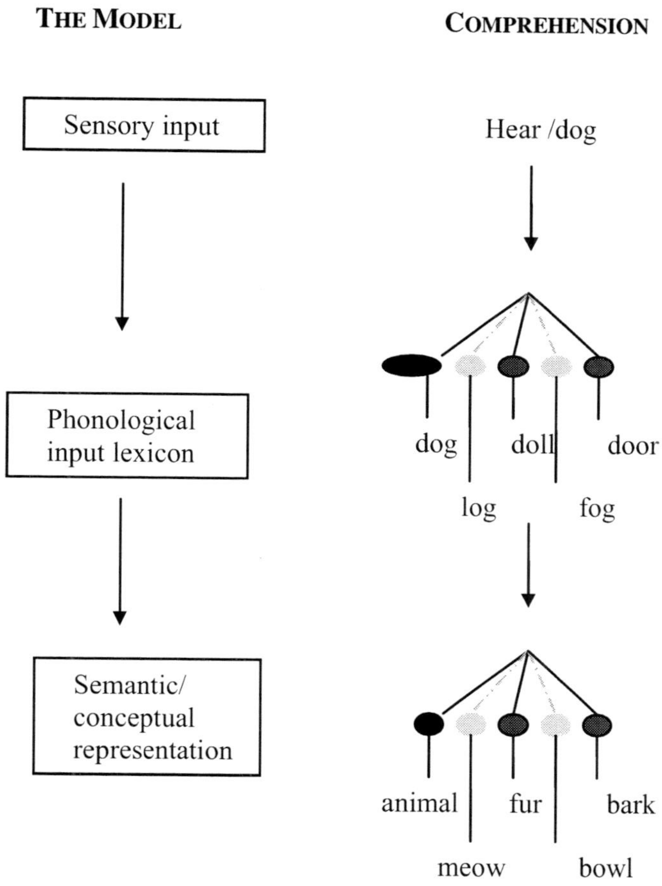

Figure 1. Cognitive psychological model of single language lexical comprehension.

SEMANTIC/CONCEPTUAL REPRESENTATION

The activation of the phonological input lexicon spreads to the semantic/conceptual representation which contains shared world knowledge, i.e. what we know about words, objects, and actions (Postler et al., 2003). The target selected in the input lexicon activates representations within the semantic/conceptual store. These representations include features of the target as well as semantically related concepts, including superordinates, coordinates, associates, and subordinates (Raymer and Gonzalez Rothi, 2001). Characteristics specific to the target word receive the strongest activation, with residual activation for less related or semantically related words (McClelland and Elman, 1986). For our target "dog", activated knowledge includes *animal* (superordinate), *fur, bark, bowl* (associates), and *meow* (for the coordinate word cat).

The semantic/conceptual store is accessed by any input modality and can access any output modality (Figure 1). Single word comprehension involves activation of the word form (input lexicon) that in turn activates that related meanings (semantic/conceptual representation) (Dell, 1988). In single word production, the semantic/conceptual representation that best captures an individual's thought activates the corresponding lexical form which then leads to activation of the corresponding phonological form (Foygel and Dell, 2000).

LEXICAL REPRESENTATIONS AND PHONOLOGICAL OUTPUT LEXICON

Activation of the semantic/conceptual store leads to the semantically and syntactically driven search of the mental lexicon for the word that best matches the intended meaning (Levelt, 1992). Assuming three levels of activation in speech production, conceptual, lexical, and phonological (Dell, 1988), the conceptual/semantic representation activates the lexical representations (see Figure 2). In the lexical component, words that relate to features identified in the conceptual store are activated. The word that best matches the features activated in the semantic/conceptual store ultimately receives the strongest activation. However, semantically related words are also activated. As shown in Figure 2, the target "fish" activates subordinates (cod, trout) as well as semantically related items (pelican, kelp).

The selection of "fish" subsequently leads to the activation and selection of /fɪʃ/, the phonological form of the target. While lexical selection involves activation of semantically related alternatives, activation in the phonological output lexicon involves activation of phonologically related alternatives particularly words with the same initial phoneme as the target (Foygel and Dell, 2000). For the target "fish", fist or foot might also be activated but to a lesser extent. Once /fɪʃ/ is selected, the word can be articulated.

SUMMARY

The process of lexical comprehension and production for a single language involves a sequence of activation and selection of forms, words, and features. Fundamentally, the organization of the bilingual lexical system has much in common with the processing of a single language. However, bilingual models of semantic access and lexical retrieval must additionally account for how words from two languages are represented and organized at the conceptual and lexical levels and how words one or both languages are accessed during language processing (Sanchez-Casas and Garcia-Albea, 2005).

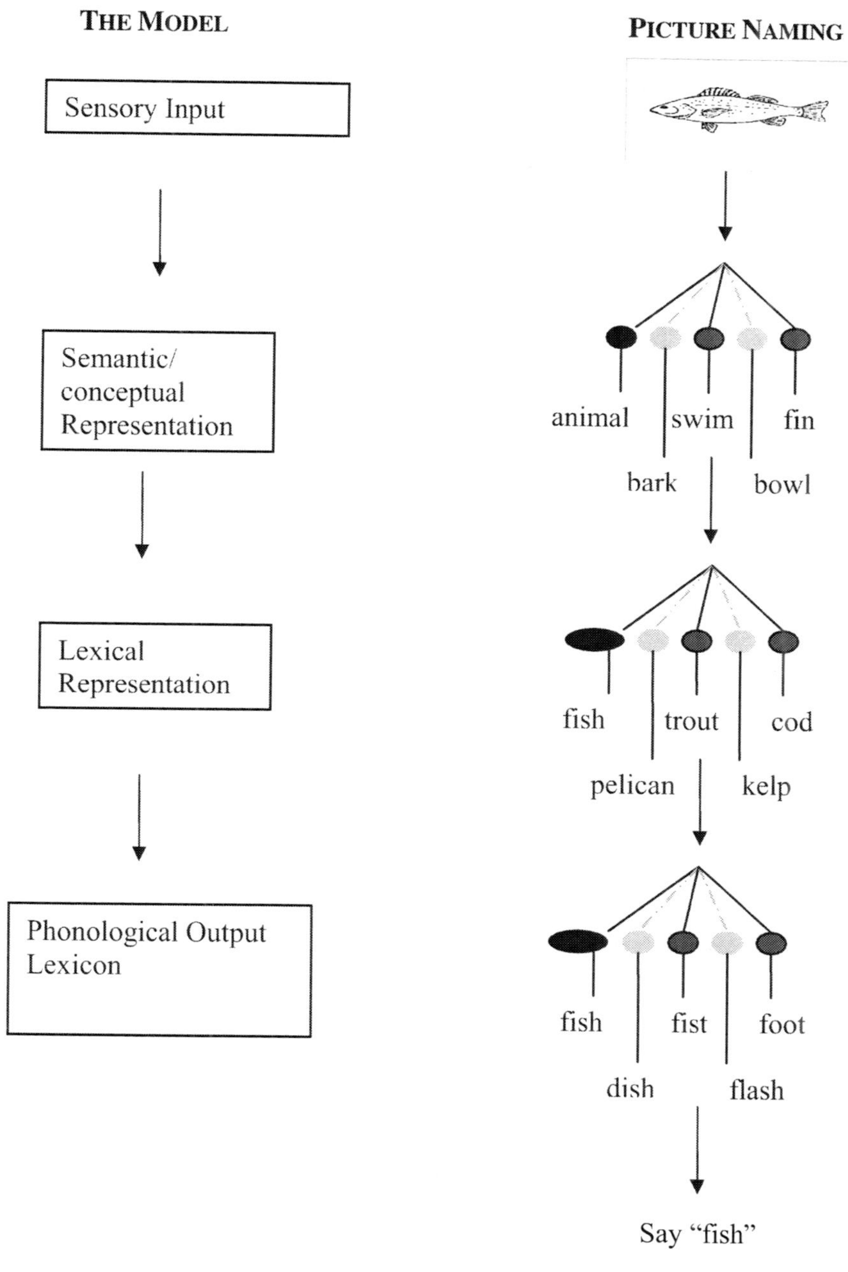

Figure 2. Cognitive psychological model of single language lexical production.

BILINGUAL SEMANTIC ORGANIZATION AND LEXICAL RETRIEVAL

Models of bilingual semantic organization and lexical retrieval attempt to articulate the interaction between multiple languages during the processes of word activation and selection. Specifically, bilingual models must account for the following: the extent to which multiple languages are represented in memory in independent and shared stores, how words access the conceptual store, and the influence of the inactive language on the active language (Keatly, 1992). Bilinguals demonstrate the ability to select only words and constructions that are appropriate given the intended language of output (Gollan and Kroll, 2001). However, bilinguals also code-switch which indicates they can maintain both languages sufficiently active to allow for rapid production and comprehension of both languages with only minor processing costs (von Studnitz and Green, 1997). Therefore, models of lexical access must account for how bilinguals maintain separate languages while retaining the ability to switch between languages in a single context. As in the unilingual process, word comprehension and production are accomplished through a process of selection and activation; however, bilingual production systems must determine whether to select elements and rules from L1, L2, or both (de Bot and Schreuder, 1993). In short, the system must be organized to determine the extent to which words in each language are active and the types of information that must be active during different kinds of tasks (Gollan and Kroll, 2001).

As with the overview of the unilingual lexicon, the discussion will be structured around a four stage model of lexical access (La Heij, 2005). Fundamentally, the structures and their functions are comparable. Activation spreads from the phonological input lexicon (word forms for recognition), to the semantic/conceptual store (meanings), lexical representations (corpus of words to represent the concept), and the phonological output lexicon (word forms for production). However, the organization of two lexico-semantic systems within a single individual creates specific questions and challenges. Specifically, to what extent are the systems shared and separate? To what extent does activation of one language concurrently activate the other language? The answers to both of these questions are complicated by a variety of linguistic and sociolinguistic factors including proficiency, language learning history, and structural similarities and differences between languages.

In the following section, I will address separately issues of word comprehension and production. First, I will review the processes as engaged for word recognition: the interaction between the input lexicon and semantic/conceptual store, or "bottom-up" processing (Costa, 2005). Then, I will discuss word production, or the interaction between the conceptual/semantic store, lexical representation and phonological output lexicon required for "top-down" processing (Costa, 2005). Finally, I will apply the models to understanding issues unique to bilinguals; specifically, differences in processing associated with level of proficiency, code-switching, and translation.

Word Comprehension or "Bottom-Up Processing"

As discussed previously, unilingual spoken word comprehension begins with the recognition of the visual or written input (phonological input lexicon) and proceeds to activation and selection of the corresponding semantic/conceptual representation, see Figure 3. At both stages multiple candidates are activated, with selection of the most strongly activated target. Multiple candidates include word forms with phonological similarity to the target. While bilingual word recognition follows fundamentally the same process, the role of the non-target language must be considered: specifically, the structure of the lexicon and conceptual representations (separate or shared) and the spread of activation in response to input (one or both languages) (Dijkstra and Van Heuvan, 2002; Grosjean, 1997).

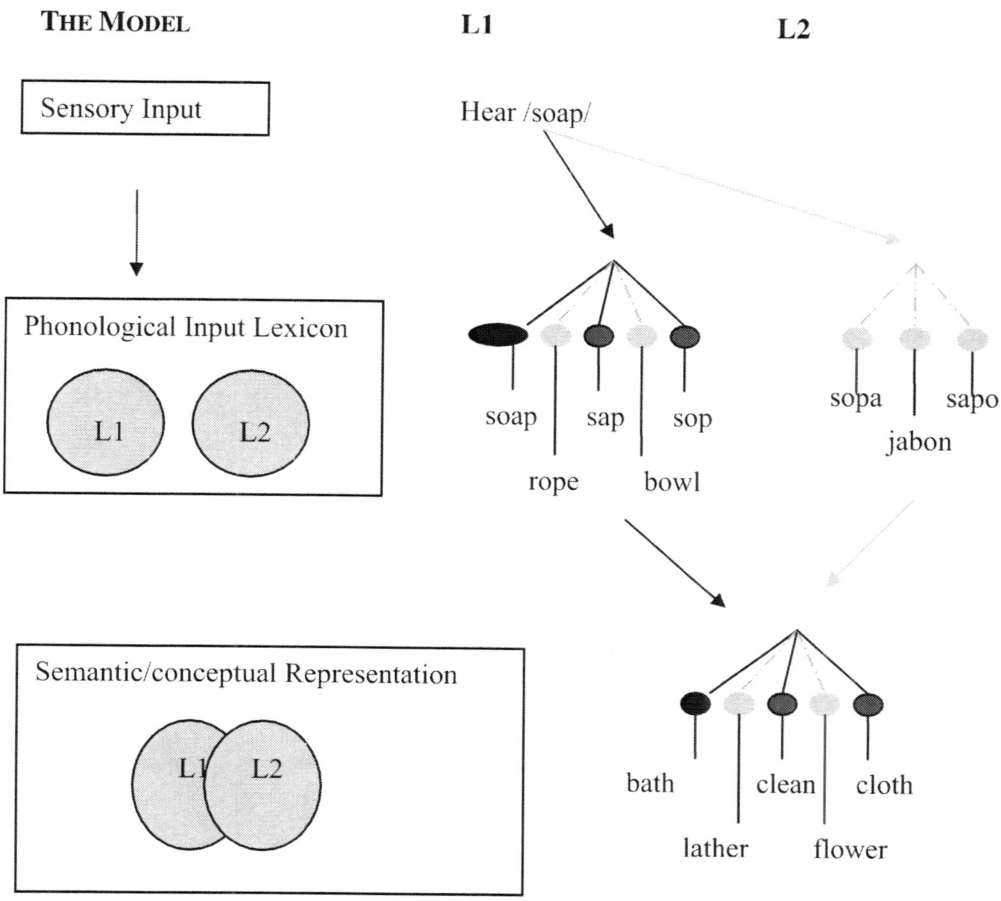

Figure 3. Cognitive psychological model of the organization, activation and selection within the bilingual lexico-semantic system for single word comprehension.

A bilingual listener hears the acoustic signal and recognizes language. Does that word immediately get assigned to the phonological input lexicon of one language, or are the two lexicons shared and activated? Two prominent models of word comprehension, the Bilingual Interactive Activation (BIA; Dijkstra, 2005) and the Bilingual Model of Lexical Access (BiMOLA; Grosjean, 1997), agree that the there is one lexicon, within which there are separate subsystems for each language (see Figure 3). According to Grosjean (1997), bilingual speakers have subsets of systems for each language, particularly for those elements unique to each language, which exist within a larger language system from which both languages may draw. This allows bilinguals to quickly access one or both languages depending on the context.

The sensory input of the word form activates the shared input lexicon. For comprehension to proceed, activation and selection of the matching target must be achieved. Selection and activation of the input lexicon may be conceptualized as language-selective or language non-selective (Dijkstra, 2005). Language selective access would indicate the language of input is recognized and only the word forms in that language are activated; the other language is inhibited (Grosjean, 1988). Language-non-selective access indicates that both lexicons are activated by linguistic input (Dijkstra and Van Heuvan, 2002). Currently, research supports the language-non-selective hypothesis with respect to form and semantic representation (Dijkstra, 2005). Evidence suggests that both languages are active and may facilitate or slow processing. For example, bilingual speakers recognize cognates more quickly than non-cognate (Dijkstra, Van Jaarsveld, and Brinke, 1998) Also, presenting a word in one language leads to faster recognition of the translation equivalent in the other language compared to unrelated words in either language (Chen and Ng, 1989). These types of findings indicate cross language facilitation which can only be accomplished if both languages are, to some extent, active in response to the linguistic input.

A sensory input enters the linguistic system and triggers activation of the phonological input lexicon. The corresponding letter strings, in either language, that match the input are activated (Dijkstra, 2005), as shown in Figure 3. Letter strings in both languages that do not match the target become inhibited, or suppressed (Dijkstra, 2005). Lewy and Grosjean (1996) refer to this process as lateral inhibition, or suppression of non-matching lexical items within a single level of processing, in this case the phonological input lexicon. The target phonological form, i.e. the one with the best match to the sensory input and subsequently the strongest activation, then proceeds to activate the semantic/conceptual store. Both the organization of the conceptual store and how it is accessed by the input lexicon must be considered.

In general, a bilingual speaker is considered to have a single semantic/conceptual store shared by both languages (Du Four and Kroll, 1995). Yet, there are indicators that the overlap is not complete and the two languages have unique conceptual representations even for common words (Francis, 2005). Concrete words may demonstrate more overlap between languages because they have more clearly defined semantic features, while abstract words may have features unique to each language (De Groot, 1992). However, word-to-referent (meaning) mapping for objects may not be as unambiguous as previously thought. Ameel, Storms, Malt, and Sloman (2005) found substantial differences in the way speakers of different languages segment stimulus space by name for both abstract and concrete concepts, (i.e. what is considered a bowl in one language may not be considered a bowl in a different language).

For the sake of this discussion, we will consider bilinguals to have a single conceptual store within which there is overlapping subsystems for each language (see Figure 3). How then does phonological input lexicon activate the conceptual store? Neither Grosjean's (1998) BiMOLA nor Dijkstra's (2005) BIA consider activation beyond the lexical level. Kroll and colleagues (Du Four and Kroll, 1995; Kroll and Curley, 1988; Kroll and de Groot, 1997; Kroll and Dussias, 2004; Kroll and Sholl, 1992) have developed the Revised Hierarchical Model to explain how the two languages access the conceptual store (see Figure 4). The model is comprised of three components: the lexicon of the first language (L1), the lexicon of the second language (L2), and a shared conceptual store. As expected, the L1 input lexicon (assumed to be the stronger language) directly accesses the conceptual store (Du Four and Kroll, 1995). L2 access to the conceptual store is dependent on level of proficiency. Early, low proficiency bilinguals experience concept mediation, e.g. activation of a lexical item in L2 input lexicon activates the comparable item in the L1 lexicon which then activates the conceptual store. As the proficiency in L2 increases, the L2 input lexicon dependence on the L1 input lexicon diminishes and the direct L2 to conceptual store connections are strengthened.

In summary, the process of word recognition involves input lexicon activation of the semantic/conceptual store. For bilinguals, this process appears to engage both languages. Lexical activation is language-non-specific, so a word presented in one language activates phonologically similar candidates in both languages. Once a specific lexeme is selected from the lexicon, the process of activating the conceptual stores depends on language proficiency and the similarities between the two languages.

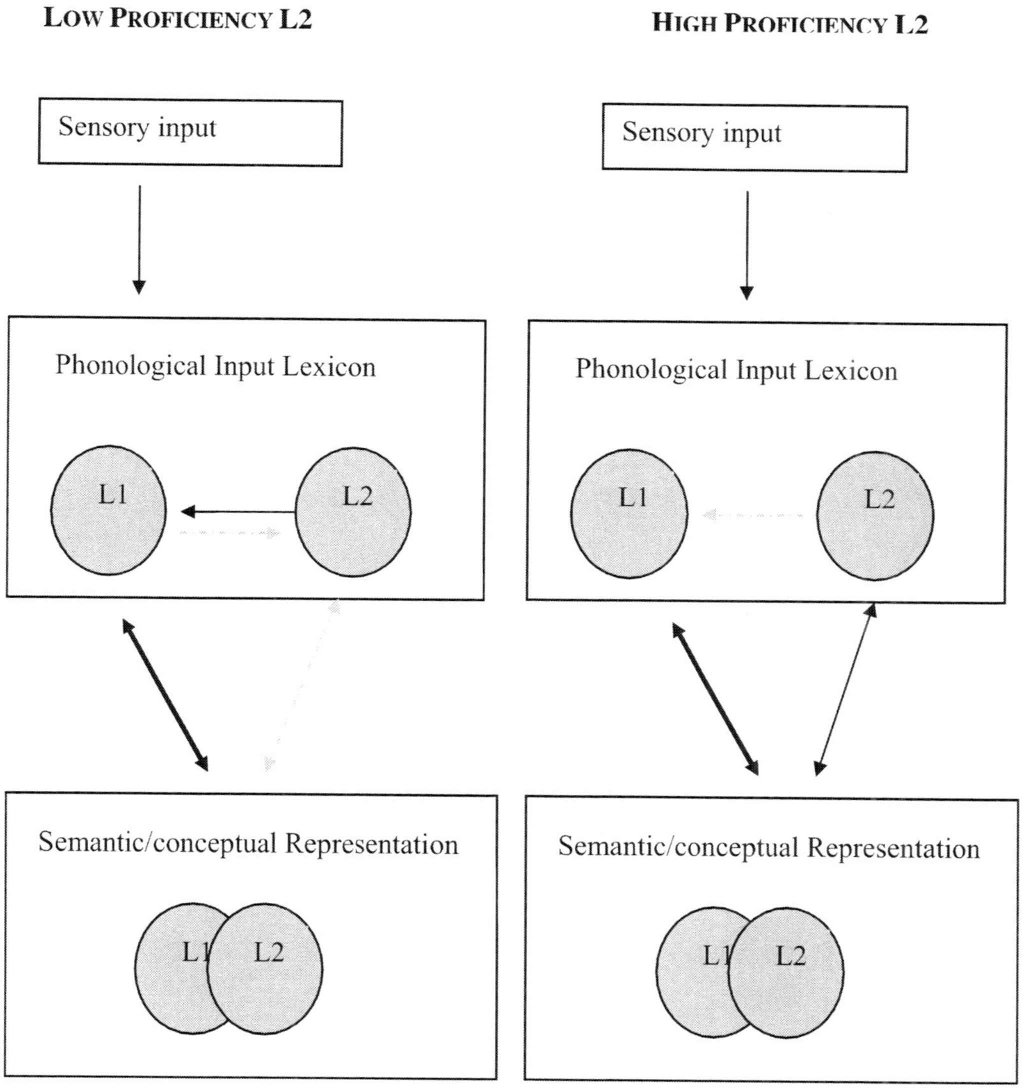

Figure 4. Concept Mediation Model explanation of process by which L2 access to conceptual stores changes with increased proficiency in L2.

Word Production or "Top-Down Processing"

As we have seen, word production involves the generation of the intended meaning (semantic/conceptual store), selection of the corresponding lexeme that best represents that meaning (lexical selection), and selection of the phonological form of the word (phonological output lexicon). The questions that arise are the following: How much is each language involved in the process of lexical selection? How much is each language activated during the process of word production in one language? To answer these questions I will use the model of speech production proposed by Albert Costa and colleagues (Costa, 2004, 2005; Costa, Miozzo, and Caramazza, 1999; Costa and Santesteban, 2004), as shown in Figure 5.

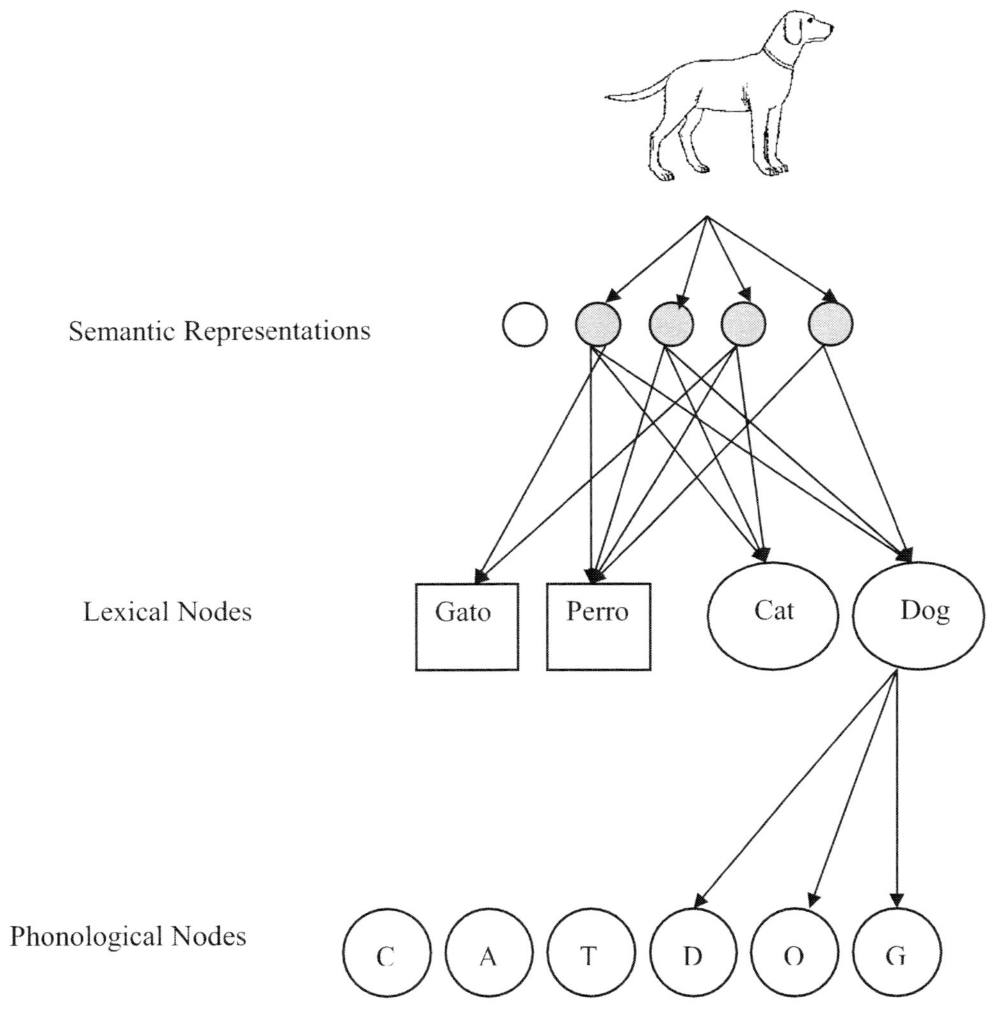

Figure 5. Albert Costa's model of bilingual single word production (Costa, 2005).

As previously discussed, speech production starts with activation of conceptual/semantic representations, spreading activation to the lexical representation, and activation of the phonological output lexicon. These stages are evident in the bilingual model (Costa, 2005) with activation spreading from semantic representations to lexical nodes to phonological nodes (see Figure 6).

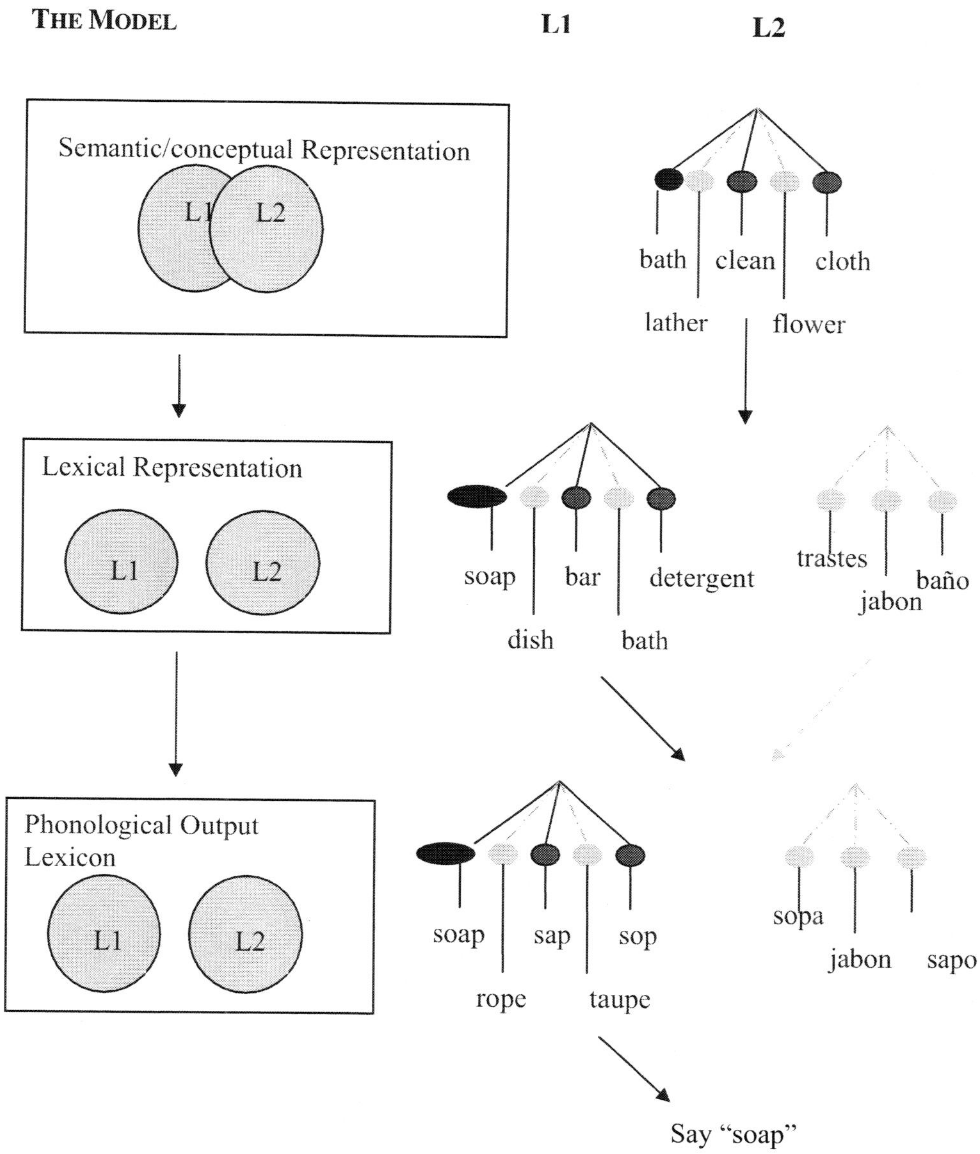

Figure 6. Cognitive psychological model of the organization, activation and selection within the bilingual lexico-semantic system for single word production.

In the first stage, the semantic/conceptual representation sends activation in parallel and to equal extents to the lexical entries in the two lexicons of the bilingual (Costa, et al 1999), i.e. the target, its translation equivalent, and semantically related items in both languages are activated to some extent. Therefore, words in both languages become competitors for selection. The word with the strongest activation, e.g. match to the semantic features of the target, is selected. Activation of the lexical representation then spreads to the phonological representation. Activation is evident in the phonological features of the selected lexical target and to a lesser extent related items in BOTH languages (Costa and Santesteban, 2004). Selection is made for the phonological form of target word in the intended response language.

In bilingual speech production, a concept is formulated and activates lexical representations in both languages; activation then spreads to phonological forms in both languages. The exact point at which a language is specified is unclear (Costa, 2005). Language selection may occur at the conceptual level (La Heij, 2005), or at a later stage in the process. Language selection is in part determined by the pragmatic and linguistic demands of the communicative context. Language mode, e.g. bilingual or monolingual context, appears to impact degree of overall activation of each language (Grosjean, 2001). Other factors unique to bilingual speech production will be considered in the following section.

FURTHER ISSUES IN BILINGUAL LEXICO-SEMANTIC PROCESSING

Semantic organization and lexical retrieval are influenced by a variety of factors. For example, research into patterns of lexical access in speakers of a single language has revealed that speed of access is influenced by a variety of stimulus variables (e.g. high frequency words are retrieved faster than low frequency words, concrete faster than abstract, words acquired early faster than those acquired later) (Beeson and Hillis, 2001). Similar variables influence lexical access for bilinguals. However, bilinguals vary tremendously in regards to age of acquisition of each language and development and attrition of a given language over time (Goggin, Estrada, and Villarreal, 1994). Therefore, understanding these variables requires considering issues of proficiency and language history. Additionally, the similarity between languages (specifically cognate status) also influences retrieval. Finally, bilinguals manifest language skill that allows for the interaction between languages, e.g. code-switching and translation that must be accounted for when modeling lexical retrieval in bilinguals.

Proficiency

Proficiency refers to level of skill in a given language. Bilinguals can vary widely in their skill in each language. Determinations of proficiency are in part dependent on the nature of the communicative task (Grosjean, 1998; Valdés and Figueroa, 1994). For example, a bilingual may be highly proficient in reading and writing in L1 and L2, but minimally proficient in spoken production in L2. However, the strength and patterns of activation throughout the lexical-semantic system are influenced by personal variables. As discussed previously, during word comprehension proficiency influences whether L2 accesses the conceptual store directly or via L1 lexical representations (Poulisse, 1997). Psycholinguistic research indicates that beginning bilinguals process language differently from fluent bilinguals. For example, Du Four and Kroll (1995) gave high and low proficiency bilinguals (English/French) a categorization task. Participants listened to the name of a category and then a list of items. They had to state if the items were/were not members of the category. The language of the category and items systematically varied. RT suggested that high proficiency bilinguals accessed the concepts directly. For low proficiency bilinguals, slower RT suggested that concepts in L2 were often (though not always) mediated through L1.

Research indicates that proficiency influences word production. The dominant or more frequently used language is more difficult to deactivate and has a stronger base activation which will influence the spread of activation and selection (de Bot and Schreuder, 1993). Within the framework of the Costa's model, implications for differences related to proficiency can be drawn. The conceptual store is shared by the two languages. For high proficiency bilinguals activation and selection would proceed as discussed previously. For low proficiency bilinguals, accessing L2 may be associated with increased activation of L1 semantic representation and lexical node. Increased activation of L1 is required to increase the activation of an L2 response. The combined L1 and L2 activation leads to selection of an L2 response.

Stimulus Characteristics

As with monolinguals, a variety of stimulus characteristics can influence the accuracy and speed with which an individual provides a response. These variables can differ between a bilingual's two languages and between monolingual and bilingual speakers of the same language. The frequency (frequency with which a word appears in a given language), familiarity (familiarity of given word for speakers of a language), and imageability (measure of the "picturability" of a word in the language) can vary across languages. For example, compare norms obtained for English by Snodgrass and Vanderwart (1980) on a corpus of 260 pictures, to those obtained on the same corpus in Spanish (Cuetos, Ellis, and Alvarez, 1999; Sanfeliu and Fernandez, 1996). In regards to age of acquisition, L2 processing appears to differ as a function of age of acquisition. For example, research shows distinct patterns of processing when comparing groups that acquired L2 before the age of 7, and after the age of 7 (Silverberg and Samuel, 2004). Additionally, stimulus variables have been shown to affect translation. Translation is faster for high frequency words, and translation is faster and better for concrete words (De Groot, Dannenburg, and van Hell, 1994).

Cognates

Activation is also influenced by the similarities and differences between languages, for example research indicates cognate words (i.e. words that have both a shared meaning and a shared phonological form, e.g. car/carro vs. manzana/apple) are processed differently than non-cognates (Friel and Kennison, 2001). Cognates are more accurately and more quickly named than non-cognates and more resistant to retrieval failures (Sanchez-Casas and Garcia-Albea, 2005). Costa et al. (2004) suggest two possible mechanisms for the cognate advantage. The unique processing of cognates may be due to shared lexical representation for cognates that is not typical of non-cognates. Conversely, the cognate advantage may be due to spreading activation to the phonological system. A target activates its semantic representation and translations (language non-specific). For cognates, activation spreads to the phonological form of the target and translation.

Code-Switching

Bilinguals are able to switch between languages within a context and from one context to another. Intrasentential code-switching (switching within a sentence) is systematic and rule governed (Myers-Scotton and Jake, 1995). Though the rules have been difficult to define, bilinguals are clear in identifying correct and incorrect code-switching (Berk-Seligson, 1986). The choice to code-switch and the manner in which it occurs is influenced by a variety of internal and external (contextual) influences. For example, proficiency influences code-switching (Costa and Santesteban, 2004). For low proficiency bilinguals, it is harder to switch from the L2 to L1, than it is to switch from L1 to L2. This asymmetry is not evident in fluent bilinguals.

Language processing models must account for the ability to suppress non-target language responses in monolingual contexts, while still allowing for activation of both languages in bilingual contexts. Within the framework of the Costa model, we can suggest implications for the mechanisms underlying code-switching. Level of activation of a given language must, to some extent be determined by the communicative context. A strictly monolingual context may lead to an overall dampening of the activation of the non-target language across all components. L1, the stronger language, may require more inhibition than L2 (Costa and Santesteban, 2004). In a bilingual context, both languages may have high levels of activation, with selection influenced by a variety of internal and external factors.

Translation

Translation involves hearing a word and saying the equivalent word in another language. Translation of single words is performed within the context of the lexicosemantic system previously discussed, i.e., using the lexical, phonological, and conceptual representations. However, the path through the lexicosemantic system is dependent on direction of translation: forward translation- L1 → L2 or backwards translation- L2 → L1. Forward translation (L1→L2), has much in common with picture naming (Kroll and Stewart, 1994). The bilingual speaker hears the acoustic signal which activates the L1 lexicon leading to activation of the conceptual store. Translation is accomplished through activation of the L2 lexicon via links between the L1 and L2 lexicons. Backward translation appears to engage a different process (Sholl, Sankaranarayanan, and Kroll, 1995). In this case, the bilingual speaker hears the acoustic signal which activates the L2 lexicon which in turn directly activates the L1 lexicon (rather than the conceptual store).

The hypothesis that L1 → L2 is conceptually mediated, while L2 → L1 is mediated at the lexical level is the result of patterns of performance on a variety of experimental tasks (Kroll and Stewart, 1994). In experiments utilizing translation tasks, findings indicate that participants are faster and more accurate when translating from L2 → L1 than when translating from L1→ L2 (Kroll and Stewart, 1994). The faster rate is attributed to the bypassing of the conceptual store. L2 → L1 translation relies on strong links between the L2 lexicon and the L1 lexicon rather than on the weak link between L2 and the conceptual store. However, as we have previously discussed, the strength of the link between L2 and the conceptual store is in part an issue of proficiency. Therefore, we can expect that as proficiency in L2 increases L2 → L1 translation becomes more conceptually mediated and performance between the two directions of translation is similar.

While it would appear that translation could be done strictly at the lexical level, research suggests that translation from L1 → L2 does engage the conceptual representations. The speed and accuracy of translation is influenced by stimulus variable (e.g. imageability, frequency, familiarity, and cognate status) associated with the semantic representation of a word (de Groot et al, 1994). Additionally, the speed at which a bilingual can translate from L1→ L2 is comparable to the speed at which they can name pictures indicating that both processes follow a similar activation process within the lexicosemantic system (Kroll and Stewart, 1994).

SUMMARY

Organization of the lexico-semantic system for two languages has much in common with that of a single language. Understanding of bilingual lexical comprehension and retrieval requires understanding how the languages are organized and activated during the selection process. In general, languages have a shared "language system" within which exist subsystems for features unique to each language. Regardless of the target language, activation of both languages is evident to an extent dependent on the communicative context. Bilinguals efficiently manipulate the lexico-semantic system to meet a variety of communicative needs, including communicating in monolingual and bilingual modes, code-switching, and translating.

REFERENCES

Ameel, E., Storms, G., Malt, B. C., and Sloman, S. A. (2005). How bilinguals solve the naming problem. *Journal of Memory and Language, 53*, 60-80.

Beeson, P. M., and Hillis, A. E. (2001). Comprehension and production of written words. In R. Chapey (Ed.), *Language Intervention Strategies in Aphasia and Related Neurogenic Communication Disorders* (4th ed.). Philadelphia, PA: Lippincott Williams and Wilkins Publishers.

Berk-Seligson, S. (1986). Linguistic constraints on intrasentential code-switching: a study of Spanish/Hebrew bilingualism. *Language in Society, 15*, 313-348.

Caramazza, A. (1997). How many levels of processing are there in lexical access? *Cognitive Neuropsychology, 14*(1), 177-208.

Caramazza, A., and Miceli, G. (1990). Structure of the lexicon: functional architecture and lexical representation. In J.-L. Nespoulous and P. Villiard (Eds.), *Morphology, Phonology, and Aphasia* (pp. 1-19). New York: Springer-Verlag.

Chen, H.-c., and Ng, M.-l. (1989). Semantic facilitation and translation priming effects in Chinese-English bilinguals. *Memory and Cognition, 17*(4), 454-462.

Costa, A. (2004). Speech production in bilinguals. In T. K. Bhatia and W. C. Ritchie (Eds.), *The Handbook of Bilingualism* (pp. 201-223). Malden, MA: Blackwell Publishers, Ltd.

Costa, A. (2005). Lexical access in bilingual production. In J. F. Kroll and A. De Groot (Eds.), *Handbook of Bilingualism: Psycholinguistic approaches* (pp. 308-325). New York: Oxford University Press.

Costa, A., Miozzo, M., and Caramazza, A. (1999). Lexical selection in bilinguals: Do words in the bilingual's two lexicons compete for selection? *Journal of Memory and Language, 41*, 365-397.

Costa, A., and Santesteban, M. (2004). Lexical access in bilingual speech production: Evidence from language switching in highly proficient bilinguals and L2 learners. *Journal of Memory and Language, 50*, 491-511.

Cuetos, F., Ellis, A. W., and Alvarez, B. (1999). Naming times for the Snodgrass and Vanderwart pictures in Spanish. *Behavior Research Methods, Instruments, and Computers, 31*(4), 650-658.

de Bot, K., and Schreuder, R. (1993). Word production and the bilingual lexicon. In R. Schreuder and B. Weltens (Eds.), *The Bilingual Lexicon* (pp. 191-214). Philadelphia: John Bejamins Publishing Co.

De Groot, A. (1992). Determinants of word translation. *Journal of Experimental Psychology: Learning, Memory, and Cognition, 18*, 1001-1018.

De Groot, A. M. B., Dannenburg, L., and van Hell, J. G. (1994). Forward and backward word translation by bilinguals. *Journal of Memory and Language, 33*, 600-629.

Dell, G. S. (1988). The retrieval of phonological forms in production: Tests of predictions from a connectionist model. *Journal of Memory and Language, 27*, 124-142.

Dell, G. S., Chang, F., and Griffin, Z. M. (1999). Connectionist models of language production: lexical access and grammatical encoding. *Cognitive Science, 23*(4), 517-542.

Dijkstra, T. (2005). Bilingual visual word recognition and lexical access. In J. F. Kroll and A. De Groot (Eds.), *Handbook of Bilingualism: Psycholinguistic Approaches* (pp. 179-201). Oxford: Oxford University Press.

Dijkstra, T., and Van Heuvan, W. J. B. (2002). The architecture of the bilingual word recognition system: from identification to decision. *Bilingualism: Language and Cognition, 5*(3), 175-197.

Dijkstra, T., Van Jaarsveld, H., and Brinke, S. (1998). Interlingual homograph recognition: Effects of task demands and language intermixing. *Bilingualism: Language and Cognition, 1*, 51-66.

Du Four, R., and Kroll, J. F. (1995). Matching words to concepts in two languages: A test of the concept mediation model of bilingual representation. *Memory and Cognition, 23*(2), 166-180.

Foygel, D., and Dell, G. S. (2000). Models of impaired lexical access in speech production. *Journal of Memory and Language, 43*, 182-216.

Francis, W. S. (2005). Bilingual semantic and conceptual representation. In J. F. Kroll and A. De Groot (Eds.), *Handbook of Bilingualism: Psycholinguistic Approaches* (pp. 251-267). Oxford: Oxford University Press.

Friel, B. M., and Kennison, S. M. (2001). Identifying German-English cognates, false cognates, and non-cognates: Methodological issues and descriptive norms. *Bilingualism: Language and Cognition, 4*(3), 249-274.

Goggin, J. P., Estrada, P., and Villarreal, R. P. (1994). Picture-naming agreement in monolinguals and bilinguals. *Applied Psycholinguistics, 15*, 177-193.

Gollan, T., and Kroll, J. F. (2001). Bilingual lexical access. In B. C. Rapp (Ed.), *A Handbook of Cognitive Neuropsychology: What Deficits Reveal About the Human Mind/Brain* (pp. 321-345). Philadelphia: Psychology Press.

Grosjean, F. (1988). Exploring the recognition of guest words in bilingual speech. *Language and cognitive processes, 3*(3), 233 - 275.

Grosjean, F. (1997). Processing mixed language: Issues, findings, and models. In A. M. B. K. de Groot, J.F. (Ed.), *Tutorials in Bilingualism: Psycholinguistic perspectives* (pp. 225-254). Mahwah, New Jersey: Lawrence Erlbaum Associates.

Grosjean, F. (1998). Studying bilinguals: Methodological and conceptual issues. *Bilingualism: Language and Cognition, 1*(2), 131-149.

Grosjean, F. (2001). The Bilingual's Language Modes. In J. Nicol (Ed.), *One Mind, Two Languages*. Malden, MA: Blackwell Publishers Ltd.

Hillis, A. E. (2001). The organization of the lexical system. In B. C. Rapp (Ed.), *The Handbook of Neuropsychology: What deficits Reveal About the Human Mind* (pp. 185-210). Philadelphia, PA: Psychology Press.

Keatly, C. (1992). History of bilingualism research in cognitive psychology. In R. J. Harris (Ed.), *Cognitive Processing in Bilinguals* (pp. 15-49). Amsterdam: Elsevier Science Publishers.

Kroll, J., and Curley, J. (1988). Lexical Memory in Novice Bilinguals: The role of concepts in retrieving second language words. In M. M. Gruneberg, P. E. Morris and R. N. Sykes (Eds.), *Practical aspects of memory: Current research and issues* (Vol. 2, pp. 389-402). New York: John Wiley and Sons.

Kroll, J. F., and de Groot, A. M. B. (1997). Lexical and conceptual memory in the bilingual: Mapping form to meaning in two languages. In A. M. B. de Groot and J. F. Kroll (Eds.), *Tutorials in bilingualism: Psycholinguistic perspectives* (pp. 169-200). Mahwah, New Jersey: Lawrence Erlbaum Associates.

Kroll, J. F., and Dussias, P. E. (2004). The comprehension of words and sentences in two languages. In T. K. Bhatia and W. C. Ritchie (Eds.), *The Handbook of Bilingualism*. Malden, MA: Blackwell Publishing Ltd.

Kroll, J. F., and Sholl, A. (1992). Lexical and conceptual memory in fluent and nonfluent bilinguals. In R. J. Harris (Ed.), *Cognitive processing in bilinguals* (pp. 191-204). San Diego: Elsevier Science Publishers.

Kroll, J. F., and Stewart, E. (1994). Category interference in translation and picture naming: Evidence for asymmetric connections between bilingual memory representation. *Journal of Memory and Language, 33*, 149 - 174.

La Heij, W. (2005). Selection processes in monolingual and bilingual lexical access. In J. F. Kroll and A. De Groot (Eds.), *Handbook of Bilingualism: Psycholinguistic Approaches* (pp. 289-307). Oxford: Oxford University Press.

Levelt, W. J. M. (1992). Accessing words in speech production: Stages, processes and representations. *Cognition, 42*, 1-22.

Lewy, N., and Grosjean, F. (1996). *A computational model of bilingual lexical access.*Unpublished manuscript.

McClelland, J. L., and Elman, J. L. (1986). The TRACE model of speech perception. *Cognitive Psychology, 18*, 1-86.

Myers-Scotton, C., and Jake, J. L. (1995). Matching lemmas in a bilingual language competence and production model: evidence from intrasentential code switching. *Linguistics, 33* 981-1024.

Norris, D. (1994). Shortlist: a connectionist model of continuous speech recognition. *Cognition, 52*, 189-234.

Postler, J., De Bleser, R., Cholewa, J., Glauche, V., Hamzei, F., and Weiller, C. (2003). Neuroimaging the semantic system. *Aphasiology, 17*(9), 799-814.

Poulisse, N. (1997). Language production in bilinguals. In A. M. B. de Groot and J. F. Kroll (Eds.), *Tutorials in Bilinguaism* (pp. 201-224). Mahwah, New Jersey: Lawrence Earlbaum Associates.

Raymer, A. M., and Gonzalez Rothi, L. J. (2001). Cognitive approaches to impairments in word comprehension and production. In R. Chapey (Ed.), *Language Intervention Strategies in Aphasia and Related Neurogenic Communication Disorders*. New York: Lippincott Williams and Wilkins.

Roelofs, A. (2003). Modeling the relation between the production and recognition of spoken word forms. In A. S. Meyer and N. O. Schiller (Eds.), *Phonetics and Phonology in Language Comprehension and Production* (pp. 115-158). Berlin: Mount de Gruyter.

Sanchez-Casas, R., and Garcia-Albea, J. E. (2005). The representation of cognate and noncognate words in bilingual memory. In J. F. Kroll and A. De Groot (Eds.), *Handbook of Bilingualism: Psycholinguistic Approaches* (pp. 226-250). Oxford: Oxford University Press.

Sanfeliu, M. C., and Fernandez, A. (1996). A set of 254 Snodgrass-Vanderwart pictures standardized for Spanish: Norms for name agreement, image agreement, familiarity, and visual complexity. *Behavior, Research Methods, Instruments, and Computers, 28*(4), 537-555.

Sholl, A., Sankaranarayanan, A., and Kroll, J. F. (1995). Transfer between picture naming and translation: a test of asymmetries in bilingual memory. *Psychological Science, 6*(1), 45 - 49.

Silverberg, S., and Samuel, A. G. (2004). The effect of age of second language acquisition on the representation and processing of second language words. *Journal of Memory and Language, 51*, 381-398.

Snodgrass, J. G., and Vanderwart, M. (1980). A standardized set of 260 pictures: Norms for name agreement, image agreement, familiarity, and visual complexity. *Journal of Experimental Psychology, 6*(2), 174-215.

Valdés, G., and Figueroa, R. A. (1994). *Bilingualism and Testing: A special case of bias.* Norwood, New Jersey: Ablex Publishing Corp.

von Studnitz, R. E., and Green, D. W. (1997). Lexical decision and language switching. *International Journal of Bilingualism, 1*(1), 3-24.

In: Speech and Language Disorders in Bilinguals ISBN 978-1-60021-560-5
Editors: Alfredo Ardila and Eliane Ramos, pp. 109-130 © 2007 Nova Science Publishers, Inc.

Chapter 6

ASSESSMENT AND TREATMENT OF BILINGUAL APHASIA AND BILINGUAL ANOMIA

Patricia M. Roberts
Audiology and Speech-Language Pathology Program
University of Ottawa
Ottawa, Ontario (Canada)
Swathi Kiran
Department of Communication Sciences and Disorders
University of Texas at Austin
Austin, Texas

INTRODUCTION

This chapter will present a general framework for looking at bilingual aphasia and will review issues relevant to the assessment and treatment of anomia in bilingual aphasic adults. Anomia is the most universal symptom in aphasia, and one which patients find frustrating. It is also one of the best studied areas in aphasia, drawing on a large body of knowledge about lexical models, lexical access, and the naming process in non-aphasic adults.

This chapter begins by defining some of the key terminology. The bulk of the chapter is devoted to a discussion of current assessment methods, especially assessment of naming impairments, and a review of studies on the rehabilitation of bilingual aphasia, with a particular focus on the assessment and treatment of naming (or word-finding) The chapter closes with a commentary on various methodological issues and steps to foster more rapid progress in the field of bilingual aphasia.

Some Definitions

Aphasia: For this chapter, "aphasia" refers only to the language impairment caused by strokes, since this is the area that has been most studied. The progressive language loss that is part of most dementias is, many authors and clinicians feel, a different disorder.

Bilingual aphasia: The term "bilingual aphasia" is generally used as a shorthand for "aphasia occurring in bilingual speaker-hearers". Although some studies of trilinguals and multilinguals are now appearing (e.g., de Bot, 2004; Goral, Levy, Obler, and Cohen, 2006; Goral and Obler, in press; Lemhöfer, Dijkstra, and Michel, 2004), we do not yet know if there are differences between bilingual and multilingual speakers with aphasia (for example, in their symptoms, prognosis, or treatment outcomes). So, for now, the term "bilingual aphasia" generally refers to multilinguals as well as to bilinguals.

Bilingualism: In this chapter, the term "bilingual" is used to describe people with a range of levels of knowledge of a second language. It is not restricted to the so-called "perfect mastery" of two languages, since it is now clear that this level may be unattainable, for a variety of reasons (Butler and Hakuta, 2006; Christophersen, 1999; Hyltenstam, 1992), including the influences, in both directions, between each language spoken (e.g., Dijkstra, del Prado, Fermin, Schulpen, Schreuder, and Baayen, 2005; Edwards, 2006; Levey, 2004; Pavlenko, 2000; Pavlenko and Jarvis, 2002; Van Hell and Dijkstra, 2002; Van Wijnendaele and Brysbaert, 2002).

We view each individual's level of bilingualism (LOB) not as a unitary thing, but as something that varies across modalities, along a continuum of proficiency within each modality. As do many other authors, we see bilingualism as multidimensional, with each individual at some level of expertise in auditory comprehension, verbal expression, reading, and writing. An overall rating of proficiency is not very informative and we should not expect high correlations between overall ratings and performance on specific tasks. Readers with expertise in aphasia recognize these modalities as part of the grid used in aphasia assessments and in planning treatment, since each modality may be differentially affected by the aphasia. It is relatively recent for these four modalities to serve as a framework for describing a bilingual speaker's level of proficiency in each language.

As Grosjean (1989) and others have said: the bilingual speaker is unlike a native speaker of either language. These two facts (bidirectional influence between languages and competency being along modality-specific continua) present problems for the assessment and treatment of aphasia, as this chapter will show.

Importance of Bilingual Aphasia

As noted by previous authors, the high incidence of bilingualism in many parts of the world (e.g., Fabbro, 2001; Harris, 1992; Paradis, 1995) and the universal presence of strokes combine to produce large numbers of bilingual adults with aphasia (Paradis, 2001). There is a professional obligation to understand the disorder, to develop treatment methods and to assess their efficacy. In 1998, Roberts found that the existing literature was "sparse in relation to the clinical importance of understanding bilingual aphasia in order to assist bilingual adults recovering from and living with their aphasia" (Roberts, 1998b, p. 145). Since 1998, there has been an increase in the number of studies of bilingual aphasia, often focusing on describing symptoms, and on language localization (e.g., Fabro, 2001; Frenck-Mestre, Anton, Roth, Vaid, and Viallet, 2005; Mechelli, Crinion, et al., 2004). There have also been a number of chapters that summarize, debate, and review issues (e.g., Paradis, 2001; Roberts, 2001, 2007). Sadly, there have been very few studies of the reliability and validity of assessment tools, or of treatment outcomes for bilingual patients. This situation mirrors that in aphasiology as a whole, where studies of language localization and the nature of aphasia outnumber validation studies of tests and treatment studies (Roberts, Code, and McNeil, 2003). We are slowly adding to our knowledge on bilingual aphasia, but need a great deal more information about valid assessment, optimal treatment methods, and determining prognosis.

Assessment of Bilingual Aphasia

To assess a patient's post-stroke naming ability, clinicians and researchers may use subtests from one of the aphasia tests available in more than one language. These include the *Aachen Aphasia Test* (Graetz, de Bleser, and Willmes, 1992; Luzzati, Willmes, and de Bleser, 1992; Miller, de Bleser, and Willmes, 1997; Miller, Willmes, and de Bleser, 2000), the *Boston Diagnostic Aphasia Examination* (Goodglass and Kaplan, 1983; Goodglass, Kaplan, and Barresi, 2000; Laine, Goodglass, Niemi, Koivuselka-Sallinen, Tuomainen, and Martilla, 1993), the *Bilingual Aphasia Test* (BAT) (Paradis and Libben 1987; Juncos Rabadan, 1994; Juncos Rabadan, Elosua de Juan, Pereiro Rozas, and Torres Maroño, 1998) and the *Multilingual Aphasia Examination* (MAE) (Elias, Elias, D'Agostino, Silbershatz, and Wolf, 1997; Benton, Hamsher, and Sivan, 1994; Rey and Benton, 1991, 1999; Rey, Feldman, Hernandez, Levin, et al., 2001; Rey, Feldman, Rivas-Vazquez, Levin, and Benton, 1999). The psychometric properties of these tests in their various languages (their initial validity, test-retest reliability, available norms etc) vary widely, from one test to another and for different language versions of the same test. For example, there are norms for the English and Spanish MAE, but not for the French or German versions, nor for most versions of the BAT.

The problem of valid assessment in aphasia is particularly acute for bilingual aphasia, but extends to some of the English-language aphasia tests as well. For example, a recent U.S. government task force that reviewed only the BDAE, from among the tests listed above, found that "The *Boston Diagnostic Aphasia Examination*, 2nd Edition (BDAE-2) met neither the reliability nor validity criterion." (Agency for Health Care Research and Quality, 2002). They further identified the need for development of better tests for communication disorders, stating: "With the increasing cultural, linguistic, and racial diversity of the U.S. population, the applicability of assessment instruments to individuals who are members of different subpopulations is of crucial importance to clinical diagnosis and the process of disability determination. Despite the existence of a large number of speech and language assessment instruments, we still lack appropriate instruments for reliably and validly assessing speech and language in many subgroups defined in terms of language, dialect, or cultural differences. Thus, future research funding and priorities should be directed at addressing these serious deficiencies." (http://www.ahrq.gov/clinic/epcsums/spdissum.htm).

To measure change over time in a given patient, or in neurologically intact adults, any of the tests listed above could be used (although the sensitivity of some of them to detect change/differences has not been demonstrated). But to compare the post-stroke ability levels and the severity of the aphasia in each language of bilingual patients (i.e. how severe is the aphasia in Russian vs. in English?), it is vital to know to what extent the versions of a given test in each language are similar in their level of difficulty (Roberts, 1998a, 1998b, 2001, 2007). As we learn more about lexical, syntactic, and phonological processing, devising tests that are equivalent across languages becomes increasingly difficult. However, some basic criteria can be met, such as selecting stimuli for single word processing tasks that are equivalent in difficulty across languages. All of the aphasia tests published in different languages must be submitted to this time-consuming, yet vital process.

To assess naming ability, the *Boston Naming Test* (Kaplan, Goodglass, and Weintraub, 1983, 2001) has been studied in quite a range of languages including, for example, French (Roberts and Doucet, 2001; Roberts, Garcia, Desrochers, and Hernandez, 2002; Thuillard-Colombo and Assal, 1992), Spanish (Allegri, Mangone, Vallavicencio, Rymberg, Taragano, and Baumann, 1997; Kohnert, Hernandez, and Bates, 1998; Ponton, Satz, Herrera, et al., 1996; Ponton, Satz, Herrera, Young, Ortiz, D'Elia, et al., 1992), "Chinese" (Cheung, Cheung, and Chan, 2004), Dutch (Marien, Mampaey, Vervaet, Saerens, and DeDeyn, 1998), Finnish (Laine, Goodglass, Niemi, Koivuselka-Sallinen, Tuomainen, and Martilla, 1993), Greek (Tsolaki, Tsantali, Lekka, Kiosseoglou, and Kazis, 2003), Korean (Kim and Na, 1999), Norwegian (Hestad, Dybing, Haugen, and Klove, 1998), and Swedish (Tallberg, 2005). In most cases problems have been found with the level of name agreement: participants provided two or more different names for a picture included in the original BNT because the authors felt there was only one acceptable name in American English. Also, in the BNT studies that provide the item difficulty for all 60 items, the difficulty levels of some pictures for speakers of other languages do not follow the supposed order of difficulty for English (although the English pictures are not in order of difficulty for many unilingual English speakers (Roberts, Garcia, Desrochers, and Hernandez, 2002; Tombaugh and Hubley, 1997). In some cases, authors have changed so many of the original stimuli (for psychometric and cultural reasons) that the test is quite different in content from the original, English-language version of the BNT (Kim and Na, 1999).

Although there is no new test designed to assess bilingual aphasia, or bilingual naming impairments, there are now a number of sets of nouns (including but not limited to the Snodgrass and Vanderwart pictures) that have been tested in a range of languages for key features such as age of acquisition, length, frequency, imageability, and name agreement in French (e.g., Chalard, Bonin, Meot, Boyer, and Fayol, 1997; New, Pallier, Brysbaert, and Ferrand, 2004), in Italian (e.g., Barca, Burani, and Arduino, 2002), Icelandic (Pind, Joergen, Jonsdottir, Gossurardottir, and Jonsson, 2000) and in Spanish (e.g., Davis and Perea, 2005; Perez and Navalon, 2005).

There are two data bases of stimuli designed for use in a range of languages. Kremin, Akhutina, Basso, Davidoff, De Wilde, Kitzing, et al. (2003) have developed a set of 269 pictures, with normative data for 90 to 130 participants for each language, who were native speakers of Dutch, English, German, French, Italian, Russian, Spanish, and Swedish. Other work is underway expanding the list of languages and the types of French and Spanish (European vs. North American dialects). Szekely, Jacobsen, D'Amico, Devescovi, Andonova, Herron, et al., (2004; see also Szekely, D'Amico, Devescovi, Federmeier, Herron, Iyer, et al., 2005) have published results from the International Picture Naming Project (pictures and data are available at: http://crl.ucsd.edu/~aszekely/ipnp/) which provides data on 520 object names and 275 verbs in American English, German, Mexican Spanish, Italian, Bulgarian, Hungarian and a Taiwanese dialect of Mandarin. These data bases will facilitate future work on naming abilities in bilingual speakers, and the design of optimally valid and reliable assessments of bilingual aphasic adults.

The difficulties of assessing naming in bilingual speakers are not solved by comparing the performance of bilingual adults to that of unilingual speakers of each language or to groups of people who are described as "native speakers", since native speakers of one language often grow up to be bilingual or multilingual. There will always be differences from one bilingual speaker to the next, differences related to their own proficiency and acquisition history for each language. But, at least, if the same stimuli can be used across studies, stimuli with known psychometric properties, some of the potential causes of variance across studies can be reduced.

Alternate Assessment Methods for Expressive Language in Bilinguals

Given the problems of name agreement, and the impossibility of predicting the level of difficulty of any given picture for any given bilingual speaker, it may be helpful to consider more divergent types of tasks, especially generative naming. Advantages of verbal fluency tasks (also called generative naming) include the fact that no materials are required for the task and it can easily be administered in various language combinations (Roberts and Le Dorze, 1997). It has been repeatedly demonstrated that generative naming tasks are very sensitive to the effects of brain damage (see Spreen and Strauss, 1998) in aphasia, dementia and following right brain damage. There are studies of this task in quite a number of different countries and languages (e.g., Cardebat, Doyon, Puel, Goulet, and Joanette, 1990; Güven and Cangökçe, 2006; Roselli, Ardila, Salvatierra, Marquez, Matos, and Weekes, 2002; Snodgrass and Tsivkin, 1995; Tombaugh, Kozak, and Rees, 1999). These (and other similar) studies provide a frame of reference for interpreting the results, although when using verbal fluency to estimate a bilingual speaker's level of vocabulary knowledge, the key point is the difference in the number of words produced in each language, and not necessarily a comparison with normative samples of speakers of each language. The number of examples produced for common natural language categories such as animals, fruits, vegetables, foods, or clothing can be examined in each language, selecting semantic categories that take into account the patient's domains of use of each language. When scores on two or more different categories are combined, test-retest variability is reduced, and sensitivity is increased (Monsch, Bondi, Butters, Salmon, Katzman, and Thal, 1992; Roberts and Le Dorze, 1997).

Furthermore, in the domain of bilingual aphasia, Roberts and Le Dorze (1998) found similar performance across the two languages of French-English bilingual adults with aphasia and their controls, a finding partially replicated by Roselli (Roselli, Ardila, Salvatierra, Marquez, Matos, and Weekes, 2002).

Another divergent approach to estimating relative abilities in each language is to examine discourse production in patients with bilingual aphasia. Comparison of discourse samples in the two languages can provide qualitative information on word finding, code switching, and the types of word retrieval disturbances. The scoring system developed by Nicholas and

Brookshire (1993) could be adapted for use with bilingual speakers. Muñoz and Marquardt (2004) examined several variables including the semantic accuracy of the utterance, the number of verbal disruptions (such as repetitions, omissions, fillers), and word retrieval errors (such as semantic errors, phonemic errors, descriptions). Munoz and Marquardt observed that two of their three bilingual aphasic patients demonstrated greater semantic accuracy and fewer paraphasias in English than in Spanish, whereas a third patient showed functional communication (very few errors) in the bilingual context.

Bilingual Aphasia Treatment Studies

Very few studies have addressed the issue of rehabilitation of language deficits in bilingual aphasia. Watamori and Sasanuma reported the effect of therapy on two patients with bilingual aphasia (Watamori and Sasanuma, 1976, 1978). One patient was a 69 year old, Japanese-English speaker, described as equally proficient but preferring to read and write in English. He suffered two CVAs and began speech therapy 2 months after the second one. He received therapy first in Japanese, from approximately 3 months post-onset (MPO) to 18 MPO, then therapy in both languages for a year. A second patient, 52 years old, probably spoke Japanese before he spoke English, although the authors note that the available information on his language history is incomplete. Starting at 3 MPO, he received six months of therapy in English.

Results revealed that the amount of recovery was greater in the trained language than the untrained language, although both patients improved to some degree in the untrained language. Specifically, Patient 1, who was assessed at 2, 14, 26 and 49 months after his stroke, demonstrated overall improvements in auditory comprehension, reading, and writing in both languages although oral production improved very little. Patient 2, who was assessed at 3, 7 and 9 months post onset, showed marginal improvements in auditory comprehension and reading but even less improvement in oral production and writing. Also, for both patients, differences in performance between the two languages in the four modalities (comprehension, reading, naming and writing) increased over time.

In both studies, it is impossible to separate the effects of the therapy early in the study from the spontaneous recovery, given how recent the strokes were. Information about language use and proficiency across modalities is incomplete, making it hard to interpret the reported scores in each language spoken by the two patients.

In another study, Sasanuma and Park (1995) examined one Korean-Japanese speaking individual (29 years old, L1-Korean, L2-Japanese, equally proficient, 2.5 months post onset) who received 36 sessions of treatment in Korean. The authors found equal levels of recovery in auditory and reading tasks in the treated and untreated language but greater improvements in Korean (the treated language) than Japanese on the oral production and writing tasks. However, it is not always the treated language that shows the greatest improvement (Roberts, 1992; Roberts, de la Riva, and Rhéaume, 1997).

Junque, Vendrell, Vendrell-Brucet, and Tobeña (1989) examined 30 Catalan-Spanish speaking individuals with aphasia. As Catalan was the more proficient language for all participants, treatment was provided in Catalan only. In all cases, improvement was greater in Catalan than in Spanish. While this study examined a fairly large number of bilingual patients, the nature of the language impairment was heterogeneous across the patients and the nature of therapy provided to the patients is relatively unclear.

Collectively, these studies provide evidence that the language of treatment influences recovery, but is not always the most important influence. Many more studies, including replications of published studies, will be needed to reveal how the many complex facets of bilingualism and aphasia interact to determine each patient's level of recovery in each language. These factors include the age of acquisition (AoA) and levels of proficiency in each modality in each language, the linguistic distance separating the patient's languages (e.g., English-Mandarin vs. Spanish-Italian), literacy levels in each language, aphasia types, the lesion size and site, the timing and intensity of therapy, and the methods used.

There are many important questions about whether treatment for bilingual aphasia generalizes across languages, to what extent, and why. Results of the few studies that have systematically examined naming treatment in individuals with bilingual aphasia show a range of patterns of crosslinguistic generalization. Hinckley (2003) provided treatment for naming deficits to a Spanish-English bilingual individual with aphasia (71 years, L1-Spanish, L2-English, 6 MPO). Using a cueing hierarchy treatment in English or Spanish did not yield crosslinguistic generalization as measured by the naming subtest of the *Bilingual Aphasia Test* (*BAT*) (Paradis and Libben, 1987). With no pre-stroke level of proficiency estimates, and the lack of studies to test the equivalency of the PALPA and the BAT in the two languages of this study (Spanish and English), the pretherapy and change scores are difficult to interpret.

In another study, Galvez and Hinckley (2003) used a cueing hierarchy with a balanced Spanish-English bilingual with transcortical motor aphasia (L1-Spanish, L2-English, late bilingual, 4 MPO). Language of treatment was alternated weekly. Overall improvement on the *BAT* was greater in Spanish than English, but naming scores on the *BAT* improved equally in the two languages.

Kohnert (2004) examined the effects of cognitive-based treatment and a lexical-based treatment on generalization in one bilingual patient with severe nonfluent aphasia (62 years old, L1-Spanish, L2-English, late bilingual, 4 MPO). Both treatments were effective in improving cognitive and language skills, measured in English and Spanish. The lexical-based therapy followed the cognitive therapy, in Spanish and then in English. Crosslinguistic (or between-language) generalization was reported for cognates (e.g., elephant/*elefante*) after the lexical therapy, but not for noncognates. Since the patient received treatment for both languages without a true control condition, it is not clear to what extent these improvements are caused by some aspect of one or both therapies or by the patient having named the pictures repetitively (Kohnert, 2004).

These bilingual aphasia treatment studies demonstrate the importance of adequately describing each patient (see also Roberts, Code, and McNeil, 2003), their language levels pre-stroke, and of using tests and stimuli that have known properties (to the extent possible). When it has not been possible to use tests or stimuli with demonstrated cross-language equivalence, authors and readers must be very cautious in the conclusions they draw from their results. As more bilingual aphasic adults are studied, patterns in treatment outcomes may emerge, but we will be able to see the patterns only if each patient is described in more detail than is currently common practice.

In a recent study, crosslinguistic generalization patterns were systematically examined in three English-Spanish bilingual individuals with aphasia (Edmonds and Kiran, 2006). Results revealed crosslinguistic generalization in all participants. However, the patterns of generalization differed across participants. The first patient (P1) in this open-ended series was pre-morbidly equally proficient in English and Spanish. Training in Spanish resulted in improved ability to name trained items (e.g., *manzana*) and within language generalization to semantically related items (e,g., *naranja*) (*manzana* means "apple" and *naranja* means "orange"). Additionally, crosslinguistic generalization was observed on untrained semantically related items (e.g., *orange*) with marginal improvement on the untrained English translation equivalents of trained Spanish items (e.g., *apple*). As predicted, no appreciable gains were observed in the Spanish and English control words (untreated and semantically unrelated to the treatment stimuli), indicating that observed improvements were due to treatment.

Patients 2 and 3 (P2 and P3) were both pre-morbidly more proficient in English than in Spanish. Whereas P2 first received treatment in English followed by Spanish, P3 received treatment in Spanish only. With English treatment, P2 showed improvements on trained items (e.g., *apple*), within-language generalization to semantically related items (e.g., *orange*) within the more proficient language but no crosslinguistic generalization. However, when treatment was shifted to Spanish (the less proficient language), improvement of trained items was observed (e,g., *naranja*), but within-language generalization to semantically related untrained items (e.g., *manzana*) was not observed. Importantly, with Spanish treatment, crosslinguistic generalization was observed for English translation equivalents and corresponding semantically related items. These results were replicated in P3, who was also more proficient in English. The main finding of this study was that crosslinguistic generalization was observed in all participants. P1, who was pre-morbidly equally proficient across languages, was trained in Spanish and showed generalization to English. P2 and P3 were pre-morbidly more proficient in English but, when trained in Spanish, showed generalization to English.

In a follow-up study by Kiran and Roberts, three additional aphasic adults, two English-Spanish speakers and one French-English speaker have been studied to date. As the *n* gradually increases, we hope to be able to make progressively more informed interpretations of why generalization within and/or between languages occurs for some patients and not for others.

Methodological Issues

To conduct a study of the effects of therapy on any component of language in bilingual aphasic adults, a number of methodological challenges must be met. Given the current state of knowledge and the variation across different bilingual speakers, it is impossible to meet all of these challenges with a high level of rigor, but researchers need to be aware of the challenges, and do everything possible to move closer to meeting them as our knowledge base expands. Readers of research need to be aware of these challenges as they evaluate the quality of published studies and try to apply published results to their own clinical work. The strategies proposed below for responding to these challenges are not "solutions", but ways to reduce the impact of factors that weaken the validity of tests and therapy studies and thus make interpretation of the results problematic.

Among the challenges in conducting studies of bilingual aphasia are the following:

1. The complexity of aphasia and our incomplete understanding of it: In reading and interpreting studies of bilingual aphasia treatment, it is vital to remember that there is great variability inherent in aphasia. The treatment studies on unilingual speakers show that a given therapy will help some patients but not others, even when these patients seem to be "the same" i.e. have a similar aphasia type and/or severity and/or time post-onset, and/or lesion location. In other studies, all patients will improve but the extent of improvement will be much greater in some patients than in others. Some unilingual patients generalize treatment gains across modalities, while others do not. Some unilingual patients generalize treatment gains to untreated words or structures, while others do not. In some cases, readers can find these disparate outcomes within a single study (e.g., Laganaro, Di Pietro, and Schnider, 2006; Nettleton and Lesser, 1991); in other cases, it is by comparing one study to another that one sees the range of outcomes. Possible explanations for the varied response to treatment include the severity of the aphasia, the exact nature of the impairment, the functional importance of spared vs. damaged regions or networks within each patient's brain and the combined effects of pre-stroke proficiency in each language and the deficits (parallel or otherwise) caused by the stroke. In studies of bilingual aphasia, if one patient or group or type of word improves and the others do not, there is a tendency to interpret results in terms of the bilingualism: early vs. late acquisition; level of proficiency, etc. The features of each patient's bilingualism are important, but they are not the only – and sometimes probably not even the most important – explanatory variables.

One way to help isolate what is due to bilingualism and what is due to the aphasia would be to include unilingual and bilingual patients in the same study. By comparing the symptoms or the treatment outcomes of one or more bilingual patients to the symptoms or outcomes of one or more unilingual patients, the patterns of deficits, improvement, and generalization (or lack thereof) can be better understood and, over a series of studies, the impact of bilingualism can be isolated. A second strategy is to use a larger number of patients in each study. The larger the number of participants, the more chance there is to see patterns and to accurately interpret results.

A third remedy is for all researchers in aphasia to provide more information about their patients (see Roberts, Code, and McNeil, 2003; Roberts, Code, Hillis, and McNeil, forthcoming). Obtaining careful pre-morbid language proficiency information is as important as the pre-treatment language assessment for these patients. In bilingual aphasia, the information provided about each patient's bilingual history and proficiency still varies widely from one article to the next and is usually incomplete. This makes it impossible to compare patients across studies, since we do not know in what ways they may be similar. The BAT contains a very thorough, detailed language history questionnaire (Paradis and Libben, 1987). Roberts and Shenker have published a somewhat shorter history form that can be used with any research participant or clinical patient (Roberts and Shenker, 2007). In Table 2, we list the information that all authors should provide about the language background of their participants. If journal reviewers and editors adopted this list (or a similar one) as part of the requirements for all papers on bilingual adults, it would contribute significantly to progress in studies of bilingualism and of bilingual aphasia. We welcome discussion and suggestions on this issue.

Finally, replications of already-published studies are needed using the same pairs of languages and different ones. Patterns of deficits or therapy effects that occur in Dutch-

English bilinguals might or might not be replicated in Punjabi-Arabic or Russian-English speakers.

As we strive to better understand cross-language generalization in aphasia treatment, it is helpful to consider the literature on cross-language generalization of gains in treatment in other disorders, where similar questions are being studied (e.g., Holm and Dodd, 2001; Jordaan, Shaw-Ridley, Serfontein, Orelowitz, and Monaghan, 2001; McNutt, 1994). Studies of response to treatment for other disorders in bilingual children and adults may have useful findings that can help in understanding bilingual aphasia treatment.

Table 1. Challenges and suggested strategies to meet them

Challenge	Mitigating strategy or response
1. the complexity of aphasia; no two patients the same	Study bilingual and unilingual patients in the same study to partially isolate effects of bilingualism vs. effects of aphasia; more complete description of each participant's language status; larger *n* in each study; replicate studies.
2. pre-stroke proficiency levels affect post-stroke performance, yet are unknowable	Estimate pre-stroke levels through combination of language history, domains of use, and self-ratings and/or family ratings of proficiency in each modality.
3. variability and unknowns in each adult's pre-stroke vocabulary	More complete descriptions of each person's proficiency; select stimuli with known psychometric properties, to the extent possible; larger *n* in each study; replicate studies; have a group of adults with similar language histories perform the experimental or therapy tasks to provide a reference range for interpreting patients' performance.
4. practice effects may affect scores on some tasks when testing two or more languages	Studies to measure this on various tests and tasks; retest in the same language to be able to compare within-language TRT changes to between-language differences. See Roberts 1998a
5. fatigue	Monitor length of sessions; look for signs of fatigue; provide breaks; ask patient !
6. cognates may make some tasks easier for pairs of languages where they exist	Control stimuli to eliminate cognate pairs or include sets of cognate words and non-cognate words, matched for length, frequency etc and compare results on the two types of words; verify cognateness by asking speakers of the pairs of languages to be used in the study.

2. *Pre-stroke levels of proficiency:* Neuroimaging studies show that cortical areas activated during lexical tasks largely overlap in a bilingual brain. But it remains unknown to what extent this gross anatomical overlap implies that the two languages are processed by the same micro level networks (Crinion et al., 2006; Roberts, 2001; Steinmetz and Seitz, 1991). AoA seems to influence localization with less overlap occurring for the two languages if one of them is acquired much later than the other (e.g., Dehaene et al., 1997; Kim et al., 1997). However, level of proficiency may be at least as important (Abutalebi, Cappa, and Perani, 2001), and cumulative exposure is also a factor (Perani, et al., 2003). We must remain cautious in interpreting "localization studies" using fMRI, given the constraints imposed on participants during the testing, the few patients and pairs of languages tested, the limited tasks performed, and the range of possible interpretations of results such as "more activation" or "less activation" in specific regions (see Van Lancker Sidtis, 2006 for a skeptical review of these and other issues about fMRI).

Table 2. Essential information for describing the language background of participants in studies of bilingual aphasia

1. List of languages the patient/participant (P) could understand;
2. Age of first regular exposure to each language identified in Question 1: classes in school; radio or TV; moved to new country or city; new friends or activities that exposed P to a new language;
3. Percent of use of each language in adulthood for at least the following domains: home life, work, socializing, reading, television/radio. A rough idea of the main language(s) used in childhood is also helpful, if P or the family can provide this. However, the farther back in time you probe, the less accurate the information MAY be, for some patients.
4. How each language was learned: relative roles of informal acquisition and classroom study.
5. Changes in overall patterns of use over P's lifetime i.e. was there a time when P used only one language? Or used a language that he has not had to use for many years?
6. Estimates of proficiency: obtained from family members and/or from P, if able.

A 7-point scale works well and is often used in studies of non-aphasic bilinguals. It works best with an added 0 (making an 8-point scale), because it seems to confuse people to rate something as a 1, yet mean "zero ability or knowledge". Several versions of this scale and various forms of instructions have been used by Roberts and by other authors. The current version developed at the University of Ottawa is provided in Appendix A.

To estimate pre-stroke levels of proficiency, some authors have used naming time (e.g., Langdon, Wiig, and Nielson, 2005); some have used the lexical decision task as a measure of language proficiency (Lemhöfer, Dijkstra, and Michel, 2004). But the most common way of providing information about likely pre-stroke levels of proficiency has been to describe the participant's language history. The information required includes: 1) language acquisition: age began learning each L, methods; 2) domains of use – a patient's family can often provide this information; 3) estimated proficiency by the patient, if the aphasia is mild enough to allow this, and/or by one or more bilingual family members. The accuracy of these self-ratings and of family ratings is unknown, but they have proved to yield "higher level" and "lower level" groups of participants in a number of studies where they have been used (Roberts and Le Dorze, 1997; Roberts and Bois, 1999). Self-ratings may be more accurate in some situations, for some levels of ability than for others (Delgado, Guerrero, Goggin, and Ellis, 1999; Dunning and Kruger, 1999; Langdon, Wiig, and Nielson, 2005).

For the rating task, a 7 point scale, with the end-points defined can be used (see Table 2 for more details on the rating). Alternatively, patients/families can rate each modality as "a little better" or "a lot better" (as in Roberts and Le Dorze, 1997, 1998). In these studies, patients and families were asked: *No one ever has exactly the same level in their two languages, but would you say that he spoke/understood/read/wrote _____ and ____ at roughly the same level or was one language better than the other?* If they say one was better, ask: *was it a LOT better, or just a LITTLE better?* One suggested addition to these ratings is to ask: Why do you say it was better, in what way was it better? This can help them think about vocabulary, grammar, accent, rate of speech, etc. and help the interviewer understand the framework that the family member or patient is using for their ratings.

3. Assessing the extent of the naming deficit: In bilingual adults post-stroke, it is impossible to know what words their pre-morbid lexicon in each language contained. It is now clear that both age of acquisition (AoA) and, probably to a lesser extent, frequency of occurrence in each language affect naming speed, lexical decision speed and accuracy, and performance on other lexical processing tasks, although the relationship between these (and other) variables is still being probed (e.g., Ghyselinck, Lewis, and Brysbaert, 2004; Johnston, and Barry, 2006 for recent reviews; Lehtonen and Laine, 2003; Voyer, 2003). In individual bilingual speakers, it is very difficult (perhaps impossible?) to know the AoA for items on naming tests or in sets of stimuli. The studies on the *Boston Naming Test* cited above demonstrate how the performance of speakers across languages and across cultures varies. An unknown number of the speakers in these studies were bilingual or multilingual. This makes interpreting the results of these studies even more problematic.

Given the complementarity principle - the use of languages in various domains and for different communication tasks based on need and exposure (Grosjean, 1998) – we can expect most speakers to have non-equivalent vocabularies in their two languages. Therefore, it is impossible to know when a particular item is not named whether this is due to the aphasia or to pre-morbid vocabulary "holes". If some words were known in both languages pre-stroke, but in the weaker language the word was acquired as an adult and/or rarely used, does this make it more vulnerable to anomia?

There is no easy solution to the problems created by the non-equivalency of the items in the test in terms of their frequency of occurrence and typical AoA for unilingual speakers and the unknown frequency of occurrence, and age-of-acquisition for each bilingual speaker. One approach is to test the stimuli to be used with patients on a group of non-aphasic bilingual speakers from the same community. For a confrontation naming task, Croft, Marshall, and Pring (2006) selected stimuli presented to 6 Bengali-English bilingual aphasic adults based on the naming latencies and name agreement obtained from a group of 20 Bengali-English speaking, non-aphasic adults. To the extent that stimuli are prepared based on known AoA, name agreement, frequency of occurrence and the other factors identified in studies of lexical access in various languages, some of the "noise" in data from bilingual studies can be reduced.

4. Practice effects and other threats to test-retest reliability: When the two languages are tested on the same day, often in the same clinical session, is there is a practice effect (see Roberts, 1998a, 2001)? Does testing on different days make a practice effect more or less likely? On the 30-item Graded Naming Test (McKenna and Warrington, 1983), some non-aphasic adults improved their score by 1 to 2 items, resulting in a change in the mean group score of 1 point (Roberts, 2003). Brain damage probably makes a practice effect less likely. Cooper and colleagues (2001) found no practice effect for patients with dementia on a category verbal fluency task. However, in aphasic adults, Roberts and Le Dorze (1994) found slight improvements in verbal fluency on retesting. Even in those patients with chronic aphasia (at least one year post-onset), the individual participants' change scores (test 2 – test 1) ranged from -6 to + 9. Note that this problem is not unique to bilingual aphasia, nor even to communication disorders. Some quite widely-used tests fail to meet acceptable levels of test-retest reliability (e.g., Philp, Lowles, Armstrong, and Whitehead, 2002). Nonetheless, it is a problem that needs to be better understood if we are to interpret differences in scores across languages, and also changes in scores from pre- to post-therapy.

5. Fatigue: Because of the effects of the stroke, fatigue during aphasia testing is often a problem. Fatigue can lead to lower scores when a patient is tested on a "bad day" or after completing other tests. Given that bilingual aphasic patients must be tested in each language, the testing is, unavoidably, longer and therefore more tiring. To mitigate this, frequent breaks and shorter blocks of testing may help.

6. Cognates: Cognates are pairs of words with the same meaning in two (or more) languages and similar pronunciation and/or spelling. There is still no consensus on how close in spelling or pronunciation a pair of words must be to count as cognates. But there is now a body of studies using different language pairs, showing consistent differences between the processing time, priming effects and task accuracy for cognates compared to non-cognates on a range of tasks (e.g., Costa, Caramazza, and Sebastian-Galles, 2000; Costa, Santesteban, and Caño, 2005; de Groot, 1993; Gollan, Forster, and Frost, 1997). If tests such as the BNT are simply translated, and administered in the patients' two languages, there is no control over the number of cognates that will arise for any given pair of languages. For French-English and Spanish-English speakers, the BNT produces approximately 20 cognates out of the 60 pictures (the exact number would depend on how "cognate" was defined and which synonyms/dialectal variants are accepted). But for other pairs of languages, there might be no cognate pairs. So, the difficulty of this test is reduced for speakers of languages with higher numbers of cognate stimuli. For language pairs where there happen to be few or no cognate stimuli, the test may be more difficult.

Moreover, cognates may have a facilitative effect on word retrieval in patients with bilingual aphasia, presumably due to the overlapping phonology across the two languages. For instance, using a picture naming task, Roberts and Deslauriers (1999) found that cognate pictures were more often correctly named in both languages than non-cognates in both normal English-French bilinguals and in 10 patients with bilingual aphasia. Likewise, Lalor and Kirsner (2001) found that a 63-year-old Italian-English bilingual individual with aphasia performed better on cognates in both languages. Cognates may also facilitate cross-language generalization in language treatment (Kohnert, 2004).

We recommend excluding cognate words from naming tests and treatment stimuli or reporting separately on the results for cognates and non-cognates.

Summary and Conclusion

As the field of bilingual aphasia grows, our understanding of the nature of bilingual aphasia is expanding. For both clinical and research purposes, there is an urgent need to develop psychometrically stronger assessment tools. Given the complex nature of bilingualism and of aphasia, and the variability across bilingual speakers, it is difficult to know why a given patient may fail a particular task, such as naming a particular picture. However, by using experimental tasks and tests that take into account what is now known about the lexicon and lexical processing, we can significantly improve the validity of studies of bilingual naming and bilingual aphasia therapy. We urge researchers to provide much more detailed and more uniform descriptions of each participant's language history and to try to control for more potentially confounding factors in the choice of stimuli, assessment tools, and therapy designs.

We urge readers to be critical in reading published studies that fail to provide key information about the participants, and call on authors to be more circumspect in drawing conclusions from their own data, given the variability inherent in both aphasia and bilingualism and the difficulty in controlling the many factors that can influence test results and treatment outcomes in bilingual aphasia.

References

Abutalebi, J. Cappa, S.F., and Perani, D. (2001). The bilingual brain as revealed by functional neuroimaging. *Bilingualism: Language and Cognition, 4*, 179-190.

Agency for Healthcare Research and Quality. (2002). *Criteria for Determining Disability in Speech-Language Disorders*. Summary, Evidence Report/Technology Assessment: Number 52. AHRQ Publication No. 02-E009, January 2002., Rockville, MD. http://www.ahrq.gov/clinic/epcsums/spdissum.htm

Allegri, R.F., Mangone, C.A., Villavicencio, A.F., Rymberg, S., Taragano, F.E., and Baumann, D. (1997). Spanish Boston Naming Test norms. *The Clinical Neuropsychologist, 11*, 416-420.

Barca, L., Burani, C., Arduino, L.S. (2002). Word naming times and psycholinguistic norms for Italian nouns. *Behavior Research Methods, Instruments, and Computers, 34(3),* 424-434.

Benton, A.L., Hamsher, K.S., and Sivan, A.B. (1994). *Multilingual Aphasia Examination, 3rd Edition (MAE)*. Iowa City: AJA Associates.

Butler, Y.G., and Hakuta, K. (2006). Bilingualism and second language acquisition. In .K. Bhatia and W.C. Ritchie (eds.). *The handbook of bilingualism* (pp. 114-144). Malden, MA: Blackwell Publishing.

Cardebat, D., Doyon, B., Puel, M., Goulet, P., and Joanette, Y. (1990). Evocation lexicale formelle et sémantique chez des sujets normaux : performances et dynamique de production en fonction du sexe, de l'âge, et du niveau d'étude. *Acta Neurologica Belgica, 90*, 207-217.

Chalard, M., Bonin, P., Meot, A, Boyer, B., and Fayol, M. (1997). Objective age-of-acquisition (AoA) norms for a set of 230 object names in French: Relationships with psycholinguistic variables, the English data from Morrison et al. (1997), and naming latencies. *European Journal of Cognitive Psychology, 15*, 209-245.

Cheung, R.W., Cheung, M-C., and Chan, A.S. (2004). Confrontation naming in Chinese patients with left, right or bilateral brain damage. *Journal of the International Neuropsychological Society, 10*, 46-53.

Christophersen, P. (1999). Two more contributions to the nativeness debate. *RASK Supplement, 9*, 117-122.

Cooper, D.B., Epker, M., Lacritz, L.,Weiner, M., Rosenberg, R.N., Honig, L., Cullum, C.M. (2001). Effects of practice on category fluency in Alzheimer's disease. *Clinical Neuropsychologist, 15*, 125-128.

Costa, A., Caramazza, A., and Sebastian-Galles, N. (2000). The cognate facilitation effect: implications for models of lexical access. *Journal of Experimental Psychology: Learning, Memory and Cognition, 26*(5), 1283-1296.

Costa, A., Santesteban, M., and Caño, A. (2005). On the facilitatory effects of cognate words in bilingual speech production. *Brain and Language, 94*, 94-103.

Crinion, J., Turner, R., Grogan, A., Hanakawa, T., Noppeney, U., Devlin, J. T., Aso, T., Urayama, S., Fukuyama, H., Stockton, K., Usui, K., Green, D. W., and Price, C. J. (2006). Language control in the bilingual brain. *Science, 312*(5779), 1537-1540.

Croft, Marshall, J., and Pring, T. (2006). Assessing noun naming impairments in bilingual aphasia. *Brain and Language, 99*, 21-22.

Davis, C.J., and Perea, M (2005). Per BuscaPalabras: A program for deriving orthographic and phonological neighborhood statistics and other psycholinguistic indices in Spanish. *Behavior Research Methods, 37*, 665-671.

De Bot, K. (2004). The multilingual lexicon: modelling selection and control. *International Journal of Multilingualism, 1*, 17-32.

De Groot, A.M.B. (1993). Word-type effects in bilingual processing tasks : Support for a mixed representational system. In R. Schreuder and B. Weltens (Eds.), *The bilingual lexicon* (pp. 27-51). Amsterdam: Elsevier.

Dehaene, S., Dupoux, E., Mehler, J., Cohen, L., Paulesu, E., Perani, D., Van de Moortele, P.F., Lehericy, S., and Le Bihan, D. (1997). Anatomical variability in the cortical representation of first and second language. *NeuroReport, 8*, 3809-3815.

Delgado, P., Guerrero, G., Goggin, J.P., and Ellis, B.B. (1999). Self-assessment of linguistic skills by bilingual Hispanics. *Hispanic Journal of Behavioral Sciences, 21(1)*, 31-46.

Dijkstra, T., del Prado M., Fermin M., Schulpen, B., Schreuder, R., and Baayen, R.H. (2005). A roommate in cream: Morphological family size effects on interlingual homograph recognition. *Language and Cognitive Processes, 20*, 7-41.

Dunning, D., and Kruger, J. (1999). Unskilled and unaware of it: how difficulties in recognizing one's own incompetence lead to inflated self-assessments. *Journal of Personality and Social Psychology, 77*, 1121-1134.

Edmonds, L. A., and Kiran, S. (2006). Effect of semantic based treatment on cross linguistic generalization in bilingual aphasia. *Journal of Speech, Language, and Hearing Research, 49*, 729-748.

Edwards, J. (2006). Foundations of bilingualism. In T.K. Bhatia and W.C. Ritchie (Eds.). *The handbook of bilingualism* (pp. 7-31). Malden, MA: Blackwell Publishing.

Elias, M.F., Elias, P.K., D'Agostino, R.B., Silbershatz, H., and Wolf, P.A. (1997). Role of age, education, and gender on cognitive performance in the Framingham Heart Study: Community-based norms. *Experimental Aging Research, 23*, 201-235.

Fabbro, F. (2001). The bilingual brain: Cerebral representation of languages. *Brain and Language, 79*, 211-222.

Frenck-Mestre, C., Anton, J.L., Roth, M., Vaid, J., and Viallet, F. (2005). Articulation in early and late bilinguals' two languages: evidence from functional magnetic resonance imaging. *Neuroreport, 16*, 761-765.

Galvez, A., and Hinckley, J. J. (2003). Transfer patterns of naming treatment in a case of bilingual aphasia. *Brain and Language, 87*, 173-174.

Ghyselinck, M., Lewis, M.B., and Brysbaert, M. (2004). Age of acquisition and the cumulative-frequency hypothesis: A review of the literature and a new multi-task investigation. *Acta Psychologica, 115*, 43-67.

Gollan, T.H., Forster, K.I., and Frost, R. (1997). Translation priming with different scripts: masked priming with cognates and non-cognates in Hebrew-English bilinguals. *Journal of Experimental Psychology: Learning, Memory, and Cognition, 23*, 1122-1139.

Goodglass, H., and Kaplan, E. (1983). *The Boston Diagnostic Aphasia Examination*. Philadelphia: Lea and Febiger.

Goodglass, H., Kaplan, E. and Barresi, B. (2000). *The Boston Diagnostic Aphasia Examination. 3rd edition*. Austin, TX: Pro-Ed.

Goral, M., Levy, E.S., Obler, L.K., and Cohen, E. (2006). Cross-language lexical connections in the mental lexicon: Evidence from a case of trilingual aphasia. *Brain and Language, 98*, 235-247.

Goral, M. and Obler, L.K. (in press) Two's company, three's a crowd? Recent advances in psycholinguistic and neurolingustic study of multilingual speakers. In A. Stavans and I. Kupferberg (Eds.), Studies in language and language education: *Essays in honor of Elite Olshtain*. Jerusalem: The Hebrew University Magnes Press.

Graetz, P., de Bleser, R., and Willmes, K. (1992). *Akense afasie test.* Lisse, The Netherlands: Swetz and Zeitlinger. (Aachen Aphasia Test)

Grosjean, F. (1989). Neurolinguists beware! The bilingual is not two monolinguals in one person. *Brain and Language, 36*, 3-15.

Grosjean, F. (1998). Studying bilinguals: methodological and conceptual issues. *Bilingualism: Language and Cognition, 1,* 131-149.

Güven, A.G., and Cangökçe, O. (2006). The role of education levels and gender on reading and phonemic (initial letter) fluency in healthy adults. Türk Psikologi Dergisi, 21 (57), 121-123 (English summary) (and 109-120, full article).

Harris, R.J. (Ed.) (1992). *Cognitive processing in bilinguals*. New York: Elsevier.

Hestad, K., Dybing, E., Haugen, P. K., and Klove, H. (1998). Using the Boston Naming Test to assess anomic difficulties in patients with dementia. [Norwegian]. Original Title Sprakforstyrrelser hos demente pasienter undersokt med Boston Naming Test. Tidsskrift for Norsk Psykologforening, 35, 322-327. English abstract in PsychInfo.

Hinckley, J. J. (2003). Picture naming treatment in aphasia yields greater improvement in L1. *Brain and Language, 87*, 171-172.

Holm A., and Dodd B. (2001). Comparison of cross-language generalisation following speech therapy. *Folia Phoniatrica et Logopaedica, 53*, 166-172.

Hyltenstam, K. (1992). Non-native features of near-native speakers: on the ultimate attainment of childhood L2 learners. In R.J. Harris (Ed.), *Cognitive processing in bilinguals* (pp. 351-368). New York: Elsevier.

Johnston, R.A., and Barry, C. (2006). Age of acquisition and lexical processing. *Visual Cognition, 13*, 789-845.

Jordaan, H., Shaw-Ridley, G, Serfontein, J., Orelowitz, K., and Monaghan, N. (2001). Cognitive and linguistic profiles of specific language impairment and semantic-pragmatic disorder in bilinguals. *Folia Phoniatrica et Logopaedica, 53*,153-165.

Juncos Rabadan, O. (1994). The assessment of bilingualism in normal aging with the Bilingual Aphasia Test. *Journal of Neurolinguistics, 8*, 67-73.

Juncos Rabadan, O. and Iglesias, (1994). Decline in the elderly's language: Evidence from cross-linguistic data. *Journal of Neurolinguistics, 8(3)*, 183-190.

Juncos Rabadan, O., Elosua de Juan, R., Pereiro Rozas, A., and Torres Marono, M. (1998). Lexical difficulties in the elderly: Basis for intervention.[Spanish].(Problemas de acceso lexico en la vejez. Bases para la intervencion. *Anales de Psicologia, 4*, 169-176.

Junque, C., Vendrell, P., Vendrell-Brucet, J. M., and Tobeña, A. (1989). Differential recovery in naming in bilingual aphasics. *Brain and Language, 36*, 16-22.

Kaplan, E., Goodglass, H., and Weintraub, S. (1983). *The Boston Naming Test*. Philadelphia: Lea and Febiger.

Kaplan, E., Goodglass, H., and Weinbraub. S. (2001). *The Boston Naming Test. 2nd edition*. Baltimore: Lippincott, Williams and Wilkins.

Kim, H., and Na, D.L. (1999). Normative data on the Korean version of the Boston Naming Test. *Journal of Clinical and Experimental Neuropsychology, 21*, 127-133.

Kim, K.H.S., Relkin, N.R., Lee, K-M., and Hirsch, J. (1997). Distinct cortical areas associated with native and second languages. *Nature, 388*, 171-174.

Kohnert, K. (2004). Cognitive and cognate-based treatments for bilingual aphasia: a case study. *Brain and Language, 91*, 294-302.

Kohnert, K. J., Hernandez, A. E., and Bates, E. (1998). Bilingual performance on the Boston Naming Test: Preliminary norms in Spanish and English. *Brain and Language, 65*, 422-440.

Kremin, H., Akhutina, T., Basso, A., Davidoff, J., De Wilde, M., Kitzing, P. et al. (2003). A cross-linguistic data bank for oral picture naming in Dutch, English, German, French, Italian, Russian, Spanish, and Swedish (PEDOI). *Brain and Cognition, 53*, 243-246.

Laganaro, M., Di Pietro, M., and Schnider, A. (2006). What does recovery from anomia tell us about the underlying impairment: the case of similar anomic patterns and different recovery. *Neuropsychologia, 44*, 534-545.

Laine, M., Goodglass, H., Niemi, J., Koivuselka-Sallinen, P., Tuomainen, J., and Martilla, R. (1993). Adaptation of the Boston Diagnostic Aphasia Examination and the Boston Naming Test into Finnish. *Scandinavian Journal of Logopedics and Phoniatrics, 18*, 83-92.

Lalor, E., and Kirsner, K. (2001). The role of cognates in bilingual aphasia: Implications for assessment and treatment. *Aphasiology, 15*(10), 1047-1056.

Langdon, H.W., Wiig, E.H., and Nielson, N.P. (2005). Dual-dimension naming speed and language-dominance ratings by bilingual Hispanic adults. *Bilingual Research Journal, 29*, 319-336.

Lehtonen, M., and Laine, M. (2003). How word frequency affects morphological processing in monolinguals and bilinguals. *Bilingualism: Language and Cognition, 6*, 213-225.

Lemhöfer, K., Dijkstra, T., and Michel, M-C. (2004). Three languages, one ECHO: Cognate effects in trilingual word recognition. *Language and Cognitive Processes, 19*, 585-611.

Levey, S. (2004). Discrimination and production of English vowels by bilingual speakers of Spanish and English. *Perceptual and Motor Skills, 99,* 445-462.

Luzzati, C., Willmes, K., and de Bleser, R. (1992). *Aachener Aphasie Test: versione italiana.* Firenze: O.S. Organizzazioni Speciali. (The Aachen Aphasia Test.)

Marien, P., Mampaey, E., Vervaet, A., Saerens, J., and De Deyn, P.P. (1998). Normative data for the Boston Naming Test in native Dutch-speaking Belgian elderly. *Brain and Language, 65*, 447-467.

McKenna, P., and Warrington, E.K. (1983). *The Graded Naming Test.* Windsor, UK: NFER-Nelson.

McNutt, J.C. (1994). Generalization of /s/ from English to French as a result of phonological remediation. *Journal of Speech Language Pathology and Audiology, 18*, 109-113.

Mechelli, A., Crinion, J.T., Noppeney, U., O'Doherty, J., Ashburner, J., Frackowiak, R.S., and Price, C.J. (2004). Structural plasticity in the bilingual brain: Proficiency in a second language and age at acquisition affect grey-matter density. *Nature*, *431*(7010), 757.

Miller, N., de Bleser, R., and Willmes, K. (1997). The English language version of the Aachen Aphasia Test, In W. Ziegler and K. Deger (Eds.), *Clinical Phonetics and Linguistics* (pp. 257-265). London: Whurr.

Miller, N., Willmes, K., and De Bleser, R. (2000). The psychometric properties of the English language version of the Aachen Aphasia Test (EEAT). *Aphasiology, 14,* 683-722.

Monsch, A., Bondi, M., Butters, N., Salmon,D., Katzman, R., and Thal, L. (1992). Comparison of verbal fluency tasks in the detection of dementia of the Alzheimer type. *Archives of Neurology, 49*, 1253-1258.

Muñoz, M.L., and Marquardt, T.P. (2004). The influence of language context on lexical retrieval in the discourse of bilingual speakers with aphasia. *Journal of Multilingual Communication Disorders, 2*, 1-17.

Nettleton, J., and Lesser, R. (1991). Therapy for naming difficulties in aphasia: application of a cognitive neuropsychological model. *Journal of Neurolinguistics*, *6*, 139-157.

New, B., Pallier, C., Brysbaert, M. and Ferrand, L. (2004). Lexique 2: A new French lexical database. *Behavior Research Methods, Instruments and Computers*, *36(3)*, 516-524.

Newman, R. S., and German, D.J. (2005). Life span effects of lexical factors on oral naming. *Language and Speech, 48*, 123-156.

Nicholas, N.E., and Brookshire, R.H. (1993). A system for quantifying the informativeness and efficiency of the connected speech of adults with aphasia. *Journal of Speech and Hearing Research*, *36*, 338-350.

Paradis, M. (1995). Bilingual aphasia 100 years later: consensus and controversies. In M. Paradis (Ed.), *Aspects of bilingual aphasia* (pp. 211-223). Tarrytown, NY: Elsevier.

Paradis, M. (2001). In R.S.Berndt (Ed). *Handbook of neuropsychology,* 2nd ed.: Vol 3: *Language and aphasia.* (pp. 69-91). Amsterdam: Elsevier Science Publishers.

Paradis, M., and Libben, G. (1987). *The assessment of bilingual aphasia*. Hillsdale, NJ: Lawrence Erlbaum Associates.

Pavlenko, A. (2000). L2 influence on L1 in late bilingualism. *Issues in Applied Linguistics, 11*, 175-205.

Pavlenko, A., and Jarvis, S. (2002). Bidirectional transfer. *Applied Linguistics*, 23, 190-214.

Perani, D., Abutalebi, J., Paulesu, E., Brambati, S., Scifo, P., Cappa, S. F., and Fazio, F. (2003). The role of age of acquisition and language usage in early, high-proficient bilinguals: an fMRI study during verbal fluency. *Human Brain Mapping, 19*(3), 170-182.

Perez, M.A., and Navalon, C. (2005). Objective-AoA norms for 175 names in Spanish: Relationships with other psycholinguistic variables, estimated AoA, and data from other languages. *European Journal of Cognitive Psychology*, *17*, 179-206.

Philp, I., Lowles, R.V., Armstrong, G.K., and Whitehead, C. (2002). Repeatability of standardized tests of functional impairment and well-being in older people in a rehabilitation setting. *Disability and Rehabilitation, 24(5)*,243-249.

Pind, J., Jonsdottir, H., Gossurardottir, H., and Jonsson, F. (2000). Icelandic norms for the Snodgrass and Vanderwart (1980) pictures: Name and image agreement, familiarity, and age of acquistion. *Scandinavian Journal of Psychology, 41(1)*, 41-48.

Ponton, M.O., Satz, P., Herrera, L., et al. (1996). Normative data stratified by age and education for the Neuropsychological Screening Battery for Hispanics (NeSBHIS): Initial report. *Journal of the International Neuropsychological Societ,. 2*, 96-104.

Ponton, M.O., Satz, P., Herrera, L., Young, R., Ortiz, F., D'Elia, L. et al. (1992). Modified Spanish version of the Boston Naming Test. *The Clinical Neuropyschologist, 6*, 334.

Rey, G.J., and Benton, A.E. (1991). Examen de afasia multilingüe. Iowa City: AJA Associates Inc.

Rey, G.J., Feldman, E., Hernandez, D., Levin, B.E., Rivas-Vazquez, R., Nedd, K J., and Benton, A.L. (2001). Application of the Multilingual Aphasia Examination-Spanish in the evaluation of Hispanic patients post closed-head trauma. *Clinical Neuropsychologist*, *15*, 13-18.

Rey, G.J., Feldman, E., Rivas-Vazquez, R., Levin, B.E., and Benton, A. (1999). Neuropsychological test development and normative data on Hispanics. *Archives of Clinical Neuropsychology*, *14*, 593-601.

Roberts, P.M. (1992, October). Therapy and spontaneous recovery in a bilingual aphasic. Paper presented to the Academy of Aphasia. Toronto, Canada.

Roberts, P.M. (1998a) . Clinical research needs and issues in bilingual aphasia, *Aphasiology*, *12*, 119-130.

Roberts, P.M. (1998b). Bilingual aphasia: some answers and more questions. *Aphasiology*, *12*, 141-146.

Roberts, P.M. (2001). Aphasia assessment and treatment in bilingual and multicultural populations. In R. Chapey (Ed.). *Language intervention strategies in adult aphasia.* 4th edition (pp. 208-232). Baltimore: Lippincott, Williams and Wilkins.

Roberts, P.M. (2007). Aphasia assessment and treatment in bilingual and multicultural populations. In R. Chapey (Ed.). *Language intervention strategies in adult aphasia.* 5th edition. Baltimore: Lippincott, Williams and Wilkins.

Roberts, P.M., and Bois, M. (1999). Picture name agreement for French-English bilingual adults. *Brain and Cognition, 40*, 238-241.

[1] Note that on page 125 of this Forum article, the theories/speculations attributed to Pitres and to Ribot are incorrect. Although this error was detected prior to publication, the rules governing the Forum format in *Aphasiology* did not allow a correction to be made, nor did they allow publication of an "erratum" notice.

Roberts, P.M., Code, C.F.S., Hillis, A.E., and McNeil, M.R. (forthcoming). Describing participants in aphasia research : Part 2. Which variables really matter?

Roberts, P.M., Code, C., and McNeil, M.R. (2003). Describing participants in aphasia research: Part 1- audit of current practice. *Aphasiology*, *17*, 911-932.

Roberts, P.M., de la Riva, J., and Rhéaume, A. (1997, May). Effets de l'intervention dans une langue pour l'anomie bilingue. Paper presented to the annual meeting of the Canadian Association of Speech-Language Pathology and Audiology. Toronto.

Roberts, P. M., and Deslauriers, L. (1999). Picture naming of cognate and non-cognate nouns in bilingual aphasia. *Journal of Communication Disorders, 32*, 1-23.

Roberts, P.M. and Doucet, N. (2001, August). Performance des adultes francophones au Boston Naming Test: réponses et variantes. Paper presented at the International Association of Logopedics and Phoniatrics (Association internationale de logopédie et phoniatrie), Montreal.

Roberts, P.M., Garcia, L.J., Desrochers, A., and Hernandez, D. (2002). Performance of proficient bilingual adults on the Boston Naming Test. *Aphasiology*, *16*, 635-645.

Roberts, P.M., and Le Dorze, G. (1994). Semantic verbal fluency in aphasia : A qualitative and quantitative study in test-retest conditions. *Aphasiology, 8*, 569-582.

Roberts, P.M., and Le Dorze, G. (1997). Semantic organization, strategy use, and productivity in bilingual semantic verbal fluency. *Brain and Language, 59*, 412-449.

Roberts, P. M., and Le Dorze, G. (1998). Bilingual aphasia: semantic organization, strategy use, and productivity in semantic verbal fluency. *Brain and Language, 65*, 287-312.

Roberts, P.M., and Shenker, R.C. (2007). Assessment and treatment of stuttering in bilingual speakers. In R.F. Curlee and E.G. Conture (Eds). *Stuttering and related disorders of fluency*, 3rd edition (pp. 183-209). New York: Thieme Medical Publishers.

Roselli, M., Ardila, A., Salvatierra, J., Marquez, M., Matos, L., and Weekes, V.A., (2002). A cross-linguistic comparison of verbal fluency tests. *International Journal of Neuroscience*, *112*, 759-776.

Sasanuma, S., and Park, H.S. (1995). Patterns of language deficits in two Korean-Japanese bilingual aphasic patients - A clinical report. In M. Paradis (Ed.), *Aspects of bilingual aphasia* (pp. 111-122). Oxford: Pergamon.

Snodgrass, J.G., and Tsivkin, S. (1995). Organization of the bilingual lexicon: categorical versus alphabetic cuing in Russian-English bilinguals. *Journal of Psycholinguistic Research, 24*, 145-163.

Spreen, O., and Strauss, E. (1998). *A compendium of neuropsychological tests: administration, norms, and commentary*, 2nd edition. New York: Oxford University Press.

Steinmetz, H., and Seitz, R.J. (1991). Functional anatomy of language processing: neuroimaging and the problem of individual variability. *Neuropsychologia*, *29*, 1149-1161.

Szekely, A., D'Amico, S., Devescovi, A., Federmeier, K., Herron, D., Iyer, G., Jacobsen, T., Arévalo, A. L., Vargha, A., and Bates, E. (2005). Timed action and object naming. *Cortex*, *41*, 7-25.

Szekely, A., Jacobsen, T., D'Amico, S., Devescovi, A., Andonova, E., Herron, D., Ching Lu, C., Pechmann, T., Pléh, C., Wicha, N., Federmeier, K., Gerdjikova, I., Gutierrez, G., Hung, D., Hsu, J., Iyer, G., Kohnert, K., Mehotcheva, T., Orozco-Figueroa, A., Tzeng, A., Tzeng, O., Arévalo, A., Vargha, A., Butler, A., Buffington, R. and Bates, E. (2004). A new on-line resource for psycholinguistic studies. *Journal of Memory and Language, 51*, 247-250.

Tallberg, I.M. (2005). The Boston Naming Test in Swedish: Normative data. *Brain and Language*, *94*, 19-31.

Thuillard-Colombo, F., and Assal, G. (1992). Boston Naming Test: French-Language adaptation and short forms / Adaptation française du Test de dénomination de Boston-versions abrégées. *European Review of Applied Psychology / Revue Européenne de Psychologie Appliquée, 42*, 67-73.

Tombaugh, T.N., and Hubley, A.M. (1997). The 60-item Boston Naming Test: Norms for cognitively intact adults aged 25 to 88 years. *Journal of Clinical and Experimental Neuropsychology, 19*, 922-932.

Tombaugh, T.N., Kozak, J., and Rees, L. (1999). Normative data stratified by age and education for two measures of verbal fluency: FAS and animal naming. *Archives of Clinical Neuropsychology, 14*, 167-177.

Tsolaki, M., Tsantali, E., Lekka, S., Kiosseoglou, G., and Kazis, A. (2003). Can the *Boston Naming Test* be used as a clinical tool for differential diagnosis in dementia? *Brain and Language*, *87*, 185-186.

Van Hell, J., and Dijkstra, T. (2002). Foreign language knowledge can influence native language performance in exclusively native contexts. *Psycholinguistic Bulletin and Review*, *9*, 780-789.

Van Lancker Sidtis, D. (2006). Does functional neuroimaging solve the questions of neurolinguistics? *Brain and Language, 98*, 276-290.

Van Wijnendaele, I., and Brysbaert, M. (2002). Visual word recognition in bilinguals: Phonological priming from the second to the first language. *Journal of Experimental Psychology: Human Perception and Performance*, *28*, 616-627.

Voyer, D. (2003). Word frequency and laterality effects in lexical decision: Right hemisphere mechanisms. *Brain and Language*, *87*, 421-431.

Watamori, T. S., and Sasanuma, S. (1976). The recovery process of a bilingual aphasic. *Journal of Communication Disorders, 9*, 157-166.

Watamori, T. S., and Sasanuma, S. (1978). The recovery processes of two English-Japanese bilingual aphasics. *Brain and Language, 6*, 127-140.

Appendix A: Self-Rating of Bilingual Proficiency

When you ask someone to rate their abilities say:

"I want to to rate your (your father's, wife's etc) knowledge of each of their languages. This might be hard to do, but I need to you give me your best estimate.

0 means you/he/she could not do it at all; no knowledge.

1 means very little ability, just a few words here and there, very poor.

7 means like a typical native speaker of that language who only speaks that language. So, 7 does not mean "perfect" mastery, or like an expert (or newscaster or author). It means, like someone with his age and education, who can only speak ____ (name the language).

All these ratings apply to how he talked before the stroke.

How would you rate P's ability to understand what people say in Lx? Ly? Lz?

How would you rate P's ability to say what he wants to say in Lx? Ly? Lz?

How would you rate P's ability to read, to understand what he read in Lx.....

How would you rate P's ability to write (not handwriting, but composing sentences, letters, whatever he had to write) in Lx? Ly? Lz

Often it is helpful to do all 4 questions for one language at a time, but some people seem to find the task easier if they compare the languages as they go through the rating task. These questions can be presented in written form, with the appropriate scale written out, for P's who can read or for their families.

Some patients who cannot understand the numbers, can do the rating task by marking the point along a solid line, with the ends of the line marked or explained verbally as meaning "can't do" and "like a native __ speaker".

In: Speech and Language Disorders in Bilinguals ISBN 978-1-60021-560-5
Editors: Alfredo Ardila and Eliane Ramos, pp. 131-149

Chapter 7

STUTTERING IN BILINGUALS

Patricia M. Roberts
Audiology and Speech-Language Pathology Program
University of Ottawa
Ontario, Canada

This chapter will provide a brief overview of concerns and questions about stuttering in bilingual speakers. The first half of this chapter will review some basic definitions and concepts about stuttering and their implications for bilingual children and adults who stutter. The second half will address some of the many unanswered questions about bilingual stuttering, focusing on those that are most relevant to clinical assessment and treatment. Readers looking for a detailed literature review, or for guidelines for clinical assessment of bilingual people who stutter and for specific treatment suggestions will find these elsewhere (Roberts and Shenker, 2007). Other authors have provided overviews of some of the cultural issues relevant to bilingual stuttering (e.g., Finn and Cordes, 1997).

Throughout this chapter I will use the word *bilingual* to refer to both bilingual individuals (two languages) and multilingual (polyglot) individuals (three or more languages). There are two main reasons for this. First, it is cumbersome to always say "bilingual and/or multilingual". Second, with so little research on stuttering in speakers of two or more languages, there is no evidence that separating bilingual from multilingual speakers is required. As noted elsewhere in this book, there are many definitions of the word *bilingual*, with some authors limiting this term to people with (ostensibly) "perfect mastery" of two languages and other authors linking the word to a specific age or manner of acquisition of the second language. In this chapter the word *bilingual* refers to individuals with some level of knowledge of two (or more) languages. As noted in other publications (e.g., Hakuta, 1986; Roberts, 2001, 2007, this volume; Roberts and Shenker, 2007), bilingualism and unilingualism are not distinct categories with all speakers being either one or the other. Rather, bilingualism is a continuum. There are degrees of bilingualism, with each individual having some level of proficiency in auditory comprehension, verbal expression, reading comprehension and written expression in each of their languages. These levels of proficiency are reached and then improve or deteriorate over time, depending on each speaker's patterns of use and exposure to each language, in each of the four modalities.

Definitions and Causes of Stuttering

The World Health Organization defines stuttering as a disorder "in the rhythm of speech in which the individual knows precisely what he wishes to say, but at the time is unable to say it because of an involuntary, repetitive prolongation or cessation of a sound" (1977, p. 202). Longer definitions, (e.g., Wingate, 1964), outline other key features of the disorder such as coping strategies, other types of disfluencies, and the psychological consequences that may accompany stuttering. The disorder first appears during early childhood, and may worsen or lessen in severity over time.

People have been aware of the disorder and have speculated about the causes of stuttering for millennia. The ancient Egyptians had a hieroglyphic symbol for the disorder (see, for example, Manning, 2001). Stuttering has been attributed to an astonishing variety of causes including malformed mouths and tongues; possession by demons; punishment by one or more deities for sins committed by the person who stutters or by their families or ancestors; child rearing practices; various forms of psychosis and neurosis; imitating others who stutter; laziness; and unwillingness to speak clearly. Happily, such wild theories and speculations about the causes of stuttering have now been rejected.

In considering the causes of stuttering, it is useful to distinguish between the fundamental or distal cause (why someone has the disorder) and the immediate or proximal cause (why someone stuttered on a particular word at a particular time) (Attanasio, Onslow, and Packman, 1998).

Recent research into the fundamental cause(s) of stuttering has identified three key facts.

1) A large percentage of people who stutter have a family history of stuttering (Poulos and Webster, 1991; Yairi, Ambrose, and Cox, 1996). However, many people who stutter have no known family history, with estimates of this number varying quite widely depending on whether family members who stuttered only briefly as young children can be identified. This points to some genetically inherited set of traits as part of the cause of stuttering for most, but not all people who stutter (PWS). One recent study estimated that genetic factors contribute more than environmental factors (70% compared to 30%) in explaining why some twins stutter (Felsenfeld et al., 2000) but identifying the exact combination of genes involved and the contribution of each will be a complex process (Felsenfeld, 2002). Genetic vulnerability to stuttering, sometimes called the genetic load, is particularly important in the roughly 30% of children who do not recover spontaneously and are, therefore, most likely to be seen by clinicians (Yairi, Ambrose, and Cox, 1996; Yairi, Ambrose, Paden, and Throneburg, 1996). Children "who stutter and have a familial history of chronic stuttering would tend to follow that pattern, and children who stutter but have a family history of recovered stuttering would tend to follow that pattern" (Yairi and Ambrose, 2005, p. 307).
2) There are differences in some motor abilities (for speech and non-speech tasks) between PWS and people who do not stutter (see Bloodstein, 1995 for a review of the older literature; more recently Chang, Ohde, and Conture, 2002; Forster and Webster, 2001; Kleinow and Smith, 2000; Maner, Smith and Grayson, 2000). In at least one study, the severity of the stuttering correlated with the severity of the

motor deficits (Jones, White, Lawson, and Anderson, 2002). The initial studies of motor abilities during speech were conducted on English-speaking PWS. New studies are appearing, replicating these findings in speakers of other languages (e.g., Hadever, Dokoza, and Saric, 2004).

3) Adults who stutter and adults who do not stutter show different patterns of brain activation during speech. Although these between-group differences are not always the same from one study to the next (e.g., Ingham, Fox et al., 2004), most of the observed differences are in regions of the brain involved in motor planning and control. In many instances, there is overactivation of areas in the right hemisphere. To what extent are these differences the consequences of stuttering and to what extent are they (part of) the causes of the stuttering? No one can yet say, but research in the next 10 years may well bring answers (for a review see Ludlow, 1999).

It is therefore now widely believed that the fundamental cause of stuttering (the reason why someone has the disorder) is neurological. In most children, developmental stuttering appears between age 2 and 4, a period in which children experience rapid neurological development, establishing neural pathways, myelinisation and dendritic growth. This neurological development makes possible significant motor development and rapid changes in language ability that also occur in this period of a child's life.

The PWS has reduced ability to plan and carry out the complex motor sequences required to produce speech. This reduced ability is, in many cases, an inherited vulnerability; in other cases, it may be the result of events during pregnancy, or birth or during early childhood when the brain pathways needed for smooth motor control of speech are being formed. It is possible that different races and ethnic groups will prove to have different incidences of the genes implicated in stuttering, just as there are ethnic differences in the genes associated with other conditions, including heart disease risk and sickle cell anemia. Researchers into the genetics of stuttering have not yet published data on this question.

Proximal Causes and Environmental Factors

When we consider stuttering in bilingual speakers and in different cultures, these neurological/genetic roots of stuttering have a number of implications. First, child-rearing practices, linguistic stimulation, and parental expectations – all culturally-influenced factors once thought to play key roles in causing stuttering – are now seen as of secondary importance in causing the disorder. As early as 1971, Van Riper pointed out that "the apparent universality of stuttering must hold some clue as to its nature….. if stuttering is to be viewed as a coordinative disorder, one in which the intricate timing of simultaneous and successive muscular contractions required for fluent utterance tends to become disrupted under stress, its universality should not surprise us." (Van Riper, 1971, p. 9). Second, when/if there is an unusually high or unusually low incidence of stuttering in a particular community, the most likely reason is genetic, not cultural.

The proximal causes of stuttering (why stuttering occurs on a particular word at a particular time) are less clearly understood. Stutters are more likely to occur on longer utterances (see Zackheim and Conture, 2003 for an excellent review of the evidence for this). There is conflicting evidence about the importance of linguistic complexity, word length, word type, phonological factors (consonant clusters, for example), and the relative proportion of stuttered consonants vs. vowels (e.g., Dworzynski, Howell, and Natke, 2003; Huinck, van Lieshout, Peters, and Hulstijn, 2004). Some studies have explored these factors in normally fluent speakers and in PWS in various languages including Spanish (Au-Yeung, Vallejo Gomez, and Howell, 2003; Carlo and Watson, 2003; Howell, et al., 2004), Portuguese (De Andrade, Sassi, and Zackiewcz, 2004; Juste and de Andrade, 2004), Dutch (Vaane and Janssen, 1978 cited in Bloodstein, 1995) and Afrikaans (Uys, 1970 cited in Bloodstein, 1995, p. 285) and in English production of children who are not native English speakers (Howell, Davis, and Au-Yeung, 2003). Are the phoneme sequences of some languages more difficult motorically and therefore more likely to trigger moments of stuttering (e.g., Jayaram, 1983)? In languages such as German and Turkish where words are much longer than they are in English and word formation processes are much different, will word length influence stuttering? No one knows. In time, patterns will emerge from this line of research, but many more studies are needed.

Some studies have identified the PWS's psychological state (nervousness, confidence, fear of consequences of not speaking well, desire to speak quickly) as a proximal cause of stuttering. Factors such as the number of listeners, the authority held by the person spoken to, and the communicative stress associated with the telephone are known to increase the frequency and/or severity of stuttering in some adolescents and adults. Many of the pioneers in the field of stuttering in the USA and England from the 1930s through the 1950s identified these sources of pressure and their impact on stuttering (See Bloodstein, 1995 for a summary of this early work). The importance of speaking well, the social, academic, and vocational consequences of not speaking well, and the degree of pressure to speak quickly all vary from one culture to another, but there has been little attention paid to cross-cultural studies of these factors in PWS.

Other factors that may vary across cultures and across sub-groups within a given linguistic group include speaking rate, the number of interruptions, and the typical/acceptable range of loudness for conversational speech. When studies are done on these factors across different languages, it will be interesting to see to what extent these factors are associated with moments of stuttering and with non-stuttered disfluencies. To date, the studies of the influence of speaking rate and interruptions (primarily in American, English-speaking children who stutter) have found conflicting results (e.g., Bernstein Ratner, 1992; Guitar and Marchinkoski, 2001; Livingston, Flowers, Hodor, and Ryan, 2000; Nippold and Rudzinski, 1995).

Even if the pragmatics of communication in a given family or cultural group involve rapid rates, frequent interruptions or speaking loudly, we cannot be sure that these factors are proximal causes of moments of stuttering for any given child. The current literature cannot support a recommendation that parents or families routinely change these features of their communication. Until the literature is clearer, clinicians should work on a case-by-case basis: identify factors that make fluent speech easier or harder for each PWS and then determine to what extent changing these behaviors might be needed for therapy to succeed. Then, if necessary, clinicians may judge it appropriate to ask/teach the client and family to make changes in the most important of these factors. This recommendation applies to all clients, not only those from "other cultures".

Why do some studies find that a particular factor such as speaking rate, interruptions, or sentence length increases the risk of stuttering while other studies fail to replicate this finding? In some cases, the small number of participants in each study, the different speaking tasks used and other methodological factors explain the contradictory findings. In other cases, the different results in different studies probably mean that some factors are important for some PWS but not for others. In studies of bilingual speakers, it is often difficult to create large groups of PWS with similar linguistic histories. Whenever a study reports data for a single speaker or for a small group, it is important for readers to be cautious in accepting their conclusions until the study has been replicated at least once.

The performance of bilingual speakers varies more widely than that of monolingual speakers. This has been found in vocabulary (Goggin, Estrada, and Villarreal, 1994; Roberts, Garcia, Desrochers, and Hernandez, 2002), and other speech and language tasks (e.g., Goldstein, 2004; Kohnert, 2004; Pena, Bedore, and Rappazzo, 2003; Tzivinikou, 2004). Also, in motor speech behaviors (e.g., Flege, Munro, and Mackay, 1995) and in other aspects of their communication, the bilingual speaker may be unlike the monolingual speakers of each of his languages (see, for example, Bhatia and Ritchie, 2004; Grosjean, 1998, 1989; Harris, 1992). Furthermore, speakers of different languages may differ in subtle ways in their motor speech in ways that are just starting to be tested. One recent study, for example, reported that Thai speakers have slower diadokokinetic rates than English speakers (Prathanee, Thanaviratananich, and Pongjanyakul, 2003). In working with bilingual children and adults who stutter, clinicians need to keep this variability in mind. It makes it harder (potentially) to diagnose mild stuttering and to separate the effects of bilingualism from the symptoms of stuttering.

LANGUAGE DEVELOPMENT AND STUTTERING: THE ONGOING DEBATE

Although stuttering is a speech disorder and not a language disorder, phonological abilities, language development, and stuttering are related to varying degrees across individual children and adults in complex ways that are not yet fully understood. There are studies reporting that the incidence of language problems in children who stutter is higher than in children who do not stutter or that children who stutter have weaker language skills than their non-stuttering peers (see for example Anderson and Conture, 2000; Arndt and Healey, 2001; Bloodstein, 1995). Some studies find differences in phonological abilities between groups of stuttering and non-stuttering children while other studies find no difference (e.g., Blood, Redenour, Qualls, and Hammer, 2003; Nippold, 2004). The lack of consensus on the relationship between stuttering and language and phonological development is demonstrated by two fairly recent quotes. On the one hand, Culatta and Goldberg (1995, p. 134) go so far as to conclude that “approximately 68% of children who stutter have other speech, language, or learning problems”. On the other hand, Watkins (2005, p. 246) states that in her longitudinal study of 89 children "there is virtually no evidence that language development is vulnerable in any significant number of young children who stutter. On the contrary, there is some hint that early precocious expressive language abilities may be a risk factor for stuttering, or may simply be a by-product of some other operating risk factor." Once again, the contradictory findings can be explained by different methodologies, different operational definitions of the abilities being assessed, small groups, unrepresentative samples, and the wide range of tasks and assessment instruments used.

From the overall pattern of results, it seems likely that there is some kind of link between language development and stuttering, at least for some children who stutter (CWS). This has a number of implications for bilingual children. The most important one is that some (often unilingual?) people have recommended that any child who shows signs of stuttering or whose family tree includes many relatives who stutter should be raised to be unilingual (for recent reviews, see Bernstein Ratner, 2004; Van Borsel, Maes, and Foulon, 2001). Although there are no published, experimental studies supporting this recommendation, it seems to have considerable intuitive appeal and the same recommendation (to limit the child to a single language) is often made when the child has other communication disorders (e.g., Thordardottir, 2006). This recommendation has been based on two lines of thought, both of which require empirical proof before speech-language pathologists should accept the idea that bilingualism is related to the incidence and/or to the persistence of stuttering in children. The first line of thought used to support the "one language limit" for children at risk for stuttering is that some groups of CWS have weaker language abilities than comparable groups of normally fluent children. Second, there is an intuitive sort of Demands and Capacities framework according to which bilingual language acquisition in these critical years places too great a strain on children, thereby causing them to stutter and/or making it less likely they will recover. So, reducing the overall linguistic-cognitive-motor speech load by requiring that the child learn only one language will reduce the risk of stuttering and/or will assist in recovery if the child already stutters. Recent studies on bilingual language acquisition are providing new insights into the process (e.g., Goldstein, 2004; Paradis and Crago, 2000). It is too early to say whether bilingual language acquisition is any more difficult for some groups or types of children than single language acquisition. In conducting and in evaluating published studies, the context of political debates, government funding of studies to support their own language education policies, and the strong emotions that bilingualism policies can trigger, are all factors to consider when interpreting the results of studies.

Recommending that a child "become unilingual" when their family and neighborhood use more than one language is a drastic step. This recommendation is upsetting for clients and families to hear, and many reject it. The available evidence that could be interpreted as supporting this recommendation is insufficient. The impact of this one language limit has never been experimentally tested. And, the studies that have found no association between language disorders/delay and stuttering further undermine the rationale for such a recommendation. Perhaps just as importantly, it would often be impossible for a family to implement this recommendation. The little boy described by Karniol (1992) continued to hear and probably to speak some English (for example, with his sister) even when his parents stopped speaking to him in English as part of an attempt to make him "a non-stuttering monolingual speaker in L1" (p. 255). This study provides – unintentionally – a demonstration of how difficult it is to limit the languages spoken to and by a young child when the community around him is not monolingual.

The Karniol (1992) article has sometimes been cited to support the idea that children who stutter should not be bilingual and/or that bilingualism increases the risk a child will stutter (e.g., Guitar, 2006, p. 177; Stahl and Totten, 1995). An examination of the article will demonstrate why it fails to provide any valid foundation for these speculations. Karniol published a diary account which documents, in anecdotal fashion, the onset, then the waxing and waning of stuttering in a boy. There is no statement about a family history for stuttering (positive or negative). There are no data on the numbers of (normal) disfluencies in Hebrew or English or on the number of stutters or on how or if the two were distinguished. The paper provides only statements like "stuttering was evident in both languages" (p. 262) or "a mild stutter consisting of part-word and whole-word repetitions, but with no struggle, returned in both languages" (p. 271). Dramatic events in the child's life, including summer camp overseas and experiencing the bombing raids of the Gulf War, mix with the normal sorting out of his language preferences during acquisition of three very different languages (Hebrew, English, and Hungarian) in the period recorded in the diaries (age 25 months to approximately 37 months). There are no data showing the eventual levels of fluency or disfluency in English or in Hebrew and no data on whether the disfluency level correlated with the child's level of knowledge of each language at any point in time. Critically, there are no data to allow the reader to determine whether or not the child still stuttered at the end of the period described in the study. Therefore, there is no way to know whether he stuttered because of the multilingual environment or whether there was a strong family history of stuttering; no way to know whether he stopped stuttering (if he did stop) through the process of unassisted recovery that occurs in approximately 70% of children who stutter or whether the changes in language use by the child and his parents contributed in any way to this recovery.

Narrative, descriptive studies cannot answer the questions about the relationship between bilingual language acquisition and stuttering in children. The field needs rigorous studies focusing on different pairs of languages and linguistic environments, and large numbers of children. Large, prospective studies of children with a family history of stuttering, some raised in bilingual conditions and others raised in monolingual conditions would provide excellent evidence, but these would be very costly and difficult to do.

Incidence of Stuttering

Studies conducted in the United States, England and Australia estimate that the incidence of stuttering (the proportion of people who at some time in their life stutter(ed)) is between 3% and 5% (Andrews, 1984; Bloodstein, 1995). A recent and rigorous study in Denmark (Mansson, 2000) found similar results. Craig and colleagues question these figures, pointing out methodological problems with many studies, and the changes in the incidence of stuttering across age groups (Craig, Hancock, Tran, Craig, and Peters, 2002; Craig and Tran, 2005). Estimating incidence is difficult, since most children who stutter recover with no help, many of them after stuttering for only a brief period. Thus, we need better, more detailed epidemiological studies.

Despite this, independent studies in 12 countries on 4 different continents, each with different methodologies and sample sizes and different levels of reliability, all found that the prevalence of stuttering in school-aged children (the number of children at any given time who stutter) varied within a narrow range. Estimates of the prevalence of stuttering in school children in 12 different countries all fall between 0.5 and 1.8% (Bloodstein, 1995, page 107). More recently, Okalidou and Kampanaros (2001) found 1 to 2% of kindergarten children were described as stuttering by their teachers in one region in Greece. Only one study (Ralston, 1981) found a prevalence rate above the 1.8% level: 4.7%. This study provides no information on the definition of stuttering used or whether the teachers who provided that data distinguished between normal disfluencies and stuttering. Its focus on political influences on language and dialect use, and its data collection methods all contributed to this high prevalence figure (and to the finding that the prevalence of stuttering in schools increased as children age, while the reverse is known to be the case in well-controlled studies).

The fact that most studies yield prevalence estimates that fall within a fairly narrow range suggests that the risk of developing stuttering is very little influenced by cultural factors, native language and, indirectly, whether most people speak one or more than one language. Unfortunately, most of the published studies fail to provide any information on the language background of the individuals in their samples, thus preventing readers from knowing whether or not bilingual speakers were included in the study or not. In the Mansson study (2000), for example, the children may have been exposed to more than one language from an early age, but this cannot be confirmed from the published descriptions of the participants. In order to see more clearly whether and/or to what extent cultural factors and/or bilingualism might contribute to triggering the onset of stuttering in vulnerable children and/or to maintaining the stuttering problem once it has appeared, the methodology of the studies will be a critical factor. Furthermore, given the methodological challenges inherent in determining what the incidence and prevalence of stuttering are in a particular region or country, we should not be too quick to accept findings of a higher or lower rate in a given cultural group on the basis of a single study.

Challenges in Conducting and Interpreting Research

Definitions of bilingualism: The fact that there is no consensus on the meaning of the word *bilingual* must be recognized. For some people *bilingual* applies only to people who learned both languages from birth, and/or to people who have high and roughly equal abilities in the two languages, while for others, the term applies to a continuum of ability acquired at any point in one's life. Perhaps because they see *bilingual* as meaning perfect mastery from birth, some authors have included in their studies adults and children who speak more than one language but have failed to report this or to provide any description of participants' language backgrounds. In some studies of stuttering, it is unclear what language the participants speak, since this information is not provided. Similarly, some studies report that all participants were "native English speakers". This is an inadequate description because some people have two native languages. Also, one can be a native speaker of one language, and speak one or more additional languages. Adequately describing the language background of participants will improve the external validity of studies and will allow replication and accurate interpretation of studies. When participants speak more than one language, clearly defining the levels of language ability in the selection criteria will also be essential.

Definitions of stuttering: Although most clinicians and researchers feel they know what stuttering is when they hear it, there is quite a wide range from one study to another in what is counted as stuttering. Some studies count only disfluencies that are judged, perceptually, to have been stuttered while other studies count stuttering-like disfluencies (SLDs) as all being stuttered. Still other studies count all disfluencies as stutters. Some count any instance of word avoidance as a stutter, even when there is no tension or repetition associated with it (e.g., Guitar, 2006, p. 185). Too often, authors fail to provide a clear definition of what was counted. This makes it impossible to compare results across studies and will mean that researchers interested in comparing results across different languages will not be able to use many of the published studies of English speakers.

Arithmetic: It may seem trivial to focus on how words, syllables, and disfluencies are counted, but unless this aspect of the methodology of a study is clearly defined, it is difficult to interpret the results, and impossible to compare results across studies.

Consider the following examples.

1) Some authors (and clinicians) count only one disfluency on a particular word, while others count each disfluent behavior separately, and allow 2 or 3 or more disfluencies to "count" during the production of a given syllable.
2) Some authors count the number of syllables spoken but others count only intended syllables, often without specifying this or stating whether revisions are counted in the total number of intended syllables.
3) Definitions of each type of disfluency. This is particularly important for interjections. Some studies count interjections only if they are non-words such as *um, er, ah*. Others count "real words", such as "well" and "like" as interjections if they have no meaning in a particular utterance. Some count interjections that are repeated as repeated (single syllable) words, while others count each interjection as a new interjection.

The following example demonstrates how different results are obtained depending on what is counted.

So *uh* I go to *like* a camp for two weeks.
It's *like it's* really cool.
We learn about *we learn about* computers and stuff.
And *um uh* we make our own web sites.
The web sites *the web sites um* | we can put whatever we want o-on (repeat part word) them.
And *and* the *uh well the* c-counsellors they *they* help us.
And then at the end we | our parents can come.
And we show them the stuff that *um* we did.
And we get | on Friday *like* we all get pizza.

T*syll*: Total syllables uttered: 103

T*int*: Total intended syllables if all repetitions, revisions and interjections are excluded: 74

T*mix*: Total intended syllables if we include revisions, but exclude interjections and repetitions: 80

IN*all*: Number of interjections if we count all types: 10

IN*nw*: Number of interjections if we count only non-words: 5 or 6

Dis*all:* Number of disfluencies if we allow more than 1 disfluency on or preceding an intended word: 21

Dis *moments*: Number of disfluencies if we count what are sometimes called "moments of disfluency" and combine all disfluencies associated with uttering an intended syllable into a single "moment": 14.

It is easy to see that different values for the number of disfluencies per 100 syllables will result from these different ways of counting both syllables and disfluencies. This sample could have 14.6 (Dis*moments*/T*syll*) or 20.4 (Dis*all*/T*syll*), or 26.3 (Dis*all*/Tmix) or 28.4 (Dis*all*/T*int*) disfluencies per 100 syllables, depending on how the counting is done.

Similarly, some authors count percent of syllables stuttered (%SS), from transcripts or using on-line counts, without defining what they have counted. Sometimes %SS is based on a perceptual judgment of unambiguous stuttering (as in the Lidcombe Program, for example). This definition of stuttering means that stuttering is not related to any particular type of disfluency. In the sample above, using this definition, there might be 0%SS, if listeners judge that all the disfluencies were said in a relaxed and "normal" manner. But, some authors use %SS as a synonym for SLDs (a very unfortunate development!). By this definition, the sample above contains 3 or 4 "stutters". Depending on how the syllables are counted, the %SS could range from 2.9 (3/103) to 5.5% (4/74).

In order to compare rates across studies and across languages, it is essential that authors explain their methods for counting syllables and define each disfluency type (until there is a consensus on what to count and how to count). When comparing one study to another, the informed reader must take the different counting methods into account.

Methodological Challenges in Conducting Research

Creating groups with similar levels of bilingualism: Many popular research designs involve comparing one group to another. For this comparison to work, the groups must be as similar as possible in all respects except the critical variable being studied. If two well-matched groups (the stuttering and control groups, for example) differ in their speech rate, level of disfluency, mean length of utterance or other features of their communication, readers can draw conclusions about the impact of stuttering. If, however, the groups are not well-matched, it becomes impossible to know if a given between-group difference is due to stuttering, or to one of the other differences between the groups, such as degree of bilingualism.

Some authors have used self ratings (Delgado, Guerrero, Goggin, and Ellis, 1999; Oscarson, 1989). Age of first exposure to each language and other details of participants' language background are also used in forming groups of participants. At present, however, there are many unanswered questions about how well age of acquisition correlates with a person's proficiency at different ages. Although self-ratings have been shown to produce groups of subjects whose mean performance reflects their mean self-ratings (e.g., Bahrick, Hall, Goggin, Bahrick, and Berger, 1994; Kohnert, Hernandez, and Bates, 1998; Roberts and Bois, 1997; Roberts and Le Dorze, 1998), individual ratings may or may not match up with each individual's performance on the experimental (or clinical) task (e.g.,Roberts, 2002;

Roberts, Garcia, Desrochers, and Hernandez, 2002). When working with young children who cannot understand or reliably carry out the rating process, parents' ratings have been used (e.g., Roberts and Hébert, 2001). When the parent does not speak one of the child's languages well, it is impossible for them to rate the child's level of proficiency in that language. There is a need for studies that will allow researchers to assign reliable "level of bilingualism" scores (LOB) to participants and that will allow clinicians to estimate pre-morbid LOBs for their patients to assess the accuracy of self-ratings.

Low power: Statistical power is "the extent to which an investigation can detect differences between groups when differences exist within the population" (Kazdin, 2003, p. 70). Studies with small numbers of participants inevitably have low power and may conclude that there is no difference between groups (stuttering vs. non-stuttering, bilingual vs. monolingual or pretreatment vs. posttreatment) when, in fact, there are differences which the study failed to find because of its low power (a Type II error). Many studies of stuttering have suffered from a lack of power (Jones, Gebski, Onslow, and Packman, 2002a, 2002b). It will be important for studies of bilinguals who stutter to avoid repeating this design error.

Challenges Ahead

There are many unanswered questions about bilingual stuttering, questions that have clinical and broader repercussions. Among the most important of these questions are the following:

1) What are the symptoms of stuttering in different languages and cultures, especially in young children who are just starting to stutter? Initial studies cited above (and, no doubt, other studies published in various languages) are finding that the symptoms of stuttering are broadly similar across languages but detailed analyses in a range of languages, especially in the months following the onset of stuttering, have not yet been done.
2) Are there any features of stuttering, especially in its early stages, that are unique to bilingual speakers or more common in bilingual than unilingual speakers? Strategies such as code-switching can be used to mask the stuttering, to avoid feared sounds and words, and will need to be studied.
3) Does exposing a child to two or more languages increase the risk that the child will develop stuttering?
4) If so, does this risk vary with the child's age, their family history of stuttering, the specific pairs of languages, or other features of the linguistic and/or cultural environment?
5) What is the range among non-stuttering speakers for various types of disfluencies labeled in studies of English-speakers as within-word and between-word or stuttering-like and other disfluencies?
6) To what extent do bilingual speakers of various levels, ages and speaking various pairs of languages fit the patterns observed in unilingual speakers of these languages? A) Are there types of disfluencies or patterns of disfluencies unique to bilingual speakers? For (probably) monolingual English-speakers, there are a number of studies on the range of disfluencies in the speech of children and adults

who do not stutter (e.g., Duchin and Mysak, 1987; Johnson, 1959, 1961; Yairi and Ambrose, 2005). There is no equivalent array of studies for other languages, although some studies are now starting to appear (e.g., De Andrade, Cervone, and Sassi, 2003; Roberts and Hébert, 2001; Ström, 1995). Common sense and experience speaking with people with different levels of proficiency both suggest that people may speak more slowly in their weaker language and/or produce more disfluencies. Alternatively, by speaking more slowly and with less spontaneity, some people probably have fewer disfluencies in their weaker language. A study by Roberts and Shenker currently underway with English-French bilingual children will provide some data on this question. The SALT language data base now includes some samples from languages other than English (for a discussion of some of the difficulties with fitting other languages into the SALT format see Thordardottir, 2005). If, and only if, the demographic data submitted with these samples include the relevant information on each child's level of bilingualism and patterns of language acquisition and use, these samples will prove extremely valuable. Initial studies also suggest that the overall level of disfluency and/or the number of SLDs produced by speakers of other languages may be higher than it is for English speakers (e.g., Roberts and Meltzer, 2004). But there may be such variability in bilingual speakers that the idea of a normal range will not be appropriate. B) What is a normal range for speaking rate in different languages for different tasks in different age groups?

7) How do bilingual speakers (who do not stutter) rate on the naturalness scale often used to rate the speech of PWS pre- and post-treatment? An interesting study by Mackey, Finn and Ingham (1997) found that speech samples were judged as less natural-sounding when the speaker and the rater did not speak the same dialect of English. Before the naturalness scale is used to rate the speech of bilingual PWS to measure stuttering severity or to measure treatment outcomes, its validity with different levels of bilingual speakers and raters must be determined.
8) How can clinicians achieve optimal results in treating bilingual speakers of different ages with different levels of proficiency in each of their languages? Is the age of acquisition of each language important? These are very complex questions that will require addressing a number of smaller questions, such as a) how should the language of treatment be selected: language spoken at home, client's level of proficiency, clinician's level of proficiency, etc. b) what is the impact, if any, of including practice activities in both/all of the client's languages? c) when should practice in different languages be introduced, for different types of therapies such as fluency shaping or stuttering modification? d) does it make any difference to the treatment outcome, attendance, dropout rate or client satisfaction to have a clinician from the same culture as the client?

Challenges for Readers, Clinicians, and Researchers

The biggest challenge for consumers of research is, perhaps, to remain appropriately skeptical as they read. Even in the age of television and other electronic media, people tend to grant printed materials such as books and scientific journals considerable crsave track chaedibility. There is a tendency to believe what one reads. Unfortunately, some very weak studies get published. Also, standards for publication in journals change over time. An article deemed suitable for publication in previous decades might not qualify using today's standards. When a poor study is published, it is important that we not cite its results as facts. For example, among the first studies of bilingual stuttering published in English were reports by Stern (1948) and by Travis, Johnson, and Shover (1937). Despite their huge flaws, these two studies are still cited by Bloodstein (1995, p. 259) as having found higher rates of stuttering in bilingual children compared to unilingual children with no statement about the quality of these studies. Being *appropriately skeptical* means having sufficient knowledge about a particular topic to compare and contrast findings from one study to another. Being appropriately skeptical also means having a good grasp of the basic principles of research methodology. One does not have to be an expert, but the concepts taught in books aimed at a broad undergraduate university level should be retained, not only by researchers, but by clinicians and by all consumers of clinical research (sample books Kazdin, 2003; Maxwell and Satake, 2006; Mitchell and Jolley, 2003).

Being appropriately skeptical means applying reasonable standards of research design and common sense to form an opinion about the credibility of each study (internal reliability, internal and external validity, etc.). If one sets impossibly high standards and looks for a perfect study, this is not an appropriate level of skepticism. No study is perfect. Therefore, setting extremely high standards would lead to rejecting all published studies. Appropriate skepticism looks for the most important strengths and weaknesses in the study, weighs their relative importance and reaches a conclusion about the overall quality and likely accuracy of the reported results.

Answering the questions raised in this chapter will take many years. Progress will be slower if researchers in bilingual stuttering repeat the methodological errors of the past such as weak research designs, failing to define "disfluencies" or "stutters" in sufficient detail to allow replication and comparison of results across studies, and incomplete descriptions of the language background of participants. Progress could be greatly accelerated if researchers learn from, and therefore do not repeat, past errors in the field of stuttering.

As we work towards understanding stuttering in bilingual speakers, the challenges may seem daunting. Some of the challenges stem from the complex nature of both bilingualism and stuttering and the gaps in our understanding of both. Some of these challenges stem from errors or weaknesses in past research. Yet, we must meet these challenges. Thousands upon thousands of bilingual children and adults who stutter will benefit as our knowledge of bilingual stuttering grows.

References

Anderson, J.D., and Conture, E.G. (2000). Language abilities of children who stutter: A preliminary study. *Journal of Fluency Disorders*, *25*, 283-304.

Andrews, G. (1984). The epidemiology of stuttering. In R.F. Curlee and W.H. Perkins (Eds.) *Nature and treatment of stuttering: New directions* (pp. 1-12). San Diego: College-Hill Press.

Arndt, J., and Healey, E.C. (2001). Concomitant disorders in school-age children who stutter. *Language, Speech, and Hearing Services in Schools, 32*, 68-78.

Attanasio, J.S., Onslow, M., and Packman, A. (1998). Representativeness reasoning and the search for the origins of stuttering: a return to basic observations. *Journal of Fluency Disorders, 23*, 265-277.

Au-Yeung, J., Vallejo Gomez, I., and Howell, P. (2003). Exchange of disfluency from function words to content words with age in Spanish speakers who stutter. *Journal of Speech, Language, and Hearing Research, 46*, 754-765.

Bahrick, H.P., Hall, L.K., Goggin, J.P., Bahrick, L.E., and Berger, S.A. (1994). Fifty years of language maintenance and language dominance in bilingual Hispanic immigrants. *Journal of Experimental Psychology: general*. 123, 264-283.

Bernstein Ratner, N. (2004). Fluency and stuttering in bilingual children. In B.Goldstein (Ed.) *Bilingual language development and disorders in Spanish-English speakers* (pp. 287–308). Baltimore: Paul H. Brookes.

Bernstein Ratner, N. (1992). Measurable outcomes in instructions to modify normal parent-child verbal interactions: implications for indirect stuttering therapy. *Journal of Speech and Hearing Research, 35*, 14-20.

Bhatia, T.K. and Ritchie, W.C. (Eds.) (2004). *Handbook of bilingualism*. Vol.15 of Blackwell Handbooks in Linguistics. Malden, MA: Blackwell Publishers.

Blood, G.W., Ridenour, V.J, Qualls, C.D., and Hammer, C.S. (2003). Co-occurring disorders in children who stutter. *Journal of Communication Disorders, 36*, 427-448.

Bloodstein, O. (1995). *A handbook on stuttering* (5th ed.). San Diego, CA: Singular.

Carlo, E.J., and Watson, J.B. (2003). Disfluencies of 3- and 5-year old Spanish-speaking children. *Journal of Fluency Disorders, 28*, 37-53.

Chang, S.E., Ohde, R.N., and Conture, E.G. (2002). Coarticulation and formant transition rate in young children who stutter. *Journal of Speec,h, Language, and Hearing Research, 45*, 676-688.

Craig, A., Hancock, K., Tran, Y., Craig, M., and Peters, K. (2002). Epidemiology of stuttering in the community across the entire lifespan. *Journal of Speech, Language, and Hearing Research, 45*, 1097-1105.

Craig, A., and Tran, Y. (2005). The epidemiology of stuttering: the need for reliable estimates of prevalence and anxiety levels over the lifespan. *Advances in Speech-Language Pathology, 7*, 41-46.

Culatta, R., and Goldberg, S.A. (1995). *Stuttering therapy: an integrated approach to theory and practice*. Boston: Allyn and Bacon.

De Andrade, C.R.F., Cervone, L.M., and Sassi, F.C. (2003). Relationship between the stuttering severity index and speech rate. *São Paulo Medical Journal, 121(2)*, 81-84.

De Andrade, C.R.F., Sassi, F.C., and Zackiewcz, D.V. (2004). Aspects of normally fluent speech in Brazilian adults. In A. Packman, A. Meltzer, and H.F.M. Peters (Eds.). *Theory, research and therapy in fluency disorders: Proceedings of the fourth World Fluency Congress on fluency disorders* (pp. 376-381). Nijmegen: Nijmegen University Press.

Delgado, P., Guerrero, G., Goggin, J.P., and Ellis, B.B. (1999). Self-assessment of linguistic skills by bilingual Hispanics. *Hispanic Journal of Behavioral Sciences, 21(1)*, 31-46.

Duchin, S.W., and Mysak, E.D. (1987). Disfluency and rate characteristics of young adult, middle-aged, and older males. *Journal of Communication Disorders, 20*, 245-257.

Dworzynski, K., Howell, P., and Natke, U. (2003). Predicting stuttering from linguistic factors for German speakers in two age groups. *Journal of Fluency Disorder,. 28*, 95-113.

Felsenfeld, S. (2002). Finding susceptibility genes for developmental disorders of speech: the long and winding road. *Journal of Communication Disorders, 35*, 329-345.

Felsenfeld, S., Kirk, K.M., Zhu, G., Statham, D.J., Neale, M.C., and Martin, N.G. (2000). A study of the genetic and environmental etiology of stuttering in a selected twin sample. *Behavior Genetics, 30*, 359-366.

Finn, P., and Cordes, A.K. (1997). Multicultural identification and treatment of stuttering: a continuing need for research. *Journal of Fluency Disorders, 22*, 219-236.

Flege, J.E., Monroe, M.J. and Mackay, I.R.A. (1995). Effects of age of second-language learning on the production of English consonants. *Speech Communication, 16*, 1-26.

Forster, D.C., and Webster, W.G. (2001). Speech-motor control and interhemispheric relations in recovered and persistent stuttering. *Developmental Neuropsychology*, 19(2),125-145.

Goggin, J.P., Estrada, P., and Villarreal, R. P. (1994). Picture-naming agreement in monolinguals and bilinguals. *Applied Psycholinguistics, 15*, 177-193.

Goldstein, B. (Ed.) (2004). *Bilingual language development and disorders in Spanish-English speakers.* Baltimore: Paul H. Brookes.

Grosjean, F. (1989). Neurolinguists beware- The bilingual is not two monolinguals in one person. *Brain and Language,36*, 3-15.

Grosjean, F. (1998). Studying bilinguals: methodological and conceptual issues. *Bilingualism: Language and Cognition, 1,* 131-149.

Guitar, B. (2006). *Stuttering: an integrated approach to its nature and treatment.*(3rd edition). Baltimore: Lippincott, Williams and Wilkins.

Guitar, B. and Marchinkoski, L. (2001). Influence of mothers' slower speech on their children's speech rate. *Journal of Speech, Language, and Hearing Research, 44*, 853-861.

Hadever, M., Dokoza, K.P., and Saric, J.P. (2004). Laryngeal dynamics in stuttering children (Original Title: Laringealna dinamika djece koja mucaju). *Hrvatska Revija za Rehabilitacijska Istrazivanja, 40(1)*, 39-44. Abstract read in English in Linguistics and Language Behavior Abstracts. October 11, 2005.

Hakuta, K. (1986). *Mirror of language: The debate on bilingualism.* New York: Basic Books.

Harris, R.J. (Ed.) (1992). *Cognitive processing in bilinguals.* New York: Elsevier.

Howell, P., Davis, S., and Au-Yeung, J. (2003). Syntactic development in fluent children, children who stutter, and children who have English as an additional language. *Child Language Teaching and Therapy, 9*, 311-337.

Howell, P., Ruffle, L., Fernandez-Zuniga, A., Gutierrez, R., Fernandez, A.H., O'Brien, M.L., Tarasco, M., Vallejo Gomez, I., and Au Yeung, J. (2004). Comparison of exchange patterns of stuttering in Spanish and English monolingual speakers and a bilingual Spanish-English speaker. In A. Packman, A. Meltzer, and H.F.M. Peters (Eds.). *Theory, research and therapy in fluency disorders. Proceedings of the 4th World Congress on Fluency Disorders* (pp. 415-422), Nijmegen: University of Nijmegen Press,.

Huinck, W.J., van Lieshout, P. H., Peters, H.F.M., and Hulstijn, W. (2004). Gestural overlap in consonant clusters: effects on the fluent speech of stuttering and non-stuttering subjects. *Journal of Fluency Disorders*, 29, 3-25.

Ingham, R.J., Fox, P.T., Ingham, J.C., Xiong, J., Zamarripa, F., Hardies, L.J., and Lancaster, J.L. (2004). Brain correlates of stuttering and syllable production: Gender comparison and replication. *Journal of Speech, Language, and Hearing Research, 47*, 321-341.

Jayaram, M. (1983). Phonetic influences on stuttering in monolingual and bilingual stutterers. *Journal of Communication Disorders, 16*, 287-297.

Johnson, W. and Associates. (1959). *The onset of stuttering: Research findings and implications*. Minneapolis: University of Minnesota Press.

Johnson, W. (1961). Measurement of oral reading and speaking rate and disfluency of adult male and female stutterers and nonstutterers. *Journal of Speech and Hearing Disorders Monograph Supplement 7*, 1-20.

Jones, M., Gebski, V., Onslow, M., and Packman, A. (2002a). Statistical power in stuttering research: A tutorial. *Journal of Speech, Language, and Hearing Research, 45*, 243-255.

Jones, M., Gebski, V., Onslow, M., and Packman, A. (2002b). Statistical power in stuttering research: A tutorial. Erratum. *Journal of Speech, Language, and Hearing Research, 45*, 493.

Jones, R.D., White, A.J., Lawson, K.H. and Anderson, T.J. (2002). Visuoperceptual and visuomotor deficits in developmental stutterers: an exploratory study. *Human Movement Science, 21*, 603-619.

Juste, F., and de Andrade, C.R.F. (2004). Distribution of disfluencies according to word class categorization in Brazilian Portuguese. In A. Packman, A. Meltzer, and H.F.M. Peters (Eds.). *Theory, research and therapy in fluency disorders: Proceedings of the 4th World Fluency Congress on fluency disorders* (pp. 369-375). Nijmegen: Nijmegen University Press.

Karniol, R. (1992). Stuttering out of bilingualism. *First Language, 12*, 255-283.

Kazdin, A.E. (2003). *Research design in clinical psychology*. 4th edition. Boston: Allyn and Bacon.

Kleinow, J. and Smith, A. (2000). Influences of length and syntactic complexity on the speech motor stability of the fluent speech of adults who stutter. *Journal of Speech, Language and Hearing Research, 43*, 548-559.

Kohnert, K. (2004). Processing skills in early sequential bilinguals. In B. Goldstein (Ed.) *Bilingual language development and disorders in Spanish-English speakers* (pp. 53-70). Baltimore: Paul H. Brookes.

Kohnert, K J., Hernandez, A.E., and Bates, E. (1998). Bilingual performance on the Boston Naming Test: Preliminary norms in Spanish and English. *Brain and Language,* 65, 422-440.

Livingston, L.A., Flowers, Y.E., Hodor, B.A., and Ryan, B.P. (2000). The experimental analysis of interruption during conversation for three children who stutter. *Journal of Developmental and Physical Disabilities, 12*, 235-266.

Ludlow, C. L. (1999). Conceptual framework for investigating the neurobiology of stuttering. In N. Bernstein Ratner and E.C. Healey (Eds.). *Stuttering research and practice: bridging the gap* (pp. 63-84). Mahwah, NJ: Lawrence Erlbaum Associates.

Mackey, L.S., Finn, P., and Ingham, R.J. (1997). The effect of speech dialect on speech naturalness ratings: A systematic replication of Martin, Haroldson, and Triden (1984). *Journal of Speech, Language, and Hearing Research, 40*, 349-360.

Maner, K.J., Smith, A., and Grayson, L. (2000). Influences of utterance length and complexity on speech motor performance in children and adults. *Journal of Speech, Language, and Hearing Research, 43*, 560-573.

Manning, W.H. (2001). *Clinical decision making in fluency disorders* (2nd ed.). San Diego: Singular-Thomson Learning.

Mansson, H. (2000). Childhood stuttering: Incidence and development. *Journal of Fluency Disorders, 25*, 47-57.

Maxwell, D.L., and Satake, E. (2006). *Research and statistical methods in communication sciences and disorders*. Toronto: Thomson Delmar Learning.

Mitchell, J., and Jolley, J. (2003). *Research design explained.* 5th edition. Toronto: Wadsworth Thomson Learning.

Nippold, M.J. (2004). Phonological and language disorders in children who stutter: impact on treatment recommendations. *Clinical Linguistics and Phonetics, 18*, 145-159.

Nippold, M.J., and Rudzinski, M. (1995). Parents' speech and children's stuttering: a critique of the literature. *Journal of Speech and Hearing Research, 38*, 978-989.

Okalidou, A., and Kampanaros, M. (2001). Teacher perceptions of communication impairment at screening stage in preschool children living in Patras, Greece. *International Journal of Language and Communication Disorders, 36*, 489-502.

Oscarson, M. (1989). Self-assessment of language proficiency: rationale and applications. *Language Testing, 6*, 1-13.

Paradis, J. and Crago, M. (2000). Tense and temporality: Commonalities and differences in French-speaking children with specific language impairment and French second language speakers. *Journal of Speech, Language and Hearing Research, 43*, 834-848.

Pena, E., Bedore, L.M., and Rappazzo, C. (2003). Comparison of Spanish, English, and bilingual children's performance across semantic tasks. *Language, Speech and Hearing Services in the Schools, 34*, 5-16.

Poulos, M.G. and Webster, W.G. (1991). Family history as a basis for sub-grouping people who stutter. *Journal of Speech and Hearing Research, 34*, 5-10.

Prathanee, B., Thanaviratananich, S., and Pongjanyakul, A. (2003). Oral diadochokinetic rates for normal Thai children. *International Journal of Language and Communication Disorders, 38*, 417-428.

Ralston, L.D. (1981). Stammering: a stress index in Caribbean classrooms. *Journal of Fluency Disorders, 6*, 119-133.

Roberts, P.M. (2001). Aphasia assessment and treatment in bilingual and multicultural populations. In R. Chapey (Ed.). *Language intervention strategies in adult aphasia.* 4th edition (pp. 208-232). Baltimore: Lippincott, Williams and Wilkins.

Roberts, P.M. (2007). Aphasia assessment and treatment in bilingual and multicultural populations. In R. Chapey (Ed.). *Language intervention strategies in adult aphasia.* 5th edition. Baltimore: Lippincott, Williams and Wilkins.

Roberts, P.M. (2002). Disfluency patterns in four bilingual adults who stutter. *Journal of Speech Language Pathology and Audiology, 26*, 5-19.

Roberts, P.M., and Bois, M. (1997). Picture name agreement for French-English bilingual adults. *Brain and Cognition, 40*, 238-241.

Roberts, P.M., Garcia, L.J., Desrochers, A., and Hernandez, D. (2002). English performance of proficient bilingual adults on the Boston Naming Test. *Aphasiology, 16*, 635-645.

Roberts, P.M., and Hébert, T. (2001, August). Le débit et les disfluidités chez des enfants francophones bilingues (Rate of speech and disfluencies in bilingual Francophone children). Paper presented at the 25th world congress of the International Association of Logopedics and Phoniatrics. Montreal.

Roberts, P.M., and Le Dorze, G. (1998). Bilingual aphasia: Semantic organisation, strategy use, and productivity in a semantic verbal fluency task. *Brain and Language*, *65*, 287-312.

Roberts, P.M., and Meltzer, A. (2004). Normal rates and disfluencies in French and English. In A. Packman, A. Meltzer, and H.F.M. Peters (Eds.). *Theory, research and therapy in fluency disorders: Proceedings of the Fourth World Congress of Fluency Disorders* (pp. 389-395). Nijmegen: Nijmegen University Press.

Roberts, P.M. and Shenker, R.C. (2007). Assessment and treatment of stuttering in bilingual children and adults. In R.F. Curlee and E.G. Conture (Eds.) *Stuttering and related disorders of fluency (3rd edition)* (pp.183-209). New York: Thieme Medical Publishers.

Stahl, V., and Totten, G. (1995). Bilingualism in young disfluent children. In C.W. Starkweather and H.F.M. Peters (Eds.) *First World Congress on Fluency Disorders: Proceedings*. The International Fluency Association, Vol. 1, 213.

Stern, E. (1948). A preliminary study of bilingualism and stuttering in four Johannesburg schools. *Journal of Logopedics, 1*, 15-25.

Ström, U. (1995). Speech rate and whole-word repetitions in the speech of three, five and seven year old finnish children. In C.W. Starkweather and H.F.M. Peters (Eds.) *First World Congress on Fluency Disorders: Proceedings*. Vol. 1, 214-217.

Thordardottir, E.T. (2005). Early lexical and syntactic development in Quebec French and English: implications for cross-linguistic and bilingual assessment. *International Journal of Language and Communication Disorders*, *40*, 243-278.

Thordardottir, E. (2006). Language intervention from a bilingual mindset. The ASHA Leader, August 15, 2006, pp. 6, 7, 20, 21.

Travis, L.E., Johnson, W., and Shover, J. (1937). The relation of bilingualism to stuttering: a survey in the east Chicago, Indiana Schools. *Journal of Speech Disorders, 12*, 185-189.

Tzivinikou, S. (2004). Developmental speech problems and bilingualism: the difficulties of identification. *International Education Journal*, *5*, 466-474.

Van Borsel, J., Maes, E., and Foulon, S. (2001). Stuttering and bilingualism: A review. *Journal of Fluency Disorders, 26*, 179-205.

Van Riper, C. (1971). *The nature of stuttering*. Englewood Cliffs, NJ: Prentice-Hall.

Watkins, R.V. (2005). Language abilities of young children who stutter. In Yairi, E. and Ambrose, N.G. (pp. 235-251). *Early childhood stuttering*. Vol 14 of *For clinicians by clinicians*. Series Editors D. Vogel and M.P. Cannito. Austin, TX: Pro-Ed.

Wingate, M.E. (1964). A standard definition of stuttering. *Journal of Speech and Hearing Research*, *29*, 484-489.

World Health Organization. (1977). Manual of the international statistical classification of diseases, injuries, and causes of death (Vol. 1). Geneva: World Health Organization.

Yairi, E., and Ambrose, N.G. (2005). *Early childhood stuttering*. Vol. 14 of *For clinicians by clinicians*. Series Editors D. Vogel and M.P. Cannito. Austin, TX: Pro-Ed.

Yairi, E., Ambrose, N.G., and Cox, N. (1996). Genetics of stuttering: a critical review. *Journal of Speech and Hearing Research*, *39*, 771-784.

Yairi, E., Ambrose, N., Paden, E., and Throneberg, R. (1996). Predictive factors in persistence and recovery: pathways of childhood stuttering. *Journal of Communication Disorders, 29*, 51-77.

Zackheim, C.T. and Conture, E.G. (2003). Childhood stuttering and speech disfluencies in relation to children's mean length of utterance: a preliminary study. *Journal of Fluency Disorders, 28*, 115-142.

In: Speech and Language Disorders in Bilinguals ISBN 978-1-60021-560-5
Editors: Alfredo Ardila and Eliane Ramos, pp. 151-160 © 2007 Nova Science Publishers, Inc.

Chapter 8

BILINGUALISM ACROSS THE LIFE-SPAN UNDER NORMAL AND ABNORMAL CONDITIONS

Alfredo Ardila
Department of Communication Sciences and Disorders
Florida International University
Miami, Florida 33199. USA

INTRODUCTION

At least half of the world population is bilingual (Grosjean, 1982). In consequence, at least half of the cases of aphasia, amnesia, dementia, etc., represent bilingual aphasias, bilingual amnesias, bilingual dementias, etc. Nonetheless, rarely these disorders are approached from a bilingualism perspective. Information, for example, about how cognition disintegrates during dementia in bilinguals; or how memory impairments are manifested if tested in L1 and L2, is extremely scarce. Moreover, excepting the specific research in the area of speech and language disturbances, it is not usual to report in published research if the participants in clinical and experimental investigation were monolinguals or bilinguals; and if bilinguals, the bilingualism characteristics.

In 1989 Hyltenstam and Obler edited the book "*Bilingualism across the Lifespan: Aspects of Acquisition, Maturity, and Loss*", with the primary purpose of analyzing "how the bilingual's two (or more) language systems interact with each other and with other higher cognitive systems, neurological substrata, and social environment" (p. 1). The book represents the most integrative attempt at the moment to understand bilingualism not just in children, but also in adult and elder individuals. Hyltenstam and Obler pointed out that whereas age-dependent language changes are relatively well-understood, life-span linguistic variations in bilinguals is rather diverse, and depend upon a diversity of factors, such as whether both languages were developed simultaneously; whether both languages were used across the life span; whether there were periods when there was not need for one of them; and whether the second language was learned in a formal classroom or acquired in an informal communication situation. Hyltenstam and Obler emphasize in the introductory chapter to the book, that "studies of mature stage bilinguals have to date not constituted a subfield within bilingualism on a par, for example, to second language acquisition" (p. 4). We think that almost 20 years later, this statement is still, to a significant degree, true.

During the last two decades, a significant effort to understand functional activity of the brain in different pathologies and under different cognitive demands has been observed (e.g., Cabeza and Kinstone, 2001). Usually, Positron Emission Tomography (PET) and functional Magnetic Resonance Imaging (fMRI) have been used as the most sophisticated available techniques for understanding the normal and abnormal functioning of the brain. No question, language has been the most frequent research topic in this regard, and several studies have studied the brain organization of oral and written language in bilinguals (e.g., Meschyan and Hernandez, 2006; Pouratian et al., 2000; Roux et al., 2004; Tam et al., 2005). Few studies, however, have analyzed the age-related brain activity changes in bilinguals. Noteworthy, currently the Center for Research in Language at University of California at San Diego is conducting an investigation that is looking at the effects of natural aging on language processes in bilingual individuals (http://crl.ucsd.edu /bilingual/aging.html). Results are not available yet, but toward the future, this type of research program can shed light on the organization of cognition under normal and abnormal conditions in bilingual individuals, and the potential effect of different pathologies in bilinguals.

In this chapter, the effect of abnormal brain conditions on bilinguals will be reviewed. Taking into account, however, that in this book there is a special chapter devoted to the question of aphasia in bilinguals (Roberts and Kiran. Assessment and Treatment of Bilingual Aphasia and Bilingual Anomia. Chapter 6), the analysis of aphasia in bilinguals will not be included. The specific idiosyncrasies of dementia in bilingual individual will be further considered. A brief mention to manifestation of some psychiatric condition in bilinguals will be presented. Finally, some general conclusions will be proposed.

Bilingualism During Normal Aging

Language is the major instrument of social communication and cognition. Language mediates not only the social relationship systems, but also the control of cognitive processes ("metacognition"), and even self-awareness and consciousness (Luria, 1966). Bilinguals use two different language systems to mediate not only their intra-personal (relation with oneself) but also their extra-personal (relations with others) life. Potential differences with monolinguals may be anticipated.

Quite often, the pattern of language use changes across the lifespan. The two languages can be associated with different social contexts and livings situations. The second language can be acquired late in life and related with working activities or migration. L1 and L2 may be used simultaneously only during certain periods of life. The two languages can be acquired early in life and maintained in active use throughout the whole life. And as a matter of fact, a significant diversity of possibilities in the pattern of use of L1 and L2 during the lifespan can be found.

Diverse cognitive changes, including changes in language abilities, are observed during aging (Craik and Bialystok, 2006). During normal aging, a bilingual person can or cannot maintain both languages in active use. L1 is often related with family life and L2 with working activities. If learned early in life, L2 may or may not be a dormant language during adult life. The most typical situation seems to be that during productive life L2 is active, but after retirement, bilinguals tend to decrease the use of L2. Many questions can arise: Is the pattern and characteristics of cognition alike in monolinguals and bilinguals? Is there a comparable pattern of aging in monolinguals and bilinguals? Do both languages present a similar rate of decline during normal and abnormal aging? Does an abnormal brain condition (e.g., a head injury) have the same effect in monolinguals and bilinguals?

Aging and general cognitive decline may have a detrimental effect in the ability to use two different languages. Aging has been related with increased interference between the two languages (Durga, 1978). Interference has been defined as the transference of elements of one language to another at various levels (phonological, grammatical, lexical and orthographical) (Berthold, Mangubhai and Batorowicz, 1997). Two different types of interference may be distinguished: *static* interference: permanent traces of one language on the other; and *dynamic* interference: transient intrusions of the other (deactivated) language (Grosjean, 1982). Alternation, or code switching, between languages occurs commonly amongst bilinguals and may take a number of different forms, including alteration of sentences, and phrases from both languages succeeding each other and switching in a long narrative (Skiba, 1997). The bilingual has to select the appropriate language and keep conversation within it. The bilingual also has to be able to switch between languages when required. The ability to select the appropriate language and switching between languages involves general executive processing and is regarded as a linguistic ability depending upon frontal lobe activity (Hernandez et al., 2001). With aging, this ability to select the appropriate language and make the correct switching when required decreases. The result is an increased mixture of both languages.

Interestingly, histopathological changes in the brain of bilingual individuals have also been reported. Mechelli et al. (2004) found that learning a second language increases the density of grey matter in the left inferior parietal cortex and that the degree of structural reorganization in this region is modulated by the proficiency attained and the age of acquisition.

Abnormal Brain Conditions in Bilinguals

For most people, bilingualism may represent a significant advantage in many regards. Questions remain about the effects of brain pathology in bilingual individuals. Unfortunately, available information is scarce. Trudeau, Colozzo, Sylvestre and Ska (2003) studied a 17-year-old French/English bilingual who had undergone a left functional hemispherectomy. Results revealed important deficits in French and English, affecting expressive and receptive language in both the written and the oral modality. The impairment pattern showed overall similarities between French and English, thus supporting the existence of a common underlying system for these two languages. However, the profiles in each language were not identical, implying that distinct subsystems may also exit.

Few studies have approached the question of specific neurological conditions, such as brain tumors, in bilinguals. Available research, however, has focused on the question of the organization of two languages in the brain, rather than in the specific cognitive disorders observed when using L1 or L2. For instance, Roux and Tremoulet (2002) studied the organization of language areas in bilingual patients using a cortical stimulation paradigm study during surgical process. All bilingual patients were native French speakers. One patient spoke four languages. The patients constituted a non-homogeneous group in terms of language proficiency or age of acquisition. Languages were evaluated and classified into three major groups, depending on proficiency and date of acquisition. Strict overlapping of language areas (for all language tasks) was found in five patients, whereas the remaining seven had at least one area that was language-specific and sometimes task specific. By the same token, Pouratian et al. (2000) investigated language representations in a proficient Spanish/English bilingual patient. The results indicated that there were cortical areas that are activated by the use of both English and Spanish languages (superior temporal sulcus, superior and middle temporal gyri, and parts of the supramarginal gyrus). In addition, language-specific areas were identified in the supramarginal (Spanish) and precentral (English) gyri. These results suggested that cortical language representations in bilingual persons may consist of both overlapping and distinct components. Roux et al. (2004) mapped the cortical areas involved in reading in mono- and bilingual patients. Reading-specific sites were preferentially found when stimulating dominant inferior parietal or posterior temporal areas. Reading arrest sites were found in many regions. In bilingual patients, if common cortical areas could be found, language- and reading-specific areas were sometimes detected, lending support to the concept that bilinguals can have relatively distinct cortical representation of their language skills.

Mendez (2000) reported a case in which a bilingual person developed an anomia in English, his most familiar language, but not in Spanish, his first-learned language. The patient was bilingual and spoke Spanish exclusively until age 7, when he began school then entirely in English. Subsequently, his entire education was in English, and this became his strongest language, both at work and at home. On the initial examination, he had a Wernicke's aphasia in both languages and was diagnosed with an acute left hemisphere stroke at the junction of the left middle cerebral and posterior cerebral arteries. Twenty days after his stroke, the patient complained of residual word-finding difficulty in English but not in Spanish. The patient estimated that prior to his stroke, fluency in Spanish was fair and in English was excellent. After his stroke, he described his fluency as reversed, that is, better in Spanish than in English. On the 60-item Boston Naming Test, however, he demonstrated significantly greater spontaneous naming difficulty in English (n=28) as compared to Spanish (n=43). Ardila (in press) reported the case of a 63 year-old woman with a history of an extensive subarachnoid hemorrhage with left temporal intracerebral hemorrhage presenting a dissociated anomia. She was a Spanish/English late bilingual; her native language was Spanish and her proficiency in English was limited. Nonetheless, during language testing an evident tendency to switch from Spanish to English was observed. Frequently, she answered in English even when the questions were presented in Spanish. Her naming ability was notoriously higher in English than in Spanish.

Dementia in Bilinguals

Communication abilities in bilingual demented patients, and language decline for L1 and L2 in dementia, are questions rarely mentioned in the dementia literature. It is well known, however, that the ability to maintain fluency in more than one language decreases with aging

(Hyltenstam and Obler, 1989). With advancing age, people may tend to retreat to a single language, regardless of a life long history of bilingualism. L2 is frequently associated with active working life, and retirement is often associated with moving to a more limited familiar environment. Moreover, older bilinguals may have increased difficulties handling two different languages due to the effects of cross-language interference. These effects in aging bilingual persons can be further exaggerated in those who develop dementia.

Mendez, Perryman, Ponton, and Cummings (1999) studied 51 patients who reported routine use of another language, as well as varying fluency in English. All patients were regularly exposed to English as a second language after age 13. Despite patients' differences in educational level, age at acquisition of English, frequency of use, and baseline fluency in English, all caregivers reported a greater preference of the patients for their original language and decreased conversation in English. Patients presented an evident tendency for words and phrases from the native language to intrude into English conversational speech. The authors found that bilingual dementia patients tended to present asymmetrical language impairment with preferential preservation and use of the first acquired language. They suggested that in dementia, recently learned information is retained the least and older, more remote information is often relatively preserved, consistent with a regression toward the predominant use of the patient's earliest language. According to Mendez and colleagues, in dementia, a retreat to the original language could result from an exacerbation of the cross-language difficulties that typically increase with age. People who are bilingual never totally deactivate either of their two languages, and this can result in interference or intrusions, particularly from the dominant language into the other one. Dementia patients tend to mix languages, and they have special problems with language separation.

General cognitive functioning has been found to be higher in demented patients if communication is carried out in L1 rather than in L2. Ekman et al (1993, 1994) studied demented persons who were born in Finland and had immigrated to Sweden (Finnish-Swedish bilinguals). They found that many of these Finnish immigrants had difficulties communicating with their Swedish-speaking caregivers, while their communication with a Finnish-speaking caregiver was adequate. The frequent misunderstanding of a person's message often leads to a one-way communication, in which the caregiver commands and interrupts the demented person. The demented Finnish immigrants functioned on a level of manifest competence that seemed far below their level of latent competence. The authors concluded that the presence of Finnish-speaking caregivers is an environmental change that would markedly enhance the demented Finnish immigrants' performance and quality of life and also reduce the costs for their care.

Mendez, Saghafi, and Clark (2004) studied two polyglot patients with semantic dementia. The first case was a 71-year-old man who experienced a slow, progressive loss of his ability to use and understand Spanish and German. The patient was a language teacher who had been fluent in Spanish and used it daily in his work. Confrontational naming in English was decreased. The patient had great difficulty understanding even common nouns in Spanish, and he was no longer able to understand any German words. On an aphasia battery, word comprehension was moderately impaired in English and severely impaired in Spanish and German. Words that were comprehended in Spanish or German were not consistently comprehended in English. His magnetic resonance imaging (MRI) studies showed anterior temporal atrophy, left greater than right. The second case was a 66-year-old man who had a 2-year history of progressive loss of the meaning of words and inability to retrieve words.

Although Spanish was his first language, he spoke English at work and knew some Polish as well. His examination was intact except for naming and recognizing famous faces. Confrontational naming in Spanish was impaired. He could not name pictures of items and made some semantic errors (e.g., "zero" for "circle"). His performance was worse in English than in Spanish, and his Polish was lost. If he comprehended a word in one language, he did not necessarily comprehend it in the other language. His MRI scan showed left anterior temporal atrophy. The authors concluded that in multilingual patients with semantic dementia, semantic anomia was progressively more impaired in their second and third languages compared to their primary languages. Words named and comprehended in one language were not consistently named and comprehended in other languages that they knew. These findings were interpreted as compatible with separate lexical semantic systems for each language.

The difficulty to select the appropriate language is observed in aging bilinguals, but becomes more severe in cases of dementia. It has been suggested that bilingual speakers with dementia, even in the early stages of deterioration, maker errors in selecting the appropriate language, and maintaining the correct language during conversational speech (Hyltenstam and Stroud, 1989, 1993, De Santi et al. 1990). There is, however, large variability in the extent of inappropriate language use, with some individuals showing more language mixing than others (Friedland and Miller, 1999). Hyltenstam and Stroud (1989) described two cases of Alzheimer's disease in bilinguals. In one of them the major problem laid mainly in the area of language choice, whereas in the other the major difficulties were observed in the ability to separate the languages. De Santi et al. (1990) concluded that the ability to make the correct language choice and keep languages separated is correlated with the overall stage of dementia. The mixture may be so significant, that if is not easy to recognize what language the patient is attempting to speak.

Finally, it is interesting that normal bilinguals can use the knowledge of two languages to increase verbal production, whereas dementia patients are unable to profit from the knowledge of two different languages. De Picciotto and Friedland (2001) studied verbal fluency abilities in 30 normal aging English-Afrikaans bilingual speakers, and six bilingual subjects with Alzheimer's disease. A semantic verbal fluency task (to find animal names) was administered in the bilingual mode, Afrikaans and English. There was no significant difference between monolingual and bilingual performance. It was observed that some normal bilingual subjects used code switching as a strategy; there was not, however, a relationship between age of acquisition, pattern of use and verbal fluency scores. In comparison, subjects with Alzheimer's disease did not make use of code switching strategies, and there was some relationship between age of acquisition, pattern of use and verbal fluency scores. In consequence, it was concluded that normal bilinguals can recur to both languages in an attempt to improve performance; demented patients were unable to use this strategy.

Psychiatric Conditions

Rarely, the question of bilingualism is mentioned in the psychiatric literature. During the early 1980s, Hughes (1981) presented a brief review of the available literature. De Zuleta (1984) suggested that bilingualism may be a significant variable in the treatment of psychotic disorders. Heinemann and Assion (1996) reported three polyglot schizophrenic patients who presented a regression to the mother tongue with acute psychosis. All of them, almost exclusively spoke in their native language during acute episodes of psychosis. No question, this is an extremely interesting observation, but it is difficult to conclude that schizophrenia breakdown is always (or at least, generally) associated with a tendency to use only (or at least, predominantly) the native language.

De Zuleta, Gene-Coss and Grachev (2001) observed that polyglot psychotic patients can present with either different or less psychotic symptoms depending on the language they use. Three schizophrenic bilingual patients were analyzed. All three patients were found to have different positive symptoms depending on the language used in the interview procedure by the same bilingual researcher. This dissociation in psychotic symptomatology may suggest different thinking strategies when using the two languages. Haasen, Yaqdiran and Mass (2000) emphasized that in bilinguals both higher and lower rates of psychotic symptoms were found when interviewed in their mother tongues, compared to being interviewed in the second language. In this study, 91 patients of Turkish origin and 50 of German origin with a paranoid-hallucinatory syndrome at admission were examined by an interviewer each of Turkish and German origins using a standardized psychopathological instrument. In spite of comparative samples, correlation of psychopathological evaluation as well as diagnostic agreement between the two interviewers was significantly higher in the German patient group. Within the Turkish patient group, correlation was higher for those with good German language knowledge than for those with poor knowledge, yet only on a few items and without an effect on diagnostic agreement. The greatest difficulties were found in the evaluation of delusions.

Glisky et al (2004) reported a psychogenic fugue in which the individual lost access not only to his autobiographical memories but also to his native German language. A series of experiments compared his performance on a variety of memory and language tests to several groups of control participants including German-English bilinguals who performed the tasks normally or simulated amnesia for the German language. Neuropsychological, behavioral, electrophysiological and functional neuroimaging tests converged on the conclusion that this individual suffered an episode of psychogenic fugue, during which he lost explicit knowledge of his personal past and his native language. At the same time, he appeared to retain implicit knowledge of autobiographical facts and of the semantic or associative structure of the German language.

CONCLUSION

Bilingualism is a heterogeneous phenomenon and patterns of language use across the life-span are diverse. Research has supported the assumption that using two or more different languages can frequently provide not only some social but also cognitive advantages. Life experiences may be associated with the use of a specific language, and life memories are also associated with the contextual language existing when the memory was acquired. The research about different intellectual disturbances in cases of brain pathology has barely approached the question of bilingualism. Nonetheless, it seems that during normal aging there is a more rapid decline of L2 than L1, and elders tend clearly to prefer using L1. In case of dementia, the cognitive defect is more severe when the demented patient is tested in L2 than when tested in L1. Similarly, psychiatric symptomatology can be not totally coincidental if the patient is tested using L1 or L2.

REFERENCES

Ardila, A. (in press). Anomia disociada en un bilingüe tardío: caso clínico [Dissociated anomia in a late bilingual: case report] . *Revista de Neurologia*, en press.

Berthold, M., Mangubhai, F., and Batorowicz, K. (1997). *Bilingualism and Multiculturalism: Study Book*. University of Southern Queensland: Toowoomba, QLD.

Cabeza, R. and Kingstone, A. (2001). *Handbook of Functional Neuroimaging of Cognition.* Cambridge, MA: The MIT Press

Craik, F.I. and Bialystok, E. (2006). Cognition through the lifespan: mechanisms of change. *Trends in Cognitive Sciences, 10*, 131-8.

crl.ucsd.edu/bilingual/aging.html

De Zulueta, F.I, Gene-Cos, N., and Grachev, S. (2001). Differential psychotic symptomatology in polyglot patients: case reports and their implications. *British Journal Medical Psychology, 74*, 277-92

de Picciotto, J. and Friedland, D. (2001). Verbal fluency in elderly bilingual speakers: normative data and preliminary application to Alzheimer's disease. *Folia Phoniatrica et Logopaedica*, 53, 145-52.

De Santi, S., Obler, L. K., Sabo-Abrahamson, H. and Goldberger, J., (1990). Discourse abilities and deficits in multilingual dementia. In Y. Joanette and H. H. Brownell (Eds.), *Discourse Ability and Brain Damage: Theoretical and Empirical Perspectives* (pp. 224-235). New York: Springer.

Durga, R. (1978). Bilingualism and interlingual interference. *Journal of Crosscultural Psychology, 9*, 401-415

Ekman, S.L., Wahlin, T.B., Norberg, A., and Winblad, B. (1993). Relationship between bilingual demented immigrants and bilingual/monolingual caregivers. *International Journal of Aging and Human Development, 37*, 37-54.

Ekman, S.L., Wahlin, T.B., Viitanen, M., Norberg, A., and Winblad, B. (1994). Preconditions for communication in the care of bilingual demented persons. *International Psychogeriatrics, 6*, 105-20.

Friedland, D. and Miller, N. (1999). Language mixing in bilingual speakers with Alzheimer's dementia : A conversation analysis approach. *Aphasiology, 13*, 4- 5, 427-444

Glisky, E.L., Ryan, L., Reminger, S., Hardt, O., Hayes, S.M., and Hupbach, A. (2004). A case of psychogenic fugue: I understand, aber ich verstehe nichts. *Neuropsychologia*, 42, 1132-47

Grosjean, F. (1982). *Life with two languages*. Cambridge, MA: Harvard University Press.

Haasen, C., Yagdiran, O., and Mass, R. (2000). [Differences between psychopathological evaluation in German and Turkish language of Turkish immigrants] *Nervenarzt, 71*, 901-5.

Heinemann, F., and Assion, H.J. (1996). [Language regression to the mother tongue in polyglot patients with acute psychosis]. *Nervenarzt, 67*, 599-601.

Hernandez, A.E., Dapretto, M., Mazziotta, J. and Bookheimer, S. (2001). Language Switching and language representation in Spanish–English bilinguals: An fMRI Study *NeuroImage*, *14*, 510–520

Hughes, G.W. (1981). Neuropsychiatric aspects of bilingualism: a brief review. *British Journal of Psychiatry*, *139*, 25-28.

Hyltenstam, K. and Obler, L.K. (1989) (eds). *Bilingualism Across the Lifespan: Aspects of Acquisition, Maturity, and Loss*. New York: Cambridge University Press

Hyltenstam, K. and Obler, L.K. (1989). Bilingualism across life span: an introduction. In: K. Hyltenstam and L.K. Obler (eds.), *Bilingualism Across the Lifespan: Aspects of Acquisition, Maturity, and Loss.* (pp. 1-12). New York: Cambridge University Press

Hyltenstam, K. and Stroud, C. (1989). Bilingualism in Alzheimer's dementia : Two case studies. In K. Hyltenstam and L. K. Obler (Eds.), *Bilingualism Across the Lifespan : Aspects of Acquisition, Maturity and Loss* (pp. 202-226) . Cambridge: Cambridge University Press

Luria, A.R. (1966). *Human brain and psychological processes*. New York: Harper and Row.

Mechelli, A., Crinion, J.T., Noppeney, U., O'Doherty, J., Ashburner, J., Frackowiak, R.S., and Price, C.J. (2004). Neurolinguistics: structural plasticity in the bilingual brain. *Nature, 431*, 75-77.

Mendez, M.F., Perryman, K.M., Pontón, M.O. and Cummings, J.L (1999). Bilingualism and dementia. *Journal of Neuropsychiatry and Clinical Neurosciences*, 11, 411-412.

Mendez, M. (2000). Language-selective anomia in a bilingual patient. Journal of *Neuropsychiatry and Clinical Neurosciences, 12*, 515-516.

Mendez, M.F., Saghafi, S., Clark, D. G. (2004). Semantic dementia in multilingual patients. *Journal of Neuropsychiatry and Clinical Neurosciences,16,* 381.

Meschyan, G. and Hernandez, A.E. (2006). Impact of language proficiency and orthographic transparency on bilingual word reading: an fMRI investigation. *Neuroimage, 29*, 1135-40.

Pouratian, N., Bookheimer, S.Y., O'Farrell, A.M., Sicotte, N.L., Cannestra, A.F., Becker, D., and Toga, A.W. (2000). Optical imaging of bilingual cortical representations: Case report. *Journal of Neurosurgery, 93*, 676-681.

Roux, F.E., and Tremoulet. M. (2002). Organization of language areas in bilingual patients: a cortical stimulation study. *Journal of Neurosurgery, 97*, 857-64.

Roux, F.E., Lubrano, V., Lauwers-Cances, V., Tremoulet, M., Mascott, C.R., Demonet, J.F. (2004). Intra-operative mapping of cortical areas involved in reading in mono- and bilingual patients. *Brain, 127*, 1796-1810.

Skiba , R. (1997). Code Switching as a Countenance of Language Interference. *The Internet TESL Journal, Vol. III, No. 10*, October, *http://iteslj.org/.*

Tham, W.W., Rickard, L.S.J., Rajapakse, J.C., Choong, L.T,, Ng, S.E., Lim, W.E., and Ho, L.G. (2005). Phonological processing in Chinese-English bilingual biscriptals: An fMRI study. *Neuroimage,* 28, 579-87.

Trudeau, N., Colozzo, P., Sylvestre, V., and Ska, B. (2003). Language following functional left hemispherectomy in a bilingual teenager. *Brain and Cognition, 53*, 384-8.

http://www.edu.bham.ac.uk/bilingualism/database/ctlnlg.htm

http://www.edu.bham.ac.uk/bilingualism/database/biweb.htm

http://www.nethelp.no/cindy/biling-fam.html

In: Speech and Language Disorders in Bilinguals ISBN 978-1-60021-560-5
Editors: Alfredo Ardila and Eliane Ramos, pp. 161-180 © 2007 Nova Science Publishers, Inc.

Chapter 9

CULTURAL AND LINGUISTIC DIVERSITY IN LANGUAGE DISORDERS

Lemmietta G. McNeilly
American Speech-Language Hearing Association
Rockville, MD USA

INTRODUCTION

Speech and Language Disorders exist within a cultural framework. Cultural and linguistic elements of the community are critically important for viewing Communication within bilingual populations. The rules and norms within a community determine whether or not a person's communication behaviors are described as exhibiting some different linguistic features or if it varies significantly from the norm that it is characterized as disordered based on the standards for the speech community. It is important to understand cultural and linguistic diversity (CLD) within the framework of linguistic competence. This chapter will provide operational definitions of CLD and the distinction between communication differences compared to communication disorders. The role of speech-language pathologists in the assessment and clinical management of individuals from bilingual populations will also be addressed in this chapter.

CULTURAL AND LINGUISTIC DIVERSITY DEFINITION

The definition of cultural and linguistic diversity includes the parameters and rules that govern specific cultural groups. Some cultures are monolingual and some are multilingual. Most cultures have rules that govern communication in informal and formal situations. The rules for communicating among friends and families may differ from the rules of communicating in formal situations among individuals who are unfamiliar to each other or who only have a professional relationship.

Cultural Differences in Communication and Learning Styles

Verbal and nonverbal communication differences exist across different cultural groups. These differences may impact the communication among individuals from culturally and linguistically different backgrounds. If misunderstood and/or misinterpreted, many of these communication differences can interfere with the establishment of rapport between clinicians and client families. If clinicians are not familiar with the different rules of communicating, they may inadvertently mistake certain communication behaviors as indicators of a language disorder.

Differences in learning style preferences can impact the assessment process and lead to inaccurate diagnoses or inappropriate treatment recommendations. Therefore, it is important for clinicians to be knowledgeable about the communicative behaviors and learning style variations cross-culturally as well as the potential impact of these differences on the service delivery process.

American English Dialects

The American Speech-Language-Hearing Association (ASHA) has published a technical report regarding the use of dialects (ASHA, 2003). It states that no dialectal variety of American English is a disorder or a pathological form of speech or language. Each dialect is adequate as a functional and effective variety of American English. Each serves a communicative function as well as a social-solidarity function. Each dialect maintains the communication network and the social construct of the community of speakers who use it. Furthermore, each is a symbolic representation of the historical, geographic, social, and cultural background of its speakers. This information provides useful guidance to the professionals in the field of speech-language-pathology regarding the provision of services to speakers of various American English dialects who wish to acquire proficiency in a dialect other than their own.

The type of English spoken in the United States is commonly referred to as American English (AE). "Languages are invariably manifested through their dialects, and to speak a language is to speak some dialect of that language.... the term dialect is defined as a neutral label to refer to any variety of a language which is shared by a group of speakers" (Wolfram, 1991). AE includes social as well as regional dialects that are systematic, highly regular, and cross all linguistic parameters (i.e., phonology, morphology, syntax, semantics, lexicon, pragmatics, and suprasegmental features).

Therefore, each represents a legitimate rule-governed language system. Dialects of AE include, but are not limited to African-American English, Appalachian English, and Standard American English (SAE). Although each dialect has distinguishing characteristics, all share a basic core of grammatical features that are common to all varieties of American English.

The existence of the various dialects is the result of historical, social, linguistic, and geographical factors. For example, due to historical and social factors, the majority of— but not all—speakers of African-American English are African American. But not all African Americans speak African-American English. There is a considerable range of language diversity within each of the different dialectal speech communities, with individual speakers varying their speech in accordance with the sociolinguistic dynamics.

SPEAKERS OF DIALECTS OTHER THAN STANDARD AMERICAN ENGLISH

ASHA's Definitions of Communication Disorders and Variations (ASHA, 1993) stipulate that "a regional, social or cultural/ethnic variation of a symbol system should not be considered a disorder of speech or language." Similarly, the Social Dialects position paper (ASHA, 1993) states that "no dialectal variety of English is a disorder or a pathological form of speech or language." Social dialects inherently are characterized by unique linguistic and cultural features that are systematic, purposeful, and meaningful, and may be found in all linguistic parameters including voice, fluency, prosody, phonology, syntax, pragmatics and semantics. Therefore, students who speak English varieties that are different from the mainstream variety within a school should not be deemed eligible for speech-language services based solely on the language difference that exist between the student and mainstream standard English speaking community.

ENGLISH LANGUAGE LEARNERS AND BILINGUAL STUDENTS

The concept of language disorders in individuals who are bilingual is complex. It is important that SLPs involved in the clinical service delivery process with individuals who speak more than one language possess competence in both languages or the services of an interpreter.

IDEA's "determination of eligibility" (Section 300.534 (b.1.ii)) addresses students who speak languages other than English. This section stipulates that "a child may not be determined to be eligible under this part if the determinant factor for that eligibility determination is limited English proficiency." For the population of students who are learning English as a second language, the linguistic features may be different from those of the mainstream population, because these features reflect the native language, the process of acquiring English, or communication strategies and behaviors of bilingual persons. These differences, which may be misdiagnosed as disorders may occur in the areas of voice, fluency or prosody as well as phonology, syntax, pragmatics, or semantics (ASHA, 1985).

A communication disorder is impairment in the ability to receive, send, process, and comprehend concepts or verbal, nonverbal and graphic symbol systems. A communication disorder may be evident in the processes of hearing, language, and/or speech. A communication disorder may range in severity from mild to profound. It may be developmental or acquired. Individuals may demonstrate one or any combination of communication disorders. A communication disorder may result in a primary disability or it may be secondary to other disabilities (Asha, 1993).

Language is defined as a ruled governed system of organized usage of the phonological, morphological, syntactical, semantic and pragmatic elements. Thus language is defined by its form, content and usage. The form is composed of the phonemes, morphemes and syntax or word order. The content refers to the actual words or nonverbal implied meaning expressed in messages. The rules of language govern how it is used with different partners across varied settings.

Language Disorders Definition

A language is described as disordered when it differs significantly from the norm for the speech community that it calls attention to itself. It has unique characteristics that are a typical in development and may miss critical components of the language. Language disorders are exhibited in phonological, morphological, syntactic, semantic and/or pragmatic components of language.

Language disorders are defined as impaired comprehension and/or use of spoken, written and/or other symbol systems. The disorder may involve (1) the form of language (phonology, morphology, syntax), (2) the content of language (semantics), and/or (3) the function of language in communication (pragmatics) in any combination.

1. Form of Language

a. Phonology is the sound system of a language and the rules that govern the sound combinations.
b. Morphology is the system that governs the structure of words and the construction of word forms.
c. Syntax is the system governing the order and combination of words to form sentences, and the relationships among the elements within a sentence.

2. Content of Language

a. Semantics is the system that governs the meanings of words and sentences.

3. Function of Language

a. Pragmatics is the system that combines the above language components in functional and socially appropriate communication.

Difference Versus Disorder

A speaker of any language or dialect may exhibit a language disorder unrelated to his or her use of the native dialect. An essential step toward making accurate assessments of communication disorders is to distinguish between those aspects of linguistic variation that represent regular patterns in the speaker's dialect and those that represent true disorders in speech and language.

Communication difference or dialect is a variation of a symbol system used by a group of individuals that reflects and is determined by shared regional, social, or cultural/ethnic factors. A regional, social, or cultural/ethnic variation of a symbol system is not considered a disorder of speech or language (Asha 1993).

BILINGUALISM

Bilingualism has been described in detail elsewhere in this book. For the purpose of discussion relative to cultural and linguistic diversity it is important to note that individuals who are bilingual that live in the United States have some unique environmental factors that impact their communication. There is no official language that is stated in the United States' constitution. In the US, American English is the primary language that is taught in schools, spoken on television, printed in newspapers and used in formal situations for conducting business in the US. Within many US communities a variety of different languages are spoken. The definition of bilingualism is the ability to speak and comprehend two languages at a level of competence that is expected for monolinguals. Multiple languages are taught as foreign languages in schools across the US including Spanish, French, and Mandarin Chinese.

CULTURAL AND LINGUISTIC DIVERSITY CONSIDERATIONS

Culturally and linguistically diverse (CLD) students exhibit cultural differences in behaviors, expectations, and belief systems. They use languages other than English; and/or use dialectal variations different from those used in the school setting. For the most part, the eligibility criteria previously stated also applies to CLD students. Special considerations must be taken in order to address the complex and interrelated issues of these populations.

Determining the eligibility for CLD students has been addressed in IDEA, the Bilingual Education Act (amended in 1974 and 1978), and court rulings in Dianna vs. Board of Education (1973), Lau vs. Nichols (1974), Larry P. vs. Riles (1977), and Martin Luther King Junior Elementary School Children vs. Anne Arbor School District Board (1979). Similarly, state laws and best practice patterns elaborated by education and health organizations have also given recommendations for addressing the specific needs of CLD students. In addition, the literature offering guidelines and recommendations is significant (Butler, 1994; Roseberry-McKibbin, 1994; Garcia, 1994; Kahmi, Pollock, and Harris, 1996; Lahey, 1990; Langdon and Saenz, 1996; Seymour and Nober, 1997).

Knowledge And Skills Needed By SLPs and Audiologists to Provide Culturally and Linguistically Competent Professional Services

Speech-language pathologists engaged in the clinical management of individuals who are bilingual need to be knowledgeable of the rules systems of the languages spoken. Awareness of geographical variations of language and knowledge of the cultural values, beliefs and practices that impact the individuals they encounter are also prerequisites.

Bilingual Speech-Language Pathologists and Audiologists

Speech-language pathologists or audiologists who present themselves as bilingual for the purpose of providing clinical services must be able to speak their primary language and to speak (or sign) at least one other language with native or near-native proficiency in lexicon (vocabulary), semantics (meaning), phonology (pronunciation), morphology/syntax (grammar), and pragmatics (uses) during clinical management.

To provide bilingual assessment and remediation services in the client's language, the bilingual speech-language pathologist or audiologist needs to possess the ability to:

1. describe the process of normal speech and language acquisition for both bilingual and monolingual individuals and how those processes are manifested in oral (or manually coded) and written language;
2. administer and interpret formal and informal assessment procedures to distinguish between communication differences and communication disorders in oral (or manually coded) and written language;
3. apply intervention strategies for treatment of communication disorders in the client's language; and
4. recognize cultural factors which affect the delivery of speech-language pathology and audiology services to the client's language community.

Competencies for Speech-Language Pathologists

The speech-language pathologist must have certain competencies to distinguish between dialectal differences and communicative disorders. These competencies include

1. recognizing all American English dialects as rule-governed linguistic systems,
2. understanding the rules and linguistic features of American English dialect(s) represented by their clientele,
3. being familiar with nondiscriminatory testing and dynamic assessment procedures, such as the following:

   - identifying potential sources of test bias,

- administering and scoring standardized tests in alternative manners,
- using observation and nontraditional interview and language sampling techniques, and
- analyzing test results in light of existing information regarding dialect use.

Additionally, clinicians have a social and ethical responsibility to provide potential clients and their families with the opportunity to objectively discuss the use of the target dialect as well as the educational and social ramifications of second dialect acquisition. Clinicians should provide individuals with sufficient information on the historical background, origin, features, and social implications of both the first and the target dialect to facilitate an informed decision. This is particularly important in the case of pediatric clients whose parents and guardians have to make decisions regarding the delivery of services.

The speech-language pathologist should also have an appreciation for the communities and cultures of speakers of AE, as well as a thorough understanding of the social attitudes toward dialect use. Just as competencies are assumed and necessary in the treatment of communication disorders, relevant competencies are also necessary in the provision of elective services to speakers from all American English dialect communities who do not present with a disorder but who wish to improve their overall use of SAE.

ASSESSMENT ISSUES

This is a critical component of the clinical management process. It is important that a SLP who is familiar with the rules of language and communication accurately assesses the individual's linguistic production and comprehension skills in both languages. Cultural issues may impact the case history interview, and the assessment and intervention process. The assessment must yield specific information so that the SLP can clearly determine if the individual's language skills are normal, disordered or different from the standard. This needs to occur for both languages. It is also important to determine which language is the primary language.

The assessment process should include complete case history interview, assessment tools in both languages, tools designed for bilingual populations, assessment of spoken and written language as well as comprehension of the languages.

Different assessment tools are used to assess formal and informal communication skills. Due to the limited number of language assessment tools for languages other than English the clinician may need to employ more criterion reference and informal measures for linguistic competence in other languages.

ASSESSMENT BIAS

According to IDEA 300.532 "Evaluation Procedures," tests selected for evaluation should not be culturally or racially discriminatory and should be administered in the child's native language. It is the speech-language pathologist's responsibility to assure that the outcome of the testing procedure measures the degree of special education the child may require rather than the child's English language proficiency. This reasoning applies both to students who speak two distinct languages and to those who speak varieties of dialects. One mechanism to avoid selecting inappropriate testing tools and procedures is to gauge possible biases. This is done by considering the following biases in tests (Taylor and Payne, 1994):

1. Situational bias addresses the pragmatic mismatches that occur between clinician and student during the testing experience. These mismatches may include "rules of who may speak to whom, appropriate elicitation procedures, appropriate language behaviors, what behavior serves as communication, and rules of production and interpretation." (Taylor and Payne, 1994, p. 97)
2. Directions or format bias refers to unfamiliarity with the testing framework. For example, students may be unfamiliar or have had little experience with some of the tasks required in tests.
3. Value bias considers how cultural experiential differences shape students' values. When a correct response in a test item depends on culturally based knowledge or acceptance different from the student's experience, then there is a mismatch.
4. Linguistic bias occurs when the test does not take into consideration the students' communication systems, such as their first languages or dialect use.

Linguistic Considerations of Bilingual Children

Clinicians should be cautious in making assumptions about bidialectal and/or bilingual children by using frameworks developed solely for monolingual populations. The following practices are recommended:

1. Measure proficiency levels for all modes of communication. It is important to know how the student is able to use the modes for social and academic purposes. Further, academic proficiencies may vary depending on subject matter, linguistic parameter (receptive, expressive, writing, reading), and pragmatics (e.g., answering a question vs. delivering an oral report) (Cummins, 1992; Mackey, 1965; Macnamara, 1969; Oller 1979).
2. Rely on information about characteristics and strategies of bilingualism, bidialectalism, and second-language learning (Damico, 1994; Duran and Chong, 1994; Eastman, 1992; Hoffman, 1991; Hakuta and D'Andrea, 1992; Krashen, 1992; Pica, 1994). These characteristics and strategies may also apply to dialectal speakers learning mainstream English. They include:

    - Transferring knowledge of rules from the native language into the second code, which, for the most part, results in successful learning. When this transfer works unsuccessfully, the student's performance will reflect rules belonging to the native language. They may look like pathologies, but they are not.
    - Making generalizations and simplifications, and using prefabricated phrases until rules are learned.
    - Losing the first language if it is not used socially or for academics.

- Avoiding situations or topics that are not linguistically comfortable.
- Relying on verbal, gestural, or other types of verification.
- Code-switching (using both codes at the same time) for different purposes.
- Stuttering because of lack of vocabulary items or need to process information in one mode before using it in another mode.

3) Identify the normal and expected behaviors of dual code learners and users, and differentiate them from disabilities. This is done first by obtaining information about the linguistic systems the student uses and comparing them to the student's performance. In this way, an attempt is made to identify expected behaviors. Only after this process has been completed can the clinician attempt to identify the residual behaviors as resulting from a disorder. A clear understanding of the systems used will facilitate making contrastive comparisons and gathering information that leads to exhaustive attempts at explaining children's behaviors.

A contrastive analysis of both languages includes some of the following parameters:

- Phonological system: the student may be pronouncing or deleting sounds using the rules and learned behaviors of another language/dialect.
- Grammar and syntax rules: the student's behaviors may reflect only the inappropriate transfer of previously learned rules. Also, inconsistent errors may appear as part of the normal learning process.
- Suprasegmentals and voice: their use may reflect the student's first language/dialect as well as cultural expectations.
- Semantic and vocabulary usage: the student may not be aware that in the second language there is only one word for a concept that uses two words in the first language.
- Dysfluent behaviors: these may appear when using a language being learned and not when using the native language (Acevedo, 1991; Bliele and Wallach, 1992; Iglesias and Anderson, 1993; LeMoine, 1994; Lowe, 1994; Merino, 1992;Tiegerman-Farber, 1995; Willis, 1992; and Wolfram, 1994).

Cultural Considerations of Bilingual Children

The clinician should use ethnographic paradigms to collect information about the child's community, past cultural experiences, and family cultures. Importantly, information about school cultures and systems to which the children have been exposed may explain their behaviors (Langdon, 1993; Langdon and Cheng, 2002; Seymour, 1981; Valdés and Figueroa, 1995). Cultural parameters may include, but are not limited to:

- Behaviors that are incongruent with conventional behaviors, including different types of eye contact, the time it takes to answer questions, and language use with adults.

- Beliefs pertaining to reasons for being tested: who should be doing the testing, how much effort should be expended on assessment exercises, etc.
- Expectations related to school and school personnel roles: what is required of the child, use of information gathered from the assessment procedures, etc.
- The degree of assimilation, including exposure to school subject matter, level of comfort with relating to new environments and persons, and adeptness at using methods to demonstrate learning.

COLLABORATING WITH INTERPRETERS/TRANSLATORS

IDEA '97 specifies that collaboration with an interpreter or translator (I/T)* is necessary to assess children when specialists do not share their primary language. Although the law does not specify the need to work with these children in their primary language, all family conferences and legal documents must be delivered in the family's primary language.

Despite these legal mandates, there has been limited literature documenting preferred strategies to implement this process. It is not unusual for a school to request assistance from anyone on the staff, including janitors or secretaries, or from family members to serve as I/Ts, just because they are bilinguals. This practice should be avoided at all costs (Langdon, 2002). The majority of these individuals have not been adequately trained to serve as an I/T.

Specific procedures should be followed when selecting an I/T. The fact that someone is bilingual does not mean that the person can fulfill the complex tasks of being an I/T who collaborates with a speech-language pathologist or audiologist. The I/T should have training in procedures followed by each professional. In addition, the communicative disorders professional should be trained on how to work effectively with an interpreter. Further information on roles and responsibilities of each team member and recommended procedures can be found in Langdon and Cheng (2002). The handbook that is a companion to this book is written specifically for the I/T (Langdon, 2002).

Training an I/T to participate in the assessment process should involve specific steps. Some stepsare highlighted here. (Cheng, Langdon, and Davies, 1991; Fradd, 1993; Langdon and Cheng, 2002; Langdon, 2002):

- The speech-language pathologist or audiologist must adequately train the I/T on specific procedures that are followed when assessing a child.
- The speech-language pathologist or audiologist, in conjunction with the administration, must provide the IT with appropriate and necessary materials, such as dictionaries or access to the Internet, to search specific references in a given language.
- All parties should have adequate time. It may take twice as long to complete a given task when the collaboration of an I/T is needed.
- The speech-language pathologist or audiologist is the professional who is ultimately responsible for providing a diagnosis and for offering suggestions to the parents, child, and other teachers.
- Three basic steps are followed during the interpreting process: briefing, interaction, and debriefing (Langdon, 2002).

*Interpreting is conveying a message presented orally from one language to another language. Translating means conveying the message from one language to the other using the written modality.

Interpreters may be used in the process, but there are specific rules of engagement that should be followed. The family members should not be used. A neutral party that is competent in the language and dialectal variation spoken by the individual is best. It is also necessary for the SLP to have a meeting with the interpreter prior to the assessment to calibrate the procedures and expectations. It is important to note that Spanish semantics varies based on the country of origin. Spanish spoken by individuals from Mexico, Puerto Rico, Columbia and Spain will have different linguistic features. Linguistic differences may be characterized in any or all of the different categories of language including phonology, morphology, syntax, semantics and pragmatics.

Intervention with Multicultural Populations

There are several issues which should be taken into consideration when attempting to design an intervention program for the culturally/linguistically diverse client. As with assessment, there are a number of cross-cultural communication and learning style differences that can impact the intervention process. Differing cross-cultural views of health and disorder as well as differing beliefs as to what constitutes the most appropriate treatment approach for addressing various conditions can also play a role. Finally, when working with the bilingual or nonstandard English client, clinicians must also determine the most appropriate language of intervention.

Management Issues for Language Disorders

The specific goals of clinical intervention with children that exhibit language disorders are determined based on the results of the assessments. The tools utilized should yield specific information across settings, audiences and languages if the child speaks more than one language. The setting will also impact the goals. If services are rendered in a school then the goals need to address educationally relevant skills. If services are rendered in outpatient facilities they need to address medical, clinical and or functional relevant skills.

The SLP delivering the services should be knowledgeable of the linguistic characteristics of the languages and/or dialectal variations spoken by the child. If the SLP is monolingual and is aware of some of the linguistic features of the language he or she needs to be knowledgeable in using an interpreter within the treatment session. It is important that the clinician and the interpreter have adequate time to meet and prepare for the session without the child being present.

The decisions regarding which language to deliver intervention in is one that should be determined by the family, SLP and other members of the interdisciplinary team. Many times the decision is based on the language or dialect that is spoken in the school or clinical facility. The decisions should emphasize the child's first or primary language. Sometimes intervention is offered in two languages using two different clinicians. If a child is linguistically compentent in the first language and has recently started speaking a second language and the results of the assessment clearly indicate that the child has not yet acquired linguistic competence in the second language then the child should not be classified as having a language disorder. This child could benefit from specific instruction in the second language but the child should not be labeled as having a language disorder in the second language.

The specific topics which are addressed by the readings referenced in this fact sheet include:

- Guidelines for determining the most appropriate language of intervention with bilingual and nonstandard English speaking clients;
- Cultural factors that impact on the intervention process;
- Implementing a culturally appropriate intervention program;
- Selecting culturally sensitive materials and activities.

Elective Services

The traditional role of the speech-language pathologist has been to provide clinical services to individuals with communication disorders. It is also within the scope of practice for speech-language pathologists to provide elective services. Given that Standard American English (SAE) is the linguistic variety used by the government, the mass media, business, education, science, and the arts in the United States, speakers of other varieties of American English may find it advantageous to be able to speak SAE. In these cases, the role of the speech-language pathologist is to assist in the acquisition of the desired competency in the second dialect without jeopardizing the integrity of the individual's first dialect. The approach of the elective service must be functional and must emphasize the appropriateness of the first and second dialects for different contexts.

Resources

There are many resources available to speech language pathologists that work with individuals and families who speak multiple languages or variations of a language. I've highlighted some in this section of the chapter. The American Speech-Language-Hearing Association website offers position statements, technical reports, knowledge and skills documents and clinical practice guidelines. Additionally there are bibliographic references organized based on assessment, intervention, bilingualism, and dialectal variations. Some of the specific topics that are addressed by the readings referenced include:

- Cultural differences in verbal and nonverbal communication;
- Cultural differences in communicative(discourse) and narrative style;
- Cultural norms for greeting and addressing individuals;
- Culturally based learning style preferences;
- Cultural differences in rules for adult-child discourse;
- Cultural differences in the conversational roles of children;

- The impact of cultural communication and learning style differences on the educational and/or clinical process.

Additionally, the Multicultural Issues Board of the American Speech-Language-Hearing Association developed a list of resources which include fact sheets and 26 different lists of suggested readings and related materials for individuals interested in obtaining a more in-depth understanding of the following issues:

- Multicultural History and Demographic Profile of the United States
- Cultural Differences in Communication and Learning Styles
- Language Attitudes and Educational Policy
- Intervention With Multicultural Populations
- Research on Multicultural Populations/Ethnography
- Service Delivery with Multicultural Populations

(These are available from the American Speech-Language-Hearing Association.)

LANGUAGE ACQUISITION

Studies involving functional imaging methodology provide a mechanism to investigate the differences in the pattern of cerebral activation associated with a subject's native language (L1) compared with a second language (L2). In 1998 a PET investigation conducted by Perani and colleagues on bilingualism, described auditory processing of stories in L1 (Italian) compared to L2 (English). The PET results illustrated the engagement of the temporal lobes and temporoparietal cortex more extensively in L1 than L2. However, in that study the Italian subjects learned L2 late and attained a fair, but not an excellent command of this language (low proficiency, late acquisition bilinguals). Thus, the different patterns of activation could be ascribed either to age of acquisition or to proficiency level. In the current study we use a similar paradigm to evaluate the effect of early and late acquisition of L2 in highly proficient bilinguals. They studied a group of Italian-English bilinguals who acquired L2 after the age of 10 years (high proficiency, late acquisition bilinguals) and a group of Spanish-Catalan bilinguals who acquired L2 before the age of 4 years (high proficiency, early acquisition bilinguals). The differing cortical responses we had observed when low proficiency volunteers listened to stories in L1 and L2 were not found in either of the high proficiency groups in this study. Several brain areas, similar to those observed for L1 in low proficiency bilinguals, were activated by L2. These findings suggest that, at least for pairs of L1 and L2 languages that are fairly close, attained proficiency is more important than age of acquisition as a determinant of the cortical representation of L2 (Perani, D et al., 1998).

ADULT LANGUAGE DISORDERS

Language disorders have been studied in bilingual adults. Comparisons have been made to language disorders in monolingual adults. There are numerous considerations when adequately assessing and designing intervention programs for bilingual adults who exhibit language disorders. Being bilingual does not exempt an adult from acquiring language disorders. The profile of how language disorders are displayed in each language is important and offers suggestions to designing intervention. The manifestation of language disorders are not exactly the same in both languages. The symptoms are not static. Changes in the symptoms presented are observable over time. On one day L1 may be more impaired than L2. The following session the reverse may occur. The differences also cross subsystems of language and are exhibited in both language comprehension and expression.

Since most people in the world know more than one language, bilingual aphasia is an important line of research in clinical and theoretical neurolinguistics. From a clinical and ethical viewpoint, it is no longer acceptable that bilingual aphasics be assessed in only one of the languages they know. Bilingual aphasic patients should receive comparable language tests in all their languages. In 2001, Fabbro studied language recovery in 20 bilingual Friulian-Italian aphasics. Thirteen patients (65%) showed a similar impairment in both languages (parallel recovery), four patients (20%) showed a greater impairment of L2, while three patients (15%) showed a greater impairment of L1. Despite the many hypotheses advanced to account for nonparallel recovery, none of them seem to provide satisfactory explanations. The study of bilingual aphasics with parallel impairment of both languages allows verification of the hypothesis whereby grammatical disorders in aphasia depend on the specific structure of each language. As far as rehabilitation programs for multilingual aphasics are concerned, several questions have been raised, many of which still need a satisfactory answer (Fabbro, 2001).

A number of constructs developed to account for the bilingual aphasia phenomena have been presented to increase understanding of language representation, processing, breakdown and rehabilitation in unilinguals as well. In particular, focus on the right-hemisphere-based pragmatic component of verbal communicative competence, the activation threshold, the control of resources, the role of emotion in second language acquisition and that of procedural vs. declarative memory, has led to the suggestion that monolinguals are in fact at one end of a continuum, with individuals who are multilingual that speak genetically unrelated languages at the other end. No function is available to the bilingual speaker that is not already available to the monolingual, unidialectal speaker. The only difference seems to be the degree of use the speaker makes of each of the relevant cerebral systems (Paradis, 2000).

Working Memory in Adults

Working memory plays a crucial role in learning a L2. Difficulties in using the phonological system, and hence, the phonological store and articulatory rehearsal, is partially responsible for the defects in language understanding in a L2. The effort required for phonological discrimination can decrease working memory capacity, thus impacting language comprehension (Ardila, 2003).

Words function as low frequency words in L2. Semantic searches require more time to complete and language processing is slower. Working memory appears to be more efficient in L1 than in L2. There are observable differences in problem solving skills in two languages within the brain of a bilingual person. Brain activation patterns during working memory tasks are more complex when the person uses the L2 than when using L1 (Ardila, 2003).

Previous research has found differences in the speed and accuracy of responses involving concrete cognate nouns and non-cognate nouns in a range of written and "on-line" tasks using neurologically unimpaired, bilingual adults. The Roberts and Deslauriers study investigated whether cognateness affects verbal confrontation naming performance in balanced French/English bilinguals (N = 15 aphasic and 15 non-aphasic subjects). Subjects in that study met selection criteria for equal proficiency, regular use, and early acquisition of both languages. Results of a picture naming test show that cognate pictures were more often correctly named in both languages than were non-cognates. Some error types and self-correction behaviors also varied with cognate status. There were similarities between the results of this study and those of previous studies of monolingual naming. Some error types and self-correction strategies appear to be unique to bilingual speakers. Theoretical questions and treatment applications arising from these findings are outlined (Roberts and Deslauriers, 1999).

Conclusion

The framework of cultural and linguistic diversity is paramount when assessing and designing clinical intervention strategies for children and adults from bilingual populations that exhibit language disorders. This chapter provides operational definitions of communication disorders, language disorders, cultural and linguistic diversity as well as dialectal variations of language. These serve as the foundation upon which a speech-language pathologist competently plans and executes clinical management of bilingual children and adults.

The assessment process is a critical component and determines what the diagnosis is and the resulting clinical management recommendations. Children from bilingual homes may exhibit language disorders in their primary language or they may only present with some linguistic features that represent the second language acquisition has not reached a level of linguistic competence.

Finally, individuals that speak variations of a language may not exhibit a disorder but their speech may be characterized by several dialectal variations of the language that are appropriate for their speech community. The family is important in the clinical process. They serve as a source of validation of the linguistic behaviors that the SLP analyzes and they are critical in successful clinical management as well. Language disorders cannot be adequately assessed or managed in the absence of the cultural and linguistic framework of the speech community.

References

Abudarham, S. (1987). Speech therapy for the child with a dual language system and/or background--Management issues in bilingualism. In S. Abudarham (Ed.), Bilingualism and the bilingual: An interdisciplinary approach to pedagogical and remedial Issues. Berkshire, UK: NFER-NELSON.

Acevedo, M. A. (1991, November). Spanish consonant acquisition among two groups of Head Start children. Paper presented at the annual meeting of the American Speech-Language-Hearing Association, Atlanta, GA.

American Speech-Language-Hearing Association. (1983). Position paper: Social dialects and Implications of the position on social dialects. Asha, 25 (9), 23-27.

American Speech-Language-Hearing Association. (1985). Clinical management of communicatively handicapped minority language populations. Asha, 27(6), 29-32.

American Speech-Language-Hearing Association. (1989, March). Bilingual speech-language pathologists and audiologists. Asha, 93.

American Speech-Language-Hearing Association. (1991a). Guidelines for speech-language pathologists serving persons with language, socio-communicative, and/or cognitive-communicative impairments. Asha, 33, (Suppl. 5), 21-28.

American Speech-Language-Hearing Association. (1992). Our multicultural agenda: We're serious. Asha, 34(5), 38- 39.

American Speech-Language-Hearing Association. (1993a). Definitions of communication disorders and variations. Asha, 35, (Suppl. 10), 40-41.

American Speech-Language-Hearing Association. (1998a). Provision of English-as-a-second-language instruction by speech-language pathologists in school settings: Position statement and technical report. Asha, 40 (Suppl. 18).

American Speech-Language-Hearing Association. (1998b). Students and professionals who speak English with accents and nonstandard dialects: Issues and recommendations. Asha, 40 (Suppl. 18).

American Speech-Language-Hearing Association. (2003). Technical Report: American English Dialects. ASHA Supplement 23.

American Speech-Language-Hearing Association. (2004). Knowledge and Skills Needed by SLPs and Audiologists to Provide Culturally and Linguistically Competent Professional Services Asha Supplement 24.

Anderson, N. and Battle, D. (1993). Cultural diversity in the development of language. In D. Battle (Ed.), Communication disorders in multicultural populations. Boston: Andover Medical Publishers.

Ardila, A. (2003). Language representation and working memory with bilinguals. Journal of Communication Disorders 36:233-40.

Bliele, K. M. and Wallach, H. (1992). A sociolinguistic investigation of the speech of African American preschoolers. *American Journal of Speech-Language Pathology, 1*(2), 54-62.

Butler, K. (1994). Cross-cultural perspectives in language assessment and intervention. Gaithersburg, MD: Aspen Publishers, Inc.

Campbell, L. (1993). Maintaining the integrity of children's home communicative variety: Speakers of Black English Vernacular. AJSLP 2(1), 11-12.

Chambers, J. K., and Trudgill, P. (1999). Dialectology (2nd ed.). Cambridge, U.K.: Cambridge University Press.

Cheng, L.L. (1999). Moving beyond accent: Social and cultural realities of living with many tongues. Topics in Language Disorders, 19(4), 1-11.

Cheng, L .L., Langdcn, H. W., and Davies, D. (1991) (Color video-28 minutes). *The art of interpreting: A dynamic process*. (color video-28 minutes). San Diego, CA: San Diego State University Department of Communication Disorders.

Clark, L.W. (1993). Faculty and student challenges in facing cultural and linguistic diversity . Springfield, IL: Charles C. Thomas.Cole, L., Holley, S.C., Taylor, O.L., Yoder, D.E., and Iglesias, A. (1989. September). Trustees of the dream. Asha, 71-75.

Courts, P.L. (1997). Multicultural literacies: Dialect, discourse, and diversity. New York: Peter Lang Publishing

Cummins, J. (1986). Empowering minority students: A framework for intervention. Harvard Educational Review, 56 , 18-36.

Cummins, J. (1992). Bilingual education and English immersion: The Ramirez report in theoretical perspective. *Bilingual Research Journal, 16*(1, 2), 91–104.

Damico, J. S. (1994). Assessment procedures with children. Paper presented at the Conference on Culturally Competent Assessment and Intervention with Hispanic and Asian/Pacific Islander Populations, Maui, Hawaii.

Damico, J., and Damico, S. (1993). Language and social skills from a diversity perspective: Considerations for the speech language pathologist. Language, Speech, and Hearing Services in Schools, 24 (4), 236-243.

Duran, E. and Chong, R. (1994). A look at second language learners with moderate to severe disabilities and autism and how they acquire English: A qualitative study. Paper presented at the Symposium on Second Language Learners in Regular and Special Education, Sacramento, CA.

Eastman, C. M. (1992). Code switching in an urban language, contact phenomenon. *Journal of Multilingual and Multicultural Development, 13* (1, 2), 1–17.

Fabbro, F. (2001). The bilingual brain: Bilingual aphasia. Brain and Language, vol. 79, n°2, pp. 201-210.

Fradd, S.H. (1993). Creating the team to assist culturally and linguistically diverse students. Tucson, AZ: Communication Skill Builders.

Garcia, S. B. (1994). Addressing cultural and linguistic diversity in special education: Issues and trends. Reston, VA: The Council for Exceptional Children.

Gutierrez-Clellen, V. and Quinn, R. (1993). Assessing narratives of children from diverse cultural/linguistic groups. Language, Speech, and Hearing Services in Schools, 24(1) , 2-9.

Gutierrez-Clellen, V.F., Pena, E., and Quinn, R. (1995) Accommodating cultural differences in narrative style: A multicultural perspective. Topics in Language Disorders,15(4).

Hakuta, K. and D'Andrea, D. (1992). Some properties of bilingual maintenance and loss in Mexican background high-school students. *Applied Linguistics,13*(1), 72–99.

Heath, S. B. (1991). Ways with words: Language, life and work in communities and classrooms. NY: Cambridge University.

Heath, S. B. (1986). Sociocultural contexts of language development. In Beyond language: Social and cultural factors in schooling language minority students. Los Angeles, CA: Evaluation, Dissemination, and Assessment Center, California State University.

Hoffman, C. (1991). *An introduction to bilingualism*. London: Longman.

Holmes, J. (2001). An introduction to sociolinguistics (2nd ed.). New York: Longman Publishing Group.

Hudson, R.A. (1980). Sociolinguistics. Cambridge, U.K.: Cambridge University Press.

Individuals with Disabilities Education Act Amendments of 1997. Washington, DC: U.S. Government Printing Office. 20 U.S.C. § 1400 *et seq.*

Iglesias, A. and Anderson, B. (1993). Communication in the home and classroom: Match or mismatch? *Topics in Language Disorders, 5* (4), 29-41.

Jimenez, B. (1987) Acquisition of Spanish consonants in children aged 3-5 years, 7 months. *Language, Speech, and Hearing Services in Schools, 18*, 357 363.

Kahmi, A. G., Pollock, K. E., and Harris, J. L. (1996). Communication development and disorders in African American children: Research, assessment, and intervention. Baltimore, MD: Paul H. Brookes Publishing Co.

Krashen, S.D. (1992). Bilingual education and second language acquisition theory. In C. Leyba (Ed.), *Schooling and language minority students: A theoretical framework.* Los Angeles: California State University.

Lahey, M. (1990). Who shall be called language disorders? Some reflection and one perspective. *Journal of Speech and Hearing Disorders, 55*, 612 620.

Langdon, H.W. (1993). Twenty-two facts about Hispanic students, clients, and their families to consider in teaching courses in communication disorders. Paper presented at the annual meeting of the California Speech-Language-Hearing Association. Palm Springs.

Langdon, H. W. (2002). *Working with interpreters to serve bilingual children and their families.* Video, ASHA.Lippi-Green, R. (1997). English with an accent: Language, ideology, and discrimination in the United States. London/New York: Rutledge.

Langdon,HW and Cheng,LL. (2002). Collaborating With Interpreters and Translators: A Guide for Communication Disorders Professionals. Eau Claire, WI: Thinking Publications.

Langdon, H.W., and Saenz, T. I. (1996). *Language assessment and intervention with multicultural students.* Oceanside, CA: Academic Communication Associates.

LeMoine, N. (1994). Serving the "language different" student: A paradigm shift. Paper presented at the annual meeting of the California Speech-Language-Hearing Association, Sacramento.

Lowe, R. J. (1994). *Phonology: Assessment and intervention applications in speech pathology.* Baltimore: Williams and Wilkins.

Mackey, W.F. (1955). *Language teaching analysis.* London: Logan.

Macnamara, J. (1969). How can one measure the extent of a person's bilingual proficiency? In L.G. Kelly (Ed.), *Description and measurement of bilingualism.* Toronto: University of Toronto Press.

McWhorter, J. (2000). Spreading the word: Language and dialect in America. Portsmouth, NH: Heinemann Publishing.

Merino, B. (1992). Acquisition of syntactic and phonological features in Spanish. In H.W. Langdon (Ed.), *Hispanic children and adults with communication disorders: Assessment and intervention.* Gaithersburg, MD: Aspen.

Miller, N. and Abudarham, S. (1984). Management of communication problems in bilingual children. In N. Miller (Ed.), Bilingualism and language disability. San Diego, CA: College-Hill Press.

Oller, J.W. (1979). *Language tests at school.* London: Longman.

Paradis, M. (2000). Generalizable Outcomes of Bilingual Aphasia Research. *Folia Phoniatrica et Logopaedica ;52:54-64.*

Perani, D., Paulesu, E., Galles, NS., Dupoux, E., Dehaene, S., Bettinardi, V., Cappa, S., Fazio, F., and J Mehler (1998). The bilingual brain. Proficiency and age of acquisition of the second language. Brain; 121; 10: 1841-52.

Perozzi, J. and Sanchez, M. (1992). The effect of instruction in L1 on receptive acquisition of L2 for bilingual children with language delay. Language, Speech, and Hearing Services in Schools, 23(4) , 348-352.

Pica, T. (1994). Questions from the language classroom: Teacher perspectives. *TESOL Quarterly, 28* (1), 49 80.Rickford, J. R. (1999). African American vernacular English. Malden, MA: Blackwell Publishers.

Rickford, J. R. (2000). Spoken soul: The story of Black English. New York: John Wiley. Taylor, O. (1971). Response to social dialects and the field of speech. In Sociolinguistics: A cross-disciplinary perspective (pp. 13-20). Arlington, VA: Center for Applied Linguistics. (ERIC Document Services No. ED 130 500).

Roberts, P. and Deslauriers, L. (1999). Picture naming of cognate and non-cognate nouns in bilingual aphasia. Journal of Communication Disorders.

Roseberry-McKibbin, C. (1994). *Multiculturism students with special language needs.* Oceanside, CA: Academic Communication Associates.

Seymour, S. (1981). Cooperation and competition: Some issues and problems in cross cultural analysis. In R. Monroe and B. Whiting (Eds.), *Handbook of cross cultural human development.* New York: Garland.

Seymour, C. M., and Nober, E. H. (1997). *Introduction to communication disorders: A multicultural approach.* Woburn, MA: Butterworth-Heinemann.

Taylor, O., and Payne, K. (1994). Culturally valid testing: A proactive approach. In K. Butler (Ed.), *Cross-cultural perspectives in language assessment and intervention.* Gaithersburg, MD: Aspen Publications.

Tiegerman-Farber, E. (1995). *Language and communication intervention in preschool children.* Needham Heights, MA: Allyn and Bacon.

Valdés, G., and Figueroa, R. (1995). *Bilingualism and testing: A special case of bias.* Norwood, NJ: Ablex Publishing Corporation

Wallace, G., Cole, T., Fairley, D., Harris, A., Hughes, C., Maiden, Y., Nunn, S., Paige, S., Sangster, A., Tebbe, L., Terry, A., and Redden E. (1997). Activities that build student leaders: Ways to promote multicultural neurogenics in the 21st century. Newsletter of the ASHA Special Interest Division 14: Communication Disorders and Sciences in Culturally and Linguistically Diverse Populations, 3(2), 13-14.

Willis, W. (1992). Families with African American roots. In E.W. Lynch and M.J. Hanson (Eds.), *Developing cross-cultural competence: A guide for working with young children and their families.* Baltimore: Paul H. Brookes Publishing Co.

Wolfram, W. (1991). Interlanguage Variation: A Review Article. Applied Linguistics. Mar 1991; 12: 102 - 106.

Wolfram, W., Adger, C.T., and Christian, D. (1999). Dialects in schools and communities. Mahweh, NJ: Lawrence Erlbaum Associates.

Wolfram, W. (1994). The phonology of a sociocultural variety: The case of African American Vernacular English. In J. Bernthal and N. Bankson (Eds.), *Child Phonology: Characteristics, assessment, and intervention with special populations.* New York: Thieme Medical Publishers.

Wong Fillmore, L. (1991). When losing a second language means losing the first. *Early Childhood Research Quarterly, 6,* 323 346.

Wyatt, T.A. (1995). Language development in African American English child speech. Linguistics and Education, 7, 7-22.

In: Speech and Language Disorders in Bilinguals ISBN 978-1-60021-560-5
Editors: Alfredo Ardila and Eliane Ramos, pp. 181-194

Chapter 10

SPEECH AND LANGUAGE ASSESSMENT IN BILINGUALS

Eliane Ramos
Department of Communication Sciences and Disorders
Florida International University
Miami, Florida 33199 USA

INTRODUCTION

The assessment of speech and language skills in bilingual children and adults has received increasing attention in both clinical and academic settings. Clinicians are faced with increasing numbers of bilingual individuals who need fair and appropriate assessments, and academic programs are hard pressed to adequately prepare these clinicians to step up to this challenge. The assessment process is far from straightforward in monolinguals, but it can become a daunting task when the complexities of bilingualism are added to it. As Grosjean stated, "working with bilinguals is a more difficult and challenging enterprise" (1998, p. 131). This chapter will systematically review the assessment process for monolinguals and describe how this process needs to be adapted for bilinguals. In doing so, an attempt will be made to include the issues raised in relevant chapters of this book to emphasize the need to incorporate research findings in clinical practice (evidence-based practice) as recommended by the American Speech-Language-Hearing Association (ASHA, 2005).

Before delving into the specifics of assessment procedures, the question of how adult bilingual populations differ from child bilingual populations must be addressed. Much attention has been devoted to child bilingualism in recent literature in communication disorders (See Bedore, Peña, Garcia, and Cortez, 2005; Genesee, Paradis, and Crago, 2004; Paradis, Crago, Genesee and Rice, 2003; Goldstein, 2004; Kayser, 1998; Paradis, 2005; Restrepo, 1998). This focus on children is probably due to the continued scrutiny school systems suffer to comply with educational legislature, which requires that a free and appropriate education must be provided to every child with a disability. The question of what is appropriate for a bilingual child must be answered before compliance can be achieved. For bilingual children with speech and language difficulties, clinicians must show that any delays are due to an underlying problem with the mechanism for acquiring speech and language skills, rather than a normal process in acquiring a second language.

It is beyond the scope of this chapter to go into the intricacies involved in making that diagnosis. However, there is one major difference between adults and children: In the case of children, whether they are simultaneous or sequential bilinguals, the clinician is dealing with a developing system, where neither of the two languages are fully acquired. Theoretically, if children show age-appropriate skills in at least one of their languages, the presence of a language disorder can be discarded. The resulting conclusion that a language disorder is present if language skills are delayed in both languages is fallacious. A number of circumstances may lead to a finding of delays in both languages without a true language disorder. Setting aside the major issue that standardized tests selected for assessments are nearly always inappropriate for testing bilingual children, these children are a special case because development of L1 may have stagnated due to lack of exposure in L1 while L2 is still being acquired, or L1 skills may have deteriorated due to attrition from L2 (Anderson, 1999; Kirshner, 1996; Kohnert, 2004; Restrepo and Kruth, 2000; Seliger and Vago, 1991). These issues are not trivial, and often play a deciding role when determining the presence of a language disorder in children. Much of a speech-language pathologist's energy and skills in assessing a bilingual child go into sorting out whether the apparent language delays found are due to a difference or a disorder.

In contrast, the presence of a disorder in adults is not usually a point of contention. Clinicians are faced with adults who were perfectly able to communicate in one or more languages in their daily lives until some major event took place. That event may have had a sudden onset, perhaps due to a stroke or a traumatic brain injury, or a more gradual onset, such as is the case with degenerative neurological disorders. The result is that the patient and/or friends and family members clearly notice a deterioration in communication ability. There is no question that a communication impairment is present. The clinician's challenge in such cases is two-fold: 1) To show that the impairment is severe enough to pose a functional limitation to the patient (e.g., see Agency for Healthcare Research and Quality report, 2002), and thus qualify clients for insurance coverage; 2) To plan for intervention, which requires a careful description of what language components have been affected and the steps that must be taken to ameliorate them or return them to as close to pre-morbid performance as possible.

These two challenges interact in very complex ways in bilingual patients. For example, what constitutes a "functional limitation" to a Spanish-English bilingual living in the U.S. whose English skills have been mostly preserved while his Spanish skills were severely affected? Is it justifiable to provide therapy in Spanish if this patient is perfectly capable of functioning in English? No doubt the clinician will want to obtain a careful case history to ascertain the roles that each language plays in this patient's life. An ethnographic approach to describe the patient's history and expected future performance would be most appropriate (e.g., Centeno, chapter 11, this volume).

In monolingual patients, describing what language components have been affected by the disorder is fairly straightforward. Clinicians can rely on their knowledge of what skills typical adult speakers of that language have and attribute any discrepancies to the disorder. With bilingual speakers, what constitutes typical performance will depend on a number of variables and may be impossible to describe. The level of proficiency achieved in each language pre-morbidly is often specific to each patient and nearly impossible to assess. Obler and Mahecha (1991) examined 156 reported cases of bilinguals with aphasia to determine patterns of impairment and recovery in each language. They found that pre-morbid levels of proficiency in each language was often missing in the files. Such a finding is not surprising given that no uniform guidelines exist for clinicians who assess bilingual patients. As we examine the assessment process, we will keep these two challenges in mind and develop recommendations on how they can be overcome.

Assessment Procedures

Case History

Every speech and language assessment must start with a detailed history, which usually includes a written case history with biographical information such as name and age as well as the medical diagnosis, medications taken, information from other professionals, and onset of problems. This information is later verified in an interview with the patient and/or family members when more detailed information can be obtained (Hedgeand Davis, 2005, Shipley and McAfee, 2004). For bilingual clients, detailed information on the bilingual history is imperative (e.g., Centeno, 2005). At the very minimum, such information should include:

Age of exposure to L2 (simultaneous or sequential)
Context in which each language was learned (e.g., L1 at home, L2 at school)
Level of education/literacy skills in each language
Language preference/dominance
Context and frequency of use of each language pre-morbidly
Estimate of language proficiency in comprehension, expression, reading, and writing
Extent of code mixing pre-morbidly

Careful gathering of the bilingual history will facilitate the diagnostic process by giving the clinician a general picture of pre-morbid skills in each language. This information will be mostly subjective and therefore not directly comparable to the objective measures obtained in assessment. Nonetheless, it will assist the clinician in estimating the degree of impairment in each language.

As suggested by Centeno (chapter 11, this volume), it is also important to ascertain the patient's "ethnic identity". Degree of language use in different contexts does not give us information about patients' feelings about the languages and degree of identification with each culture. This information may be difficult to obtain from family members if the patient is not able to provide it him/herself, but it will be crucial in determining the "functional disability" associated with the language loss. It will also be a determining factor in selecting language of intervention and maintaining high levels of motivation towards achieving therapy goals.

In addition to the obvious advantages to the assessment and intervention process for individual patients, careful documentation of the bilingual history will be an invaluable resource for future research. Access to such detailed history will allow better studies of extent of loss and recovery patterns in each of a bilingual's language.

Screening

Ideally, a screening should be a quick measure of performance on speech, language, and cognitive abilities designed to guide more in-depth assessment of identified areas of impairment. Unfortunately, given the time and remuneration constraints placed on most speech-language pathologists in health care settings, it is usually the case that the entire assessment is nothing more than a screening, often performed at bedside, because it must be completed in 30 minutes or less. There are obvious problems with this practice whether patients are monolingual or bilingual. Such quick and superficial assessments can identify general areas of impairment, but they provide little guidance in establishing intervention goals. In addition, assessment protocols are site specific, i.e., designed by practicing clinicians for their individual sites. There is usually no validation of the areas assessed and how they are assessed. For bilingual patients, there are even more shortcomings. If two languages, rather than one, are to be assessed within that same allotted time period, it is obvious that some areas will be left out of the protocol. Additionally, when a patient is lucky enough to be evaluated by a bilingual clinician, that clinician will likely translate the protocol (often in real time, rather than ahead of time) into the intended language without consideration for the appropriateness of the translated items for the patient's language and culture.

In general, screenings contain several areas within cognition and communication that must be checked off as either "within normal limits" or impaired. Areas of cognition include orientation (to person, place, time, and situation), memory (immediate, short-term, and long-term), attention, problem solving, executive function, processing speed, deficit awareness, and judgment. Areas of communication include speech intelligibility, auditory comprehension (object recognition, yes/no questions, and commands), verbal expression (word fluency, automatic speech, naming, and conversation), pragmatics, writing, and reading. Each of these areas can be assessed with a few specific tasks (e.g., number recall for short-term memory) which are often designed by individual clinicians, or determined by informal observation (e.g., processing speed).

It should be clear by the sheer number of skills assessed in such a short period of time that a quick screening cannot substitute for a full in-depth assessment. In addition, the lack of homogeneity in selecting test items and the subjectivity of what constitutes "within normal limits" performance poses serious questions as to the validity and reliability of these protocols. Nevertheless, this is common practice in many health care settings where speech-language pathologists are employed. It is hoped that conscientious bilingual clinicians will at the very least follow a consistent protocol that can be translated ahead of time and checked for linguistic and cultural appropriateness. By having family members present during administration of the protocol, some information can be obtained about what test items the family member believes the patient would have been able to do pre-morbidly.

The following sections describe components of a thorough speech, language, and cognitive assessment that need to be adapted to bilingual populations. Such in-depth assessments should always follow a quick screening. However, clinicians who are unable to perform a comprehensive assessment during a diagnostic session often can incorporate assessment tasks into therapeutic sessions (diagnostic therapy). Such practice can ensure that current research findings will be incorporated into clinical practice and make intervention more efficient and efficacious.

Language Assessment

Clinicians working with patients with neurogenic disorders are familiar with formal tests designed to assess the language abilities of this population. Some of the tests most commonly used include the Porch Index of Communicative Ability (PICA, Porch, 1981), the Western Aphasia Battery (WAB, Kertesz, 1982), and the Boston Diagnostic Aphasia Examination (BDAE, Goodglass and Kaplan, 1983). For bilingual patients, the Bilingual Aphasia Test (Paradis, Hummel, and Libben, 1989) is available. This test is available in over 60 languages and is designed to be used in conjunction with the book "Assessment of Bilingual Aphasia" (Paradis, 1987). Some tests have been translated into other languages and can be used with monolingual speakers of those languages or given in two different versions for bilingual speakers. Examples include the Multilingual Aphasia Examination (Benton, Hamsher, and Sivan, 1994), the Boston Naming Test (Kaplan, Goodglass, and Weintraub, 1983), and the previously mentioned Boston Diagnostic Aphasia Examination, and Western Aphasia Battery.

Formal language tests are useful for helping clinicians arrive at a differential diagnosis, but they do not provide the in-depth analysis necessary to plan intervention goals effectively. In addition, tests that are translated and/or adapted into other languages may help to identify deficits in each of the patient's languages, but they do not take into consideration the intricate relationships between languages and the unique organization of the bilingual brain. This volume provides us with insight into this uniqueness at different levels of language access and processing. Each of these levels can be examined in individual patients to obtain a clearer picture of the deficits present and hopefully to plan intervention goals that may take advantage of the peculiarities of the bilingual experience. Each level is described in the following sections.

The Lexical/Semantic Level

Muñoz (chapter 5, this volume) reviewed lexical and semantic organization and retrieval in bilinguals. Clinicians working with patients with neurogenic language disorders must have a clear understanding of the different levels of representation for the lexical and semantic systems. That separation is particularly relevant for bilingual patients. As pointed out in the chapter, bilinguals have one semantic (conceptual) system and two lexical systems (one for each language). The degree of separation and overlap between the lexical systems is still under debate (see Du Four and Kroll, 1995), but there seems to be clear overlap of cognate words (words with shared meaning and similar phonological form) (e.g., Costa and Santesteban., 2004). This peculiarity of the bilingual lexical system coupled with frequency and familiarity effects on word retrieval and recognition (more frequent and more familiar words are more easily/quickly accessed and recognized than less frequent/less familiar words) have important clinical consequences worth exploring in assessment.

Bilingual patients with aphasia will show either impairment or preservation of cognate clusters in both languages due to this shared representation/store of cognates (Lalor and Kirsner, 2001). Naming and word retrieval tests do not test cognates, but this information can be extremely useful for intervention planning. For example, work on cognates is likely to stimulate stronger activation of the semantic store, which in turn can activate related semantic concepts and respective lexical entries (see Muñoz, chapter 5, this volume for models of lexical/semantic activation).

Word frequency effects can also be used to facilitate word retrieval in bilinguals. Lalor and Kirsner (2001) found that low frequency words in one language with high frequency translations in the other language facilitated recognition in an English-Italian bilingual patient with aphasia even in non-cognates (e.g., "rooster" in English versus "gallo" in Italian). Decisions on which language to use for intervention should take into consideration word frequency in each language, always moving from the most frequent to the less frequent translation equivalent. Obviously, word familiarity must also be taken into consideration when examining word frequency effects. An unbalanced bilingual may not be familiar enough with certain words that are considered high frequency in one of his/her languages. In addition, as pointed out by Muñoz (chapter 5, this volume), less proficient bilinguals may not have direct access from L2 lexical items to the semantic system, that is, they may rely on translating from L2 to L1 before accessing semantics. Though it is not clear what role these variables will play in intervention efficacy, the careful clinician will need to monitor them closely.

In summary, a basic understanding of how the bilingual brain accesses and processes lexical and semantic information will lead to more accurate assessments, which in turn will lead to more efficacious and efficient intervention. However, as Centeno (chapter 11, this volume) points out, we must look beyond the intricacies of language representation in the bilingual brain and take into consideration the effects of cultural and psychoemotional variables in individual patients. Most bilinguals will associate each of their languages with different contexts, and different words are likely to be used in each context. Keeping in mind the "functional" emphasis of speech and language intervention, clinicians must also delineate which words in which language must be addressed in therapy to fulfill each individual patient's communication and psychoemotional needs.

The Syntactic Level

For a long time, researchers believed that the syntax of each of a bilingual's languages was sealed in separate modules that never interacted. Today, we know that even syntax is susceptible to the effects of bilingualism. Grosjean (1989) noted that a bilingual "cannot be decomposed into two separate parts…rather, he or she has a unique and specific linguistic configuration" (p.6). That assertion seems to be true for all aspects of language, including syntax. This interaction may occur in subtle ways, such as in becoming more flexible in judging the grammaticality of sentences as compared to monolilnguals (e.g., Chan, 2004; Hartsuiker, Pickering, and Veltkamp, 2004) or using different strategies to identify the subject of a sentence (Bates, Devescovi, and D'Amico, 1999). Hartsuiker, Pickering, and Veltkamp (2004) also found that bilingual subjects are likely to use sentence constructions in one language that parallel constructions recently used in the other language.

Why is it important to be aware of these interactions? As pointed out by Fabbro (2001), bilingual patients with aphasia must be tested in both of their languages, because many of these patients show patterns of impairment that differ in each language. However, we must keep in mind that by testing each language separately, we are assuming that the two languages are completely independent from each other. In doing so, we may overlook the fact that some response patterns shown by these patients may be due to language interaction/interference, rather than the language impairment.

Regardless of how much interaction there may be between the two languages, it seems clear that the profile of grammatical deficits in each language will depend on the specific structure of those languages (Fabbro, 2001). Therefore, the speech-language pathologist will need to be knowledgeable about the structure of each language.

Much current research has been dedicated to find a common basic component that is affected in both languages of a bilingual aphasic. Diego et al. (2004) examined the use of regular and irregular verb morphology in Spanish-Catalan bilingual aphasics. They argued that in spite of superficial differences, the common deficit lies in morphosyntactic processing, independently of language and the regularity of the forms.

Using syntactic theory, some researchers have argued that the common deficit can be found in the hierarchical structure of syntactic trees or in trace-deletion applied to moved constituents within the tree. Friedman (2001) studied productions of 14 Hebrew/Arabic bilingual aphasics for tense and agreement verb inflection, subordination, interrogatives, and verb movement. Analysis of results pointed to an underlying deficit in high nodes of the syntactic tree, while lower nodes seemed to be unaffected.

Grodzinsky (2000) proposes a complex theory where traces of syntactic movement are deleted in aphasia (Trace-Deletion Hypothesis). In very simplified terms, whenever there is a constituent movement in syntax, a trace is left in the originating site of the constituent which allows us to recover the role of the moved constituent. For example, in passive voice sentences such as "the boy was pushed by the girl", a trace is left in the object position of the verb "push" that allows us to understand that "boy" is the object and not the subject of the sentence. In bilingual aphasics, then, trace-deletion would be the culprit in both languages, though its surface manifestation might differ in each language.

Though such theories seem highly abstract and still too young to be useful in clinical practice, they show much promise for the assessment and intervention of aphasic patients. Once we identify the underlying deficit, assessment will become a matter of describing how the deficit manifests itself in each language, and intervention may become more efficient if we are able to address a common deficit in both languages at the same time.

The Pragmatic Level

The most complex achievement for bilinguals at the pragmatic level is the ability to code-switch between languages. Unfortunately, code-switching is also one of the most difficult abilities to assess. As seen in chapter 4 (Basnight-Brown and Altarriba, this volume), code-switching ability is highly dependent on speakers' proficiency in each language. Highly proficient bilinguals can code-switch seamlessly in what Basnight-Brown and Altarriba (chapte 4, this volume) described as a third grammar, which is a combination of two language structures. Though highly unpredictable, code-switched utterances are grammatical in the sense that they occur at appropriate points in the utterance and do not violate the rules of either language (e.g., Heredia and Altarriba 2001; Myers-Scotton and Jake, 1995).

Given how code-switching varies depending on language proficiency, disruptions should occur when there are deficits to one or both languages of a bilingual patient. It is also possible that code-switching will be absent in cases when one language is disproportionately more affected than the other. This level of assessment will be highly subjective. The clinician will need to rely on reports of pre-morbid language proficiency and code-switching behavior and compare it to careful observation and analysis of spontaneous language use. Such observation should include the patient's interactions with friends and family members who may be monolingual in each of the patient's language (where little or no code-switching should occur) as well as bilinguals (where code-switching should occur). The assessment may include a checklist indicating whether or not code-switches were judged as appropriate by the clinician and the interlocutors.

Few studies of code-switching abilities in disordered bilingual populations are available. Hyltenstam and Stroud (1989) observed that bilingual patients with Alzheimer's disease show difficulty in selecting the correct language and maintaining the two languages separate. De Santi, Obler, Sabro-Abrahamson, and Goldberger (1990) noted that these difficulties may start at very early stages of dementia and progress to a point where the listener will not be able to determine which language is being used. In a study of conversational discourse in four Spanish-English bilinguals with aphasia, Muñoz, Marquardt, and Copeland (1999) found that the subjects were able to match each of their languages to the appropriate context. However, they also noted that these subjects code-switched significantly more often than normal subjects, suggesting a dependence on using both languages to communicate effectively.

Perhaps it is more important to determine whether or not a patient can utilize code-switching as a strategy to overcome language deficits than to determine whether this ability has suffered any impairment. It is well known that bilingual children actively code-switch to fill lexical gaps in their vocabulary (Grosjean, 1982). A patient that can use this strategy has a better chance of establishing effective communication than a monolingual patient. In addition, because of levels of lexical activation (see Muñoz, chapter 5, this volume), it is possible that by encouraging code switching, a clinician can facilitate access and retrieval of the other language as well. Code-switching may well be the greatest tool in the arsenal of bilingual patients with neurogenic disorders and it should be used in intervention on a regular basis to its fullest extent.

Cognitive Assessment

In a recent position statement, the American Speech-Language-Hearing Association (ASHA, 2005) delineated the roles of speech-language pathologists in evaluating and treating communication disorders associated with cognitive impairments. The document recognized that impairments in areas of cognition such as attention, perception, memory, organization, and executive function can affect social interaction, self regulation, learning, academic, and vocational performance, all areas in which speech-language pathologists can intervene. Traditionally, speech-language pathologists have approached non-verbal cognitive abilities as a separate entity from linguistic abilities. This approach may lead clinicians to believe that cultural-linguistic variations need not be taken into consideration when assessing cognitive abilities. This section will revisit some cognitive effects of bilingualism raised elsewhere in this volume that are relevant to the assessment process and should be carefully considered by clinicians working with bilingual populations with cognitive impairments.

Ardila and Ramos (chapter 12, this volume) point out that there are both "positive" and "negative" cognitive effects associated with bilingualism. The words "negative" and "positive" are used here within quotation marks to alert the reader to the fact that negative or positive effects observed on task-specific performance in research studies and assessment tools may or may not translate into negative or positive effects on functional aspects of communication. However, when administering an assessment tool, clinicians are usually comparing a patient's performance to that of normal populations and not to what is functional in communication. Any "deficits" noted may be truly a result of the cognitive impairment or simply a reflection of the unique way in which the bilingual brain processes and stores information. Understanding this uniqueness will make the diagnostic process much more accurate. On the other hand, even "positive" effects that may not give normal bilinguals any functional advantage, may be used to capitalize on a patient's ability to compensate for the cognitive impairment and thus be made functional.

Moving from what is most relevant for assessment purposes to what is most relevant for intervention planning, let's start with "negative" effects that must be considered when administering a cognitive assessment protocol. Some of the relevant "negative" effects identified in Ardila and Ramos (chapter 12, this volume) are: decrease in verbal fluency, interference between languages, calculation ability, and biographical and working memory.

Decrease in verbal fluency is a particularly important effect to keep in mind as most assessment tools in speech-language pathology will test patients' ability to provide an appropriate number of members of a superordinate category. Repetition tasks are also affected in bilinguals and very common in these assessment tools. As reviewed in Ardila and Ramos, it is not clear why bilinguals should perform more poorly in these tasks and there are no guidelines as to how much variability to expect when comparing bilinguals to monolinguals. However, small variations should be expected and disregarded. In addition, patients should be given the opportunity to respond in either or both languages to optimize performance. Interference between languages may be responsible for some of this decreased performance. Therefore, allowing patients to freely switch between languages may be helpful.

The ability to perform arithmetic calculations is extremely important in daily living activities and often assessed by speech-language pathologists to determine functional disability. Several studies (see Ardila and Ramos, chapter 12, this volume) have shown that bilinguals are more accurate in performing arithmetic calculations in their first language, even after long periods of functioning in L2. Patients should be allowed to use their preferred language when given such tasks. If intervention in this area is deemed necessary, the preferred language should also be used in intervention.

Working memory is often assessed by speech-language pathologists using word and number series to be recalled. Digit-span tasks seem to be highly dependent on the language being tested, with both advantages and disadvantages noted for bilinguals (see Ardila and Ramos, chapter 12, this volume). Translated test items are extremely inappropriate for testing recall of words and digits, due to the differences in the length of the phonological units to be recalled. Long-term memory may also be affected in bilinguals when biographical memory is enlisted. Bilinguals are more accurate in recalling events in their lives in the language in which the event was originally experienced. Speech-language pathologists often inquire about biographical information as a way to assess patients' orientation and executive functioning. It is important to match the language of the original experience with the language of report to ensure optimal recall.

Positive effects of bilingualism may well give bilingual patients an advantage in softening the extent of impairment incurred, but such effects would be nearly impossible to measure in terms of functional advantage. They can be extremely useful, however, in facilitating compensatory strategies to deal with the observed impairments. In fact, the three advantages identified in Ardila and Ramos (chapter 12, this volume) are highly relevant for therapeutic success: Learning new cognitive strategies, getting better insight of one's language, and increasing cognitive control are all skills that usually need to be taught to monolingual patients, but may be readily available to bilingual patients. It is not within the scope of this chapter to review intervention procedures, but providing a prognosis for improvement is part of the assessment process, and these bilingual advantages should be considered when arriving at a prognosis.

Speech Assessment

Speech-language pathologists familiar with the different types of dysarthrias and apraxia of speech will have no difficulty identifying them in bilingual populations. Dysarthrias are most accurately identified by obtaining a speech sample to identify the speech characteristics associated with each type of dysarthria such as intonational patterns, voice quality, consonant and vowel distortions, etc. Bilingual clinicians who are familiar with the characteristics of each of these parameters in the patient's language and dialect will readily identify the abnormal patterns associated with dysarthrias. Apraxia of speech may be more difficult to identify, especially if it appears concurrently with dysarthrias. Clinicians are more likely to use formal tests to diagnose apraxia of speech. Some aphasia batteries include sections for identifying apraxia and there are some tools designed specifically for that purpose, such as the Apraxia Battery for Adults (Dabul, 1986) and the Comprehensive Apraxia Test (DiSimoni, 1989).

It is important to keep in mind that translating tests of apraxia of speech will make them invalid. One of the key components in these tests is the number of syllables assessed in each test item, which will not be kept constant when translations are used. Identifying the key component in test items and keeping that component constant in a test *adaptation* may be appropriate, but it takes specialized skill to successfully complete such adaptations. Gathering a spontaneous speech sample and analyzing it carefully for types of errors will be a much more valid assessment procedure.

Monolingual English speaking clinicians assessing speakers of English as a second language should be familiar with speech patterns associated with the patients' first language. Speakers of English as a second language will also use universal phonological simplification processes that are common to most English learners regardless of first language background. See Yavas and Goldstein (1998) for a review of such speech patterns. Bilingual clinicians must also be familiar with the dialectal variations of the patient's first language to avoid erroneously identifying normal dialectal differences as part of the patient's speech disorder. Goldstein and Iglesias (2001) found that a significant number of normally developing English/Spanish bilingual children were identified as having a speech disorder due to dialectal differences that were unfamiliar to the diagnosing clinicians. In adults, the effects of dialectal variation in the diagnosis of speech disorders has not been studied, but it may also pose special challenges in the identification of speech disorders in this population.

Conclusion

Whether a speech-language pathologist is assessing a bilingual or a monolingual patient, the goal is to determine whether a functional limitation is present and if so, to determine the extent of that limitation and the steps that must be taken to overcome it. As seen in this chapter, that goal is especially challenging when the patient is bilingual. A careful history and a description of the patient's pre-morbid abilities in each language must be obtained. Every step of the assessment process must take that description into consideration along with results of formal assessment tools, and clinical observations. More importantly, an in-depth understanding of the bilingual mind is crucial for accurately interpreting any assessment data. Obviously, our understanding of the bilingual mind is only as good as what current research can tell us. Much research still needs to be done before we can fully understand bilingualism. Nevertheless, we also have a lot of information on which to rely. Bilingualism will affect most aspects of the assessment process, from the gathering of a case history, to language, cognitive, and speech assessment. By evaluating each of these areas systematically against the information available, clinicians can provide more accurate assessments and more efficient and efficacious treatment. Given that half of the world's population is bilingual, most clinicians will be faced with this challenge at one time or another. It is our moral and ethical responsibility to rise to that challenge to the best of our ability.

References

Agency for Healthcare Research and Quality. (2002). Criteria for determining disability in speech-language disorders. *U.S. Department of Health and Human Services.* www.ahrq.gov.

American Speech-Language- Hearing Association. (2005). Evidence-Based Practice in Communication Disorders [Position Statement]. Available at http://www.asha.org/members/deskrefjournals/deskref/deafult.

American Speech-Language- Hearing Association. (2005). Roles of speech-language pathologists in the identification, diagnosis, and treatment of individuals with cognitive-communication disorders. Position statement: *ASHA supplement*, 25.

Anderson, R. (1999). Loss of gender agreement in L1 attrition: Preliminary results. *Bilingual Research Journal, 23*, 389-407.

Bates, E., Devescovi, A., and D'Amico, S. (1999). Processing complex sentences: A crosslinguistic study. *Language and Cognitive Processes, 14*, 68-123.

Bedore, L. M., Peña, E. D., García, M., and Cortez, C. (2005). Conceptual versus monolingual scoring: When does it make a difference? *Language, Speech, and Hearing Services in Schools. 36*, 188-200.

Benton, A. L., Hamsher, K. deS., and Sivan, A. B. (1994). *Multilingual Aphasia Examination* (3rd ed.). Iowa City, IA: AJA Associates Inc.

Centeno, J. G. (2005). Working with bilingual individuals with aphasia: The case of a Spanish-English bilingual client. *American Speech-Language-Hearing Association Division 14 - Perspectives on Communication Disorders and Sciences in Culturally and Linguistically Diverse Populations, 12*, 2-7.

Chan, A. Y. W. (2004). Syntactic transfer: Evidence from the interlanguage of Hong Kong Chinese ESL learners. *The Modern Language Journal, 88*, 54-74.

Costa, A., and Santesteban, M. (2004). Lexical access in bilingual speech production: Evidence from language switching in highly proficient bilinguals and L2 learners. *Journal of Memory and Language, 50*, 491-511.

Dabul, B. (1986). *Apraxia battery for adults*. Austin, TX: PRO-ED.

Diego, R. B. de, Costa, A., Sebastian-Galles, N., Juncadella, M., Caramazza, A. (2004). Regular and irregular morphology and its relationship with agrammatism: Evidence from two Spanish-Catalan bilinguals. *Brain and Language, 91*, 212-222.

De Santi, S., Obler, L. K., Sabo-Abrahamson, H. and Goldberger, J., (1990). Discourse abilities and deficits in multilingual dementia. In Y. Joanette and H. H. Brownell (Eds). *Discourse Ability and Brain Damage: Theoretical and Empirical Perspectives* (pp. 224-235). New York: Springer.

DiSimoni, F. G. (1989). *Comprehensive apraxia test*. Dalton, PA: Praxis House.

Du Four, R., and Kroll, J. F. (1995). Matching words to concepts in two languages: A test of the concept mediation model of bilingual representation. *Memory and Cognition, 23*(2), 166-180.

Fabbro, F. (2001). The bilingual brain: Bilingual aphasia. *Brain and Language, 79*, 201-210.

Friedmann, N. (2001). Agrammatism and the psychological reality of the syntactic tree. *Journal of Psycholinguistic Research, 30*, 71-90.

Genesee, F., Paradis, J., and Crago, M. B. (2004). *Dual language development and disorders: A handbook on bilingualism and second language lea*rning. Baltimore: Brookes.

Goldstein, B. (2004.). Bilingual Language Development and Disorders in Spanish-English Speakers. Baltimore: Brookes.

Goldstein, B. and Iglesias, A. (2001). The effect of dialect on phonological analysis: Evidence from Spanish-speaking children. *American Journal of Speech and Language Pathology, 10*, 394-406.

Goodglass, H., and Kaplan, E. (1983). *Boston diagnostic aphasia examination*. Malvern, PA: Lea and Febinger.

Grosjean, F. (1982). *Life with two languages*. Cambridge, MA: Harvard University Press.

Grosjean, F. (1989). Neurolinguists, beware! The bilingual is not two monolinguals in one person. *Brain and Language*, 36, 3-15.

Grosjean, F. (1998). Studying bilinguals: Methodological and conceptual issues. *Bilingualism: Language and Cognition, 1,* 131-149.

Gordzinsky, Y. (2000). The neurology of syntax: Language use without Broca's area. *Behavioral and Brain Sciences, 23*, 1-71.

Hartsuiker, R.J., Pickering, M.J., and Veltkamp, E. (2004). Is syntax separate or shared between languages? Cross-linguistic syntactic priming in Spanish-English bilinguals. *Psychology Sciences,.15*, 409-14.

Hedge, M. N. and Davis, D. (2005). *Clinical Methods and Practicum in Speech-Language Pathology*. Clifton Park, NY: Thomson Delmar Learning.

Heredia, R.R., and Altarriba, J. (2001). Bilinguals language mixing: Why do bilinguals code switch? *Current Directions in Psychological Science, 10,* 164-168.

Hyltenstam, K. and Stroud, C. (1989). Bilingualism in Alzheimer's dementia: Two case studies. In K. Hyltenstam and L. K. Obler (Eds) *Bilingualism Across the Lifespan :*

Aspects of Acquisition, Maturity and Loss (pp. 202-226) . Cambridge: Cambridge University Press.

Kaplan, E., Goodglass, H., and Weintraub, S. (1983). *The Boston Naming Test.* Philadelphia: Lea and Febiger.

Kayser, H. (1998). *Assessment and Intervention Resource for Hispanic Children.* San Diego: Singular.

Kertesz, A. (1982). *Western aphasia battery.* Orlando, FL: Grune and Stratton.

Kirshner, C. (1996). Language attrition and the Spanish-English bilingual: A case of syntactic reduction. *The Bilingual Review, 21*, 123-129.

Kohnert, K. (2004). *Processing skills in early sequential bilinguals. Bilingual language development and disorders in Spanish-English speakers.* Baltimore: Brookes

Lalor, E. and Kirsner, K. (2001). The role of cognates in bilingual aphasia: Implications for assessment and treatment. *Aphasiology, 15*, 1047-1056.

Muñoz, M. L., Marquadt, T. P., and Copeland, G. (1999). A comparison of codeswitching patterns of aphasic and neurologically normal bilingual speakers of English and Spanish. *Brain and Language*, 66, 249-274.

Myers-Scotton, C., and Jake, J. L. (1995). Matching lemmas in a bilingual language competence and production model: evidence from intrasentential code switching. *Linguistics, 33*, 981-1024.

Obler, L. K. and Mahecha, N. R. (1991). First language loss in bilingual and polyglot aphasics. In H. W. Selinger and R. M. Vago (eds.), *First language attrition.* New York: Cambridge University Press.

Paradis, J. (2005). Grammatical morphology in children learning English as a second language: Implications of similarities with specific language impairment. *Language, Speech, and Hearing Services in Schools, 36,* 172-187.

Paradis, J., Crago, M., Genesee, F., and Rice, M. (2003). French-English bilingual children with SLI: How do they compare with their monolingual peers? *Journal of Speech, Language, and Hearing Research, 46*, 113-127.

Paradis, M. (1987). *The assessment of bilingual Aphasia.* Hillsdale, NJ: Lawrence Erlbaum Associates Inc.

Paradis, M., Hummel, K., and Libben, G. (1989). *The bilingual aphasia test.* Hillsdale, NJ: Lawrence Erlbaum Associates Inc.

Porch, B. E. (1981). *Porch index of communicative ability* (3rd ed.). Palo Alto, CA: Consulting Psychologists Press.

Restrepo, M. A. (1998). Identifiers of predominantly Spanish-speaking children with specific language impairment. *Journal of Speech, Language, and Hearing Research, 41,* 1398-1411.

Restrepo, M. A., and Kruth, K. (2000). Grammatical characteristics of a Spanish-English bilingual child with specific language impairment. *Communication Disorders Quarterly, 21*, 66-76.

Seliger, H. W. and Vago, R. M. (1991). The study of first language attrition: an overview. In H. W. Selinger and R. M. Vago (eds.), *First language attrition.* New York: Cambridge University Press.

Shipley, G. K. and McAfee, J. G. (2004). *Assessment in speech-language pathology: A resource manual.* Clifton Park, NY: Thomson Delmar Learning.

Yavas, M. and Goldstein, B. (1998). Phonological assessment and treatment of bilingual speakers. *American Journal of Speech and Language Pathology, 7,* 49-60.

In: Speech and Language Disorders in Bilinguals ISBN 978-1-60021-560-5
Editors: Alfredo Ardila and Eliane Ramos, pp. 195-212

Chapter 11

Considerations for an Ethnopsycholinguistic Framework for Aphasia Intervention with Bilingual Speakers

José G. Centeno
Department of Speech, Communication Sciences and Theatre
St. John's University,
Jamaica, New York 11439 USA

Bilingual adults seeking speech-language services may exhibit a variety of communication deficits, such as speech impairments or neurologically-based acquired disorders, as discussed in earlier chapters of this volume. Yet, recent demographic counts of the U.S. population suggest prominent numbers of adult bilinguals, especially elderly, with acquired communication impairments. Approximately, 47 million (17.9%) individuals in the U.S. speak a language other than English at home, an increase of 15 million people since 1990 (U.S. Census Bureau, 2002; 2003). Also, there are close to 46 million (16.2%) people in the country aged 60 years and over (U.S. Census Bureau, 2002). Because aging is consistently associated with the occurrence of strokes (Chapey and Hallowell, 2001), an integrated look at the preceding demographic data leads us to expect a considerable number of bilingual elderly, who are users of a foreign language in addition to English, in post-stroke rehabilitation.

There is great paucity, however, in the empirical evidence and clinical discussions on effective methods in bilingual aphasia treatment (Roberts, 2001). The development of realistic management techniques for bilingual aphasic elders is imperative. Like diagnostic procedures relying on valid tools (see Ramos, ch.10, and Roberts and Kiran, ch. 6, this volume), treatment of bilingual aphasic speakers would similarly require the use of effective strategies that would facilitate language rehabilitation. Contemporary treatment perspectives with monolingual aphasic individuals may provide valuable grounds to develop bilingual aphasia interventions. Current clinical philosophy views aphasia as a social phenomenon whose realistic treatment should aim to enhance communicative interactions between patients and their human environments (e.g., Elman, 2005; LaPointe, 2003; Life Participation

Approach to Aphasia [LPAA] Project Group, 2001; Simmons-Mckie, 2001). Further, because the processes supporting functional communication and language recovery depend on multiple factors, aphasia intervention requires a broad multi-disciplinary theoretical foundation that looks at language rehabiliation beyond strictly linguistic domains and incorporates additional operations underlying effective communication, such as sociolinguistic, cognitive, psycholinguistic, and psychoemotional phenomena (Byng, Parr, and Cairns, 2003; Code, 2001).

Translated to bilingual contexts, aphasia intervention would critically depend on insightful frameworks that can explicate the multi-faceted aspects of bilingualism relevant to language rehabilitation with adult bilinguals. Indeed, bilingualism is a complex phenomenon. Accumulating evidence from different lines of inquiry suggests that understanding bilingualism requires a multidimensional construct that would connect "ethnographic data from social aspects of bilingualism with psycholinguistic data from more cognitively-oriented research" (Walters, 2005: 2; also see Ellis, 2002). Thus, accounts of bilingualism relevant to aphasia treatment would need to integrate language structure, psycholinguistic processing, interactional contexts, affective dispositions, and neurocognitive substrates participating in language learning, processing, and use in dual-language users (see Green, 2005; Paradis, 2004; Pavlenko, 2005; Walters, 2005).

Hence, an intervention framework for bilingual aphasic individuals grounded in the interaction between culture and its impact on linguistic and cognitive processing may not be an implausible theoretical approach. Cultural experiences shape language acquisition and use and cognitive representations, or schemas, of members of all ethnic communities (Quinn and Holland, 1987; Salzmann, 1993; Zentella, 2005). Crucially, in this framework, the use of ethnographic descriptions is warranted. Ethnography, the study of cultural influences on the behavior, beliefs, practices, and knowledge of an ethnic group (Mertens, 1998), is an important methodology in qualitative research that has been useful in speech-language pathology. Because ethnography enhances the collection of authentic, contextualized social data to describe sociocultural phenomena (Damico and Simmons-Mackie, 2003), ethnographic data have been extremely useful to gain deeper insights on the complexities of communication in both research and clinical practice in neurogenic communication disorders in both monocultural and multicultural populations (e.g., Guendouzi and Müller, 2006; Simmons-Mackie and Damico, 1999; Wallace, 1997). Hence, in an ethnopsycholinguistic approach, ethnographic observations would provide the data to link overt sociocultural and linguistic practices with possible covert psycholinguistic operations.

It is worth adding that sociolinguistics, broadly speaking, the study of the interaction between language use and society at both individual (micro) and societal (macro) levels (Coulmas, 1997), often overlaps with ethnography in scope and a clear separation between both approaches is not always clear (see Salzmann, 1993). In this chapter, however, an ethnographic perspective is taken and specific sociolinguistic dimensions will be highlighted wherever pertinent.

This chapter aims to provide the conceptual foundations to support an ethnopsycholinguistic (EPL) framework for aphasia therapy with bilingual individuals in which ecologically valid communication enhancement in bilingual aphasic clients reflects the inextricable connections between cultural norms and their cognitive and linguistic implications. Several caveats are necessary. First, because communication and cognitive skills in bilingual adults, as in all individuals, depend on individual living trajectories throughout life (Pavlenko, 2005), discussions will include pertinent acquisitional phenomena in younger bilinguals. Second, while drawing from some of the theoretical principles predicated earlier in this book, content of this chapter will also complement such principles as it integrates some of those notions with additional phenomena into a multidimensional ethnographic perspective. Finally, Hispanic individuals in the U.S. will be used as a case illustration throughout this chapter for various reasons. Discussing how the proposed framework applies to the ethnographic characteristics of each ethnic group in the U.S. is not possible in one single chapter. In addition, demographically, Hispanics represent both the largest minority group and the group with the most prominent demographic growth in the U.S. (National Alliance for Hispanic Health, 2004; U.S Census Bureau, 2002). They similarly constitute the most common ethnic group in speech-language caseloads, as suggested by pediatric contexts (Roseberry-McKibbin, Brice, and O'Hanlon, 2005). Principles based on Hispanics discussed in this chapter are expected to be adapted to the particular circumstances of other bilingual groups in the U.S.

This chapter is structured in four sections to discuss the proposed interaction among culture, language, and cognition in an EPL therapy program with aphasic bilinguals. Specifically, the first section will address the relationship between ethnography and group diversity, as intrinsic group heterogeneity plays a critical role in ethnographic analysis. The next two sections will highlight some important cultural determinants of language use and psycholinguistic processing in adult bilinguals; namely, the interplay between sociocultural/sociolinguistic contexts and bilingual development/communication, and between sociocultural contexts and cognition. The final section will integrate the three preceding conceptual strands into an EPL perspective for aphasia intervention with bilingual speakers. The sections in this chapter represent conceptual clusters to illustrate the target framework. As linguistic and cognitive phenomena sometimes are not easily separable, some material in the following sections may overlap theoretically.

ETHNOGRAPHY OF CULTURAL AND LINGUISTIC DIVERSITY IN THE U.S.

Each cultural or ethnic group in the U.S. (e.g., white, Black, Native American, Hispanic, and so forth) is defined in terms of the shared cultural bonds among its members, such as language, ancestry, and religion. While ethnic groups culturally differ among each other, there is also internal diversity within each group as each one consists of various communities that may differ in countries of origin (e.g., Blacks may be from Africa, the Caribbean, and the U.S. [African Americans], or tribes or native groups of ancestry (e.g., Native Americans may be Indians [Navajo, Sioux, etc.], Eskimos, and Aleus) (see Battle, 2002). Further, members of each group differ along many life experiences (e.g., SES, occupations, educational history, etc.) and extent of cultural identity with the group. The combined effect of both inter- and intra-group dynamics makes "culture" a dynamic and fluid phenomenon. Understanding cultural heterogeneity in the country, therefore, requires the careful examination of cultural diversity across and within the various ethnic groups (Battle, 2002; Centeno, 2007; Rodriguez and Olswang, 2002).

Cultural heterogeneity is best understood in terms of demographic characteristics, acculturation, and the impact of societal attitudes on minority individuals (Centeno, 2007, in press-a; Phinney, 2003; Rodriguez and Olswang, 2002). As illustrated by Hispanics in the country, regarding demographic characteristics, Hispanics, also identified as Latinos(as), differ in ancestry. Mexican-Americans (66.9%) constitute the largest group followed by Central Americans and South Americans (14.3%), Puerto Ricans (8.6%), Cubans (3.7%), and other Hispanics (6.5%) (U.S. Census Bureau, 2002). These groups tend to identify with their homeland countries hence preferring to be identified by their national origin (e.g., Mexican, Puerto Rican, Cuban, etc.) (Zentella, 1997). Hispanics similarly represent varied levels of schooling, life experiences, and socioeconomic circumstances (Centeno, 2005; Zentella, 1997). Linguistically, their language skills reflect different dialectal varieties of Spanish consistent with their countries of ancestry, and, like all bilingual populations in the U.S., exhibit varying degrees of bilingualism with a wide range of receptive and expressive skills in their first (L1) and second (L2) languages (Spanish and English, respectively) (Centeno, 2005; 2007).

In terms of acculturation, heterogeneity in Hispanics in the U.S. reflects the complex interplay among race, ethnicity, and acculturation in a minority context (Trimble, 2003). Race is a biogenetic condition resulting in physical features whereas ethnicity, or ethnic identity, is a psychological state or a sense of affiliation to an ethnic group (Mertens, 1998; Phinney, 2003). Cultural or ethnic identity formation occurs gradually over time through the process of acculturation as an individual experiences changes in cultural practices and symbols, including language, values, beliefs, and overall lifestyle. Acculturation differs from assimilation. While acculturation involves changes towards another culture without completely losing the original cultural traits, assimilation results in complete absorbtion into another culture (Trimble, 2003). In contrast to earlier models viewing acculturation as a unidirectional phenomenon leading to full assimilation, recent understandings describe acculturation as a multidimensional process in which elements of both original and new cultures are internalized and maintained (Brozgold and Centeno, in press; Trimble, 2003).

The factors that determine a person's acculturative strategies are complex and beyond the scope of this chapter (see Brozgold and Centeno, in press, and Zentella, 1997, for a discussion). In general, cultural identification is not a uniform phenomenon within members of an ethnic group; its development depends on many personal and societal elements. At the personal level, several variables have been reported to be important determinants in acculturation, such as age, gender, generation, urban vs. rural locations, socioeconomic circumstances, and length of residence in the new country (Brozgold and Centeno, in press; Centeno, 2007; Hidalgo, 1993; Torres, 1997). For example, Salas-Provance, Erickson, and Reed (2002) showed that less educated, low income, and/or older Hispanic individuals tended to hold folk beliefs regarding health practices, such as using *curanderos* (healers) and home remedies, whereas youngest generations and individuals with more years of education and/or access to the mainstream majority culture tended to be unsupportive of folkore. Further, the language choice of the middle and younger generations was English relative to the preferred use of Spanish by their older counterparts. In fact, this latter finding has great significance in the assessment of individual acculturative traits because language is the most frequent measure of acculturation (Marin, Organista, and Chun, 2003).

At the societal level, the process of acculturation is also dependent on the attitudinal disposition from the larger majority group towards minority individuals, such as discrimination and prejudice (Centeno, 2007; Hidalgo, 1993; Zentella, 1997). Racial, socio-economic, and political elements participate to create a "hierarchy of prestige" among the different subgroups of an ethnic group, as reported on Hispanics in the U.S. (Zentella, 1997: 175). Immigrant groups that are similar to the mainstream society of the U.S. in physical appearance, social class, and language receive a more favorable reception than those that look and act differently (Goldstein, 2004). Hispanics in the U.S. have not escaped from this bias. Often, whiter, wealthier, better educated, English-dominant Latinos(as) gain access to more prestigious occupational and social levels in the mainstream U.S. society than Hispanics that are darker and have less education and income (Zentella, 1997).

Hence, the complexity in describing diversity in ethnic groups should alert us against the use of generalizing stereotypes that collectively unify all members of an ethnic group as a homogeneous community. All efforts that obscure individual differences in terms of experiential history and personalities, such as the use of labels (e.g., Hispanic, Latino(a), and so forth), should be avoided as we tailor clinical services to each bilingual client. We now turn to how the preceding cultural diversity interacts with language learning and performance in bilingual speakers.

Sociolinguistic and Ethnographic Considerations of Language Acquisition and Communication in Adult Bilinguals

Bilinguals are a special sociolinguistic cohort. First, bilingual individuals are linguistically heterogeneous because their language gains depend on each learner's individual sociolinguistic contexts of L1 and L2 use throughout life. Rather than being monolinguals in each language, differences in communication environments (i.e., home, school, and work) and language socialization routines across languages (i.e., conversation and reading and writing modalities) make bilingual speakers' overall linguistic knowledge summative in nature with both languages complementing each other (Centeno, in press-a; Centeno and Obler, 2001b; Grosjean, 2004). Second, bilingual speakers' discourse is sociolinguistically characterized by special expressive features reflecting individual acquisition history in each language and discourse routines typical of language-contact situations (e.g., having an L1 accent when using L2, mixing both languages in one utterance, and using L1 sentence structure when speaking in L2) (Centeno, 2005; Romaine, 1995).

Hence, understanding and assessing language proficiency in adult bilinguals is a challenge for the longer multimodality history in L1 and L2 that they have accumulated relative to bilingual children. Bilingual adult clients attending speech-language clinics, as all other adult bilinguals, may have acquired their bilingual skills in either *simultaneous* or *sequential* contexts, the two broad definitions often used to describe bilingual development (see Centeno, in press-a, for a review). Simultaneous bilingualism, or *bilingualism as a first language* or *bilingual first language acquisition* (De Houwer, 1995; Meisel, 1990), refers to the early regular exposure to both L1 and L2 in children before age three. In contrast, sequential (*successive or consecutive*) bilingualism occurs when the learner is exposed to L2 after there has been considerable development in L1 (Romaine, 1995). In a sequential context, older children and adults acquire L2 skills in naturalistic environments, as *second language acquisition* (SLA), or in the classroom, as *foreign language* (FL) learning (Centeno, in press-a; Ritchie and Bhatia, 1996).

The number of definitions of bilingualism is extensive as bilingual development may occur in multiple ways and L1-L2 proficiency profiles may similarly be extremely diverse (see Hamers and Blanc, 2000, for a discussion). Linguistic heterogeneity in bilinguals has received considerable attention for its challenges in both research and clinical practice (e.g., Centeno, in press-a; Grosjean, 2004; Roberts, 2001; Roseberry-McKibbin et al., 2005). What is crucial to understand is that linguistic gains in bilingual speakers reflect a complex interplay of many factors, including age, language socialization practices, educational opportunities, and motivation, for each bilingual speaker throughout life (Centeno, in press-a; Jia, Aaronson, and Wu, 2002).

In terms of age, children tend to outperform adults in final linguistic gains. While adult L2 learners may bring more mature and experienced linguistic and cognitive skills and strategies to the learning process, research evidence irrefutably confirms that final L2 achievements in young L2 learners tend to be better (Hyltenstam and Abrahamsson, 2003). Although there are exceptional adult sequential learners who have mastered native-like L2 skills, those individulas may represent a neurospsychologically distinctive cohort of talented and motivated individuals, fortunately afforded the social and educational opportunities for L2 learning (Centeno, in press-a; Novoa, Fein, and Obler, 1988; Schneiderman and Desmarais, 1988).

Bilingual development, however, represents a complex reality in addition to maturational constraints. Because there is a close link between spoken and written language (Harris, 2003), the dynamic interaction between conversational routines and literacy experiences in the language socialization practices of bilingual environments warrant attention (Zecker, 2004; Zentella, 2005). This oral-literate interdependence is shaped by the specific sociocultural context of each bilingual learner, including socioeconomic factors, home literacy practices, educational opportunities, and rural vs.urban life experiences (Harris, 2003; Zentella, 2005).

Such relationships acquire a particular dimension in the special living contexts of some minority bilingual individuals in the country. Some bilingual minority speakers in the U.S. may exhibit restrictions in both L1 and English (L2) from limited educational exposure in their country of origin and a lack of stimulation in L1 in the U.S. not to the same extent as in their native origin; their L2 skills similarly are compromised for socioeconomic factors and social circumstances that isolate the bilingual immigrant group from an intensive exposure to English (Baetens Beardsmore, 1986; Centeno and Eng, 2005; Pavlenko, 2000).

Understanding routine expressive features in bilingual discourse similarly is crucial in aphasia intervention with bilinguals. Depending on their bilingual or monolingual communication modes, bilingual individuals may use both languages in an utterance (code-mixing or code-switching), employ particular vocabulary items from one language when speaking in the other language (borrowing), or show L1 or L2 syntactic patterns when speaking in the other language (transfer). They may also exhibit L1 limitations, such as a reliance on simple verb tenses rather than using the expected complex verb structures, due to loss of L1 mastery (attrition), pronounce sounds in one language under the influence from the other (phonetic transfer), or use linguistic features of another speech community, such as African American English (AAE), with whom they routinely interact (dialectal influences) (Centeno, 2005, 2007, in press-a; Zentella, 1997; also see Basnight-Brown and Altarriba, ch. 4, this volume for related discussion).

Hence, a Spanish-English bilingual who says "The girl was getting ready *porque su boyfriend la estaba esperando*" [the girl was getting ready because her boyfriend was waiting for her] and "You *was* here yesterday" [you were here yesterday] is using appropriate expressions reflecting his/her daily linguistic routines. In the first utterance, both languages are mixed in one utterance following the grammatical rules of each language whereas, in the second, the bilingual speaker has produced an utterance resulting from frequent interactions with AAE-speaking neighbors (Centeno, 2007). Expressions of this sort constitute typical linguistic forms in the expressive repertory of individuals from sociolinguistic environments of language contact. Like language choices made due to acculturation factors, described above, these expressive features similarly constitute part of bilingual speakers' cultural identity as they represent these speakers' daily expressive realities in their social communication networks (Zentella, 1997; 2005)

The preceding discussion underscores that bilingual speakers' linguistic development is a multidimensional process in which sociocultural, personal, and societal variables interact. In general, bilingual speakers demonstrate strengths and weaknesses in each language that are directly tied to their social and educational language experiences (Manuel-Dupont, Ardila, Rosselli, and Puente, 1992). Thus, understanding language proficiency and performance in each bilingual individual requires the examination of how the preceding forces intersect at the individual level to determine linguistic gains in each language. Additionally, the speaker's extent of use of the expressive features in bilingual discourse is part of the proficiency analysis to examine possible communicative strategies during communication.

In the next section, we explore some possible ways in which language learning circumstances and language use in bilingual speakers may have an impact on their cognitive processing.

Ethnopsychological Considerations in Adult Bilingualism

Differences in language socialization practices between L1 and L2 generally result in contrasting communication scenarios in which each language is used for different communicative purposes and involves different linguistic skills, as suggested by the previous discussion. Such contextual variability, in turn, represents differences in cognitive demands and sociocultural environments between the two languages that ultimately impact on processing strategies, intellectual skills, and long-lasting mental representations associated with each language. In this section, the complex interplay among cultural experiences, language practices, and cognition in bilingual environments is explored by surveying variables and interactions suggested by research on cognitive dimensions in language proficiency and psychosocial factors in language processing.

As highlighted in the previous section, language proficiency is a multidimensional phenomenon whose definition requires the specification of the linguistic features being measured and their contextual settings of use. In this regard, Bialystok (2001) offers an approach which distinguishes a complexity hierarchy in the various dimensions of language proficiency and their corresponding differences in cognitive requirements. According to Bialystok, language proficiency may be viewed in terms of three broad communication domains of increasing complexity, including oral (auditory comprehension and speaking), literate (reading and writing), and metalinguistic levels (language analysis), with progressively higher levels of linguistic and cognitive demands. Each of these levels of language-cognition interactions conceals great internal variability. Cognitively speaking, increasing linguistic demands call for different levels of analysis, attention, and control. For example, within the oral domain, a bilingual speaker experiences varying linguistic and cognitive demands when conversing as compared to giving a lecture. Similarly, for literacy tasks, reading and writing at different levels of competence (e.g., beginning vs. fluent reading), for different purposes (e.g., studying vs. perusing), and different genres (e.g., email vs. essay) require different levels of language proficiency and cognitive operations.

In this perspective, as development proceeds, mental representations of knowledge become more explicit and more structured, influenced by the learner's environmental circumstances. Hence, varying formal (e.g., academic tasks) and informal use (e.g., conversational discourse) of L1 and L2 would lead to differences in how language is processed and overtly used. For example, Snow, Cancino, De Temple, and Schley (1991) reported that bilingual students showed a stronger ability to provide formal definitions, an academic task, in the language of instruction (i.e., L2) than in the home language (i.e., L1), an informal, conversational language. These findings led the authors to argue that the language used at home enhanced conversational skills but did not seem to facilitate those processing skills called upon for decontextualized, classroom-related language tasks (also see Centeno and Eng, 2005).

Hence, the social and educational realities defining every bilingual learner's encounter with language must not be ignored. As bilinguals, like any other individual, move from oral to higher-language processes, such as literacy and metalinguistic levels, the social conditions and educational expectations in the home as well as the quality of literacy instruction influence overall language gains and concomitant cognitive skills (also see Ardila, Roselli, and Ostrosky-Solís, 1992; Bialystok, 2001). In the case of bilinguals, especially in situations of underprivileged minority environments, the preceding interactions have critical importance. Besides examining home and social language practices, possible limitations in the academic programs in minority communities must be considered. Racial/ethnic minorities continue to receive limited quality education resulting from several factors, such as inequalities in funding allocation, classroom supplies, and teacher certification (Ryan et al., 2005). In addition to hindering the development of language-related cognitive strategies, poor academic experiences, often interacting with stringent socioecomic circumstances (Centeno and Eng, 2005), can similarly impact nonverbal cognitive areas, such as memory (e.g, digit span) and visuospatial recall (e.g., block design) (Ardila et al., 1992). Essentially, because cognitive abilities, be it verbal or non-verbal processing, are highly trained skills that are culture- and education-dependent, those with many more years of cognitive training in the skills adaptive for and valued by the majority social group will outperform those with some or no formal training in those areas (Ardila et al., 1992; Ogbu, 2002).

Besides social and educational influences, information processing in bilingual individuals may also be viewed as a culturally-determined psychosocial process. Language, in addition to its strictly linguistic dimensions (e.g., vocabulary, grammatical structure, etc.), represents a powerful psychosocial phenomenon through which individuals experience and internalize their culture (Hamers and Blanc, 2000). Language, culture, emotions, and thought are intertwined across the lifespan of bilingual speakers (Brozgold and Centeno, in press; Pavlenko, 2005; also see Van Lancker and Pachana, 1998). Each language, including its conceptual representations and affective responses, becomes deeply linked to the sociocultural world and associative relationships represented by personal interactions, settings, and themes "lived" in each language (Pavlenko, 2005; Pérez-Foster, 1998).

To understand how these complex interactions impact information processing in bilingualism, ethnopsychological fluctuations in bilingual speakers must be acknowledged as bilinguals' language use practices, language dominance, and cultural identity may vary over time. For example, during early stages of bilingualism, when bilinguals tend to rely on their L1, their code switching mostly tends to involve L1 intrusions when speaking in L2. However, for those early bilinguals whose L2 becomes the dominant language, their code switching would tend to consist of L2 intrusions as they use their L1 thus suggesting that changes in language dominance play an important role in how bilinguals acces their two languages (Heredia, 1997; Heredia and Altarriba, 2001; Heredia and Brown, 2004; also see Basnight-Brown and Altarriba, ch. 4, this volume).

Understanding how language dominance and the preferential use of certain linguistic elements intersect may additionally be illuminated by examining cognitive and interactional factors in bilingual discourse. For example, in those situations of restricted use of L1, as in minority environments in which L1 is overpowered by the majority's L2, bilingual speakers experience attritional L1 loss. In these scenarios, bilinguals tend to favor the use of simplified verb forms (e.g., present indicative [yo como/I eat]) rather than complex verb forms (e.g., conditional [comería/I would eat]) because simple verb tenses are cognitively less complex and more frequently employed in routine conversational interactions in L1 (Silva-Corvalán, 1991). Thus, linguistic attrition and fluctuations in language dominance, as suggested by the above findings, would result in the weakening of both linguistic and cognitive abilities in the language that is less frequently employed or restricted in use (also see Montrul, 2002).

Finally, understandings of cognitive processing in bilingual speakers have similarly benefited from memory studies highlighting the possible interactions between culture, language, and emotions. Schrauf and Rubin (2000) examined the extent long-term memory for personal past, or autobiographical memory, was encoded in a language-specific manner in bilingual Spanish-English speakers. Findings showed that autobiographical memories were encoded in the language in which they were experienced; memories experienced in Spanish or English were retrieved in the language the event took place. Moreover, Altarriba (2003) adds an affective dimension to the way bilinguals process experienced episodes in their two languages. When assessing mental representations of words in Spanish-English bilinguals, Altarriba found that emotion words in Spanish (L1), unlike their English (L2) counterparts, were more easily associated with contexts or specific episodes in which the words were coded. Altarriba argues that contextual differences in the use of both languages may explain these findings. Spanish may be used in private, more intimate settings allowing more emotional expression compared to English which may be used for occupational and educational purposes. However, emotionality, like linguistic skills, may change with acculturation. Schrauf and Rubin (2004) report that, for some bilinguals with many years of residence in the L2 (U.S.) culture, acculturative forces may have influenced their ability to rate their autobiographical memories in L2 as having more intense emotional accompaniment than those in L1.

Taken together, research points to the participation of various factors and processes in the language-cognition interaction in bilinguals, including language socialization practices, language dominance, and language-emotion connections in each language. These factors seem to be molded by fluctuations in individual communication domains, SES, and acculturation as they shape the extent and nature of the linguistic input and concomitant cognitive demands in each language.

In sum, the complex interconnections among cultural diversity, language, and cognition in bilingual speakers offer intriguing conceptual bases for aphasia intervention. Although the ways such interactions operate is still in explorative stages and require further empirical specification, the plausibility of such preliminary understandings, however, may be assessed clinically in the treatment of bilingual aphasic individuals.

An Ethnopsycholinguistic Intervention Framework for Bilingual Clients with Aphasia

This chapter aims to propose an ecologically-valid, theoretically-grounded approach to therapy with bilingual aphasic speakers which acknowledges the interplay among culture, language, and cognition. The preceding discussion underscores three important principles. First, because bilinguals are linguistically and culturally diverse, complex relationships among cultural, linguistic, and cognitive factors warrant individual examination as differences in sociocultural histories among bilingual speakers would impact language learning and associated cognitive abilities in contrasting ways. Second, concomitant factors shaping linguistic and cognitive practice and performance must be considered, including SES, sociopolitical and educational contexts of language acquisition, and acculturation. Third, language proficiency may not be fully understood without the realistic knowledge of sociolinguistic scenarios of bilingual acquisition and the typical expressive routines in bilingual discourse.

Clearly, ethnographic observations, collected during assessment, would provide the evidence on the preceding sociocultural and linguistic practices in order to account for possible psycholinguistic processes and, in turn, develop suitable intervention contexts. In addition to the standard intake information collected on all aphasic clients (i.e., medical, social, occupational, and educational factors), knowledge of each bilingual patient's ethnographic and sociolinguistic history is imperative. Specifically, a questionnaire should be designed to explore ethnic identity (through the patient's social networks and expressed feelings about his/her two languages and their cultures), language acquisition history (i.e., age of initiation of L2 experiences, contexts [e.g., home, school, work] and modalities [e.g., speaking, writing, reading, and listening comprehension] of L1 and L2 use), and pre-morbid dominance (i.e., proficiency ratings based on family reports and, if possible, self-reports) (Brozgold and Centeno, in press; Centeno, 2005, in press-a). Similarly, information on the extent of pre-morbid use of typical expressive features in bilingual discourse by patients, such as language mixing, having an L1 accent when speaking in L2, and so forth, should be collected from close relatives and, if possible, from the patients themselves.

Using the collected ethnographic and sociolinguistic data, optimal intervention contexts can be developed to maximally cull cognitive-linguistic resources and promote communication utilizing the linguistic resources available to the client. Thus, the proposed EPL perspective would bring together language (i.e., target linguistic stimuli and multi-modality stimulation), cognitive strengths (e.g., attention, representational schemata, and memory), communication contexts (e.g., interlocutors, themes, and settings), and motivation (i.e., conversational engagement) into an integrated paradigm that would stimulate linguistic and psycholinguistic resources, consistent with the ethnographic history of each bilingual client with aphasia.

This approach is in line with cognitive bases for bilingual aphasia rehabilitation and psychoemotional principles in mental health intervention with bilingual populations. Motivation and affect may strengthen a memory trace physiologically inhibited in the bilingual aphasic speaker by the cerebral insult (Paradis, 2004). Similarly, because emotion words appear to be encoded in L1 and L2 differently and emotional scripts associated with each language may change with acculturation (Altarriba, 2003; Schrauf and Rubin, 2004), knowledge of contexts of acquisition, acculturation, and emotional connections to each language seem necessary for appropriate language and topic selection and enhance recall during therapy (see Altarriba, and Morier, 2004; Brozgold and Centeno, in press). Further, reinforcing basic information processing skills (i.e, attention, perception, categorization, and so forth) may enhance language improvement in bilingual speakers with aphasia (Kohnert, 2004). Finally, intensive multi-modality stimulation has been hypothesized to facilitate access to preserved abilities and reactivate physiologically inhibited skills in either language of a bilingual aphasic person as well as more general cognitive processes (Gil and Goral, 2004).

Although bilingual patients with aphasia may recover either or both languages after a stroke (Paradis, 2004; also see Roberts and Kiran, ch. 6, this volume), intervention strategies based on the above principles may be implemented either bilingually or monolingually. Drawing from a therapy rationale developed for bilingual children (i.e., Kohnert and Derr, 2004), Kohnert (2005) proposes that bilingual aphasic individuals, just like bilingual children, may benefit from either bilingual or monolingual intervention. In the former strategy, cognitive underpinnings common to both languages, such as the use of lexical cognates (e.g., rose-rosa, plate-plato), would maximize cognitive interconnections between the two languages and, in turn, progress in both languages. In the latter strategy, each language is treated separately by targetting unique features of the language and, hence, addressing non-overlapping areas between the languages. Treatment gains may generalize to the nontreated language (also see Kiran and Edmonds, 2004).

Similarly, Paradis (2004) advances a translation-based intervention format, grounded in neurolinguistic operations underlying bilingual language processing. Based on a review of the literature, Paradis proposes that translation, a metalinguistic task, would simultaneously activate cognitive and linguistic operations in both languages inhibited by the aphasia by encouraging the patient to make cross-linguistic semantic and syntactic associations necessary for the translation task. Because metalinguistic knowledge is not affected by aphasia and translational abilities are less impaired than other linguistic skills in aphasia, translation may provide a useful compensatory technique for therapy. Even in those situations when there is no exact translation equivalence, the metalinguistic analysis involved in the problem-solving may be a plausible approach to simultaneously engage the patient's linguistic and cognitive resources in both languages and facilitate the production of the target expression using the most available linguistic means.

Kohnert's (2005) and Paradis' (2004) theoretical possibilities may be explored by adapting them to a multi-modality approach which utilizes all functional linguistic resources. The speech-language pathologist, having collected sufficient ethnographic and sociolinguistic information, creates realistic communication contexts for the patient, based on meaningful pre-morbid experiences to address the particular aphasic problem (e.g., agrammatism, anomia, semantic paraphasias, etc.). Realistic communication formats interconnect language stimuli (i.e., nouns, verbs, phrases, idiomatic expressions, and so forth), topics of conversation (i.e., family, work, daily routines, etc.), and available interlocutors (i.e., siblings, espouse, children, aide, and so forth) in rich thematic scenarios that would highlight past experiences, and, in turn, evoke memories, stimulate related language, and enhance motivation in the client (also see Altarriba and Morier, 2004; Centeno, 2005; Harris, 1997). Although a multi-modality method would stimulate language and cognition using all sensory channels of communication, dyadic interactions should take primacy, as conversational communication would enhance social engagement.

Hence, an EPL approach is consistent with current social perspectives to aphasia intervention. Specifically, the *Life Participation Approach to Aphasia* (LPAA), developed by the American Speech-Language-Hearing Association (ASHA) to define the philosophy of clinical practice and research in aphasia (LPAA Project Group, 2001), stresses the re-engagement of the aphasic person in life as the ultimate goal of aphasia services. Broadly speaking, the LPAA focuses on real-life goals and intervention strategies grounded in personal and environmental factors impacting the interaction between aphasic individuals and their social environment. In this manner, intervention aims to engage aphasic individuals in communicative exchanges and enabling experiences, rather than focusing on deficit-oriented techniques targeting specific linguistic skills.

There is much research still needed in bilingual aphasia therapy. The limited studies available have largely examined isolated linguistic skills without exploring the possible role of ethnographic-psycholinguistic interactions. Unanswered questions and conflicting evidence still remain (see Paradis, 2004). Studies have shown that treatment can help both treated and untreated languages, that the treated language may improve more than the untreated language, or that both languages may improve simultaneously (see Fabbro, 1999, Paradis, 2004; Roberts, 2001, for review). Also, there is a large number of confounding variables whose separate effects on intervention remain unsolved, such as age of L2 acquisition, pre-morbid language proficiency, and spontaneous recovery, among others (see Gil and Goral, 2004; Paradis, 2004).

Examining the interconnections between typical ethnographic language practices and their accompanying psycholinguistic mechanisms may not be an implausible notion, particularly knowing that access to linguistic forms by aphasic speakers may be enhanced by the forms' high frequency of occurrence in pre-morbid discourse routines (e.g., Centeno, in press-b; Centeno and Obler, 2001a). Also, the interconnections of memory, emotions, and language through the use of autobiographical retellings during speech therapy may have a faciliating role (Harris, 1997; also see Centeno, 2005). Given that bilingualism is a complex multidimensional phenomenon in which psycholinguistic processing may be intertwined with ethnographic language practices and psychoemotional factors (Altarriba, 2003; Ellis, 2002; Pavlenko, 2005; Walters, 2005), an ethnopsychological perspective for aphasia treatment of bilingual patients may be a viable approach that deserves clinical exploration, particularly in these changing demographic times.

ACKNOWLEDGMENTS

I gratefully acknowledge the editorial comments on earlier versions of this paper provided by Jeanette Altarriba, Alfredo Ardila, Dana M. Basnight-Brown, Aneta Pavlenko, and Eliane Ramos.

REFERENCES

Altarriba, J. (2003). Does *cariño* equal liking? A theoretical approach to conceptual nonequivalence between languages. *International Journal of Bilingualism, 3*, 305-322.

Altarriba, J., and Morier, R. (2004) Bilingualism: Language, emotions, and mental health. In T.J. Bhatia and Ritchie (Eds.), *The handbook of bilingualism* (pp. 250-280). Malden, MA: Blackwell.

Ardila, A., Rosselli, M., and Ostrosky-Solís, F. (1992). Socioeducational. In A. E. Puente and R. J. McCaffrey (Eds.), *Handbook of neuropsychological assessment: A biopsychosocial perspective* (pp. 181-192). New York: Plenum.

Baetens Beardsmore, H. (1986). *Bilingualism: Basic principles* (2nd ed.).San Diego: College-Hill.

Battle, D. (2002). Communication disorders in a multicultural society. In D. E. Battle (Ed.), *Communication disorders in multicultural populations* (3rd ed., pp. 3-31). Boston: Butterworth-Heinemann.

Bialystok, E. (2001). *Bilingualism in development: Language, literacy, and cognition.* Cambridge: Cambridge University Press.

Brozgold, A., and Centeno, J. G. (In press). Sociocultural, societal, and psychological aspects of bilingualism: Variables, interactions, and therapeutic implications in speech-language pathology. In J. G. Centeno, R. T. Anderson, and L. K. Obler (Eds.), *Communication disorders in Spanish speakers: Theoretical, research, and clinical aspects.* Clevedon, UK: Multilingual Matters.

Byng, S., Parr, S., and Cairns, D. (2003). The science or sciences of aphasia? In I. Papathanasiou and R. De Bleser (Eds.), *The sciences of aphasia: From therapy to theory* (pp. 201-224). Oxford: Pergamon.

Centeno, J. G. (2005). Working with bilingual individuals with aphasia: The case of a Spanish-English bilingual client. *American Speech-Language-Hearing Association Division 14 - Perspectives on Communication Disorders and Sciences in Culturally and Linguistically Diverse Populations, 12*, 2-7.

Centeno, J. G. (2007). From theory to realistic praxis: Service-learning as a teaching method to enhance speech-language pathology services with minority populations. In J. Hellebrandt and A. Wurr (Eds.), *Learning the language of global citizenship: Service-learning in applied linguistics* (pp. 190-218). Bolton, MA: Anker.

Centeno, J. G. (In press-a). Bilingual development and communication: Implications for clinical language studies. In J. G. Centeno, R. T. Anderson, and L. K. Obler (Eds.), *Communication disorders in Spanish speakers: Theoretical, research, and clinical aspects.* Clevedon, UK: Multilingual Matters.

Centeno, J. G. (In press-b). Canonical features in the inflectional morphology of Spanish-speaking individuals with agrammatic speech. *Advances in Speech-Language Pathology.*

Centeno, J. G., and Eng, N. (2005). Bilingual speech-language pathology consultants in culturally diverse schools: Considerations on theoretically-based consultee engagement. *Journal of Educational and Psychological Consultation, 16*, 333-347.

Centeno, J. G., and Obler. L. K. (2001a). Agrammatic verb errors in Spanish speakers and their normal discourse correlates. *Journal of Neurolinguistics, 14*, 349-363.

Centeno, J. G., and Obler, L. K. (2001b). Principles of bilingualism. In M. Pontón and J. L. Carrión (Eds.), *Neuropsychology and the Hispanic patient: A clinical handbook* (pp. 75-86), Mahwah, NJ: Lawrence Erlbaum.

Chapey, R., and Hallowell, B. (2001). Introduction to language intervention strategies in adult aphasia. In R. Chapey (Eds.), *Language intervention strategies in aphasia and related neurogenic communication disorders* (4th ed., pp. 3-17). Baltimore, MD: Lippincott Williams and Wilkins.

Code, C. (2001). Multifactorial processes in recovery from aphasia: Developing the foundations for a multilevel framework. *Brain and Language, 77*, 25-44.

Coulmas, F. (1997). Introduction. In F. Coulmas (Eds.), *The handbook of sociolinguistics* (pp. 1-11). Cambridge, MA: Blackwell.

Damico, J. S., and Simmons-Mackie, N. N. (2003). Qualitative research and speech-language pathology: A tutorial for the clinical realm. *American Journal of Speech-Language Pathology, 12*, 131-143.

De Houwer, A. (1995). Bilingual language acquisition. In P. Fletcher and B. MacWinney (Eds.), *The handbook of child language* (pp. 219-250). London: Basil Blackwell.

Ellis, N. C. (2002). Frequency effects in language processing: A review with implications for theories of implicit and explicit language acquisition. *Studies in Second Language Acquisition, 24*, 143-188.

Elman, R. (2005). Social and life participation approaches to aphasia intervention. In L. L. LaPointe (Ed.), *Aphasia and related neurogenic language disorders* (3rd ed., pp. 39-50). New York: Thieme.

Fabbro, F. (1999). *The neurolinguistics of bilingualism: An introduction.* East Sussex, UK: Psychology Press.

Gil, M., and Goral, M. (2004). Nonparallel recovery in bilingual aphasia: Effects of language choice, language proficiency, and treatment. *International Journal of Bilingualism, 8*, 191-219.

Goldstein, B. A. (2004). Bilingual language development and disorders: Introduction and overview. In B. A. Goldstein (Ed.), *Bilingual language development and disorders in Spanish-English speakers* (pp. 3-20). Baltimore: Paul H. Brookes.

Green, D. W. (2005). The neurocognition of recovery patterns in bilingual aphasics. In J. F. Kroll and A. M. B. de Groot (Eds.), *Handbook of bilingualism: Psycholinguistic approaches* (pp. 516-530). New York: Oxford University Press.

Grosjean, F. (2004). Studying bilinguals: Methodological and conceptual issues. In T. K. Bhatia and W. C. Ritchie (Eds.), *The handbook of bilingualism* (pp. 32-63). Malden, MA: Blackwell.

Guendouzi, J. A., and Müller, N. (2006). *Approaches to discourse in dementia.* Mahwah, NJ: Lawrence Erlbaum.

Hamers, J. F., and Blanc, M. H. A. (2000). *Bilinguality and bilingualism* (2nd ed.). Cambridge University Press.

Harris, J. L. (1997). Reminiscence: A culturally and developmentally appropriate language intervention for older adults. *American Journal of Speech-Language Pathology, 6,* 19-25.

Harris, J. L. (2003). Toward an understanding of literacy issues in multicultural school-age populations. *Language, Speech, and Hearing Services in the Schools, 34,* 17-19.

Heredia, R. R. (1997). Bilingual memory and hierarchical models: A case for language dominance. *Current Directions in Psychological Science, 6,* 34-39.

Heredia, R. R., and Altarriba, J. (2001). Bilingual language mixing: Why do bilinguals code-switch? *Current Directions in Psychological Science, 10,* 164-168.

Heredia, R. R., and Brown, J. M. (2004). Bilingual memory. In T. K. Bhatia and W. C. Ritchie (Eds.), *The handbook of bilingualism* (pp. 225-249). Boston: Blackwell.

Hidalgo, M. (1993). The dialectics of Spanish language royalty and maintenance on the U.S.-Mexico border: A two-generation study. In A. Roca and J. M. Lipsky (Eds.), *Spanish in The United States: Linguistic contact and diversity* (pp.47-74). Berlin: Mouton de Gruyter.

Hyltenstam, K. and Abrahamsson, N. (2003). Maturational constraints in SLA. In C. Doughty and M. Long (Eds.), *Handbook of second language acquisition* (pp. 539-588). Malden, MA: Blackwell.

Jia, G., Aaronson, D., and Wu, Y. (2002). Long-term language attainment of bilingual immigrants: Predictive variables and language group differences. *Applied Psycholinguistics, 23,* 599-621.

Kiran, S., and Edmonds, L. A. (2004). Effect of semantic naming treatment on crosslinguistic generalization in bilingual aphasia. *Brain and Language, 91,* 75-77.

Kohnert, K. (2004). Cognitive and cognate-based treatments for bilingual aphasia: A case study. *Brain and Language, 91,* 294-302.

Kohnert, K. (2005). Cognitive-linguistic interactions in bilingual aphasia: Implications for intervention. *American Speech-Language-Hearing Association Division 2 - Perspectives on Neurophysiology and Neurogenic Speech and Language Disorders, 15,* 9-14.

Kohnert, K. and Derr, A. (2004). Language intervention with bilingual children. In B. A. Goldstein (Ed.), *Bilingual language development and disorders in Spanish-English speakers* (pp. 315-343). Baltimore: Paul H. Brookes.

LaPointe, L. L. (2003). Functional and pragmatic directions in aphasia therapy. In I. Papathanasiou and R. De Bleser (Eds.), *The sciences of aphasia: From therapy to theory* (pp. 163-172). Oxford: Pergamon.

Life Participation Approach to Aphasia Project Group. (2001). Life participation approach to aphasia: A statement of values for the future. In R. Chapey (Ed.), *Language intervention strategies in adult aphasia* (4th ed., pp. 235-245). Baltimore, MD: Lippincott, Williams and Wilkins.

Manuel-Dupont, S., Ardila, A., Rosselli, M., and Puente, A. E. (1992). Bilingualism. In A. E. Puente and R. J. McCaffrey (Eds.), *Handbook of neuropsychological assessment: A biopsychosocial perspective* (pp. 193-210). New York: Plenum.

Marin, G., Organista, P. B., and Chun, R. M. (2003). Acculturation research: Current issues and findings. In G. Bernal, J. E. Trimble, A. K. Burlew, and F. T. L. Leong (Eds.), *Handbook of racial and ethnic minority psychology* (pp. 208-219). Thousand Oaks, CA: Sage.

Meisel, J. (1990). *Two first languages: Early grammatical development in bilingual children.* Dordrecht: Foris.

Mertens, D. M. (1998).*Research methods in education and psychology: Integrating diversity with quantitative and qualitative approaches.* Thousand Oaks, CA: Sage.

Montrul, S. (2002). Incomplete acquisition and attrition of Spanish tense/aspect distinctions in adult bilinguals. *Bilingualism: Language and Cognition, 5,* 39-68.

National Alliance for Hispanic Health. (2004). *Delivering health care to Hispanics: A manual for providers.* Washington, DC: Estrella Press.

Novoa, L., Fein, D., and Obler, L. K. (1988). Talent in foreign languages: A case study. In L. K. Obler and D. Fein (Eds.), *The exceptional brain: Neuropsychology of talent and special abilities* (pp. 294-303). New York: Guilford.

Ogbu, J. U. (2002). Cultural amplifiers of intelligence: IQ and minority status in cross-cultural perspective. In J. Fish (Ed.), *Race and intelligence: Separating science from myth* (pp. 241-280). Mahwah, NJ: Lawrence Erlbaum.

Paradis, M. (2004). *A neurolinguistic theory of bilingualism.* Amsterdam: John Benjamins.

Pavlenko, A. (2000). Access to linguistic resources: Key variables in second language learning. *Estudios de Sociolingüistica, 1,* 85-106.

Pavlenko, A. (2005). Bilingualism and thought. In J. F. Kroll and A. M. B. de Groot (Eds.), *Handbook of bilingualism: Psycholinguistic approaches* (pp. 433-453). New York: Oxford University Press.

Pérez-Foster, R. (1998). *The power of language in the clinical process: Assessing and treating the bilingual person.* Northvale, NJ: Jason Aronson.

Phinney, J. S. (2003). Ethnic identity and acculturation. In K. M. Chun, P. B. Organista, and G. Marín (Eds.), *Acculturation: Advances in theory, measurement, and applied research* (pp. 63-82). Washington, DC: American Psychological Association.

Quinn, N., and Holland, D. (1987). Culture and cognition. In D. Holland and N. Quinn (Eds.), *Cultural models in language and thought* (pp. 3-42). Cambridge: Cambridge University Press.

Ritchie, W. C., and Bhatia, T. K. (1996). Introduction. In W. C. Ritchie and T. K. Bhatia (Eds.), *Handbook of second language acquisition* (pp. 1-46). San Diego, CA: Academic Press.

Roberts, P. M. (2001). Aphasia assessment and treatment for bilingual and culturally diverse clients. In R. Chapey (Ed.), *Language intervention strategies in aphasia and related neurogenic communication disorders* (4th ed., pp. 208-234). Baltimore, MD: Lippincott, Williams and Wilkins.

Rodriguez, B. L., and Olswang, L. B. (2002). Cultural diversity is more than group differences: An example from the Mexican American community. *Contemporary Issues in Communication Science and Disorders, 29,* 154-164.

Romaine, S. (1995). *Bilingualism* (2nd ed.). Oxford: Blackwell.

Roseberry-McKibbin, C., Brice, A., and O'Hanlon, L. (2005). Serving English language learners in school settings: A national survey. *Language, Speech, and Hearing Services in Schools, 36,* 48-61.

Ryan, E., L., Baird, R., Rivera Mindt, M., Byrd, D., Monzones, J., and Morgello, S. (2005). Neuropsychological impairment in racial/ethnic minorities with HIV infection and low literacy levels: Effects of education and reading level in participant characterization. *Journal of the International Neuropsychological Society, 11*, 889-898.

Salas-Provance, M. B., Erickson, J. G., and Reed, J. (2002). Disabilities as viewed by four generations of one Hispanic family. *American Journal of Speech-Language Pathology, 11,* 151-162.

Salzmann, Z. (1993). *Language, culture, and society: An introduction to linguistic anthropology.* Boulder, CO: Westview Press.

Schneiderman, E. I., and Desmarais, C. (1988). A neuropsychological substrate for talent in second language acquisition. In L. K. Obler and D. Fein (Eds.), *The exceptional brain: Neuropsychology of talent and special abilities* (pp. 103-126). New York: Guilford.

Schrauf, R. W., and Rubin, D. C. (2000). Internal languages of retrieval: The bilingual encoding of memories for the personal past. *Memory and Cognition, 28,* 616-623.

Schrauf, R. W., and Rubin, D. C. (2004). The 'language' and 'feel' of bilingual memory: Mnemonic traces. *Estudios de Sociolingüistica, 5 (1),* 21-40.

Silva-Corvalán. C. (1991). Spanish language attrition in a contact situation with English. In H. W. Seliger and R. Vago (Eds.), *First language attrition* (pp. 151-171). Cambridge: Cambridge University Press.

Simmons-Mackie, N. (2001). Social approaches to aphasia intervention. In R. Chapey (Ed.), *Language intervention strategies in aphasia and related neurogenic communication disorders* (4th ed., pp. 246-268). Baltimore, MD: Lippincott, Williams and Wilkins.

Simmons-Mackie, N., and Damico, J. S. (1999). Qualitative methods in aphasia research: Ethnography. *Aphasiology, 13,* 681-687.

Snow, C. E., Cancino, H., de Temple, J., and Schley, S. (1991). Giving formal definitions: A linguistic or metalinguistic skill? In H. Bialystok (Ed.), *Language processing in bilingual children* (pp. 90-112). Cambridge University Press.

Torres, L. (1997) *Puerto Rican discourse: A sociolinguistic study of a New York suburb.* Mahwah, NJ: Lawrence Erlbaum.

Trimble, J. E. (2003). Introduction: Social change and acculturation. In K. M. Chun, P. B. Organista, and G. Marín (Eds.), *Acculturation: Advances in theory, measurement, and applied research* (pp. 3-13). Washington, DC: American Psychological Association.

U.S. Census Bureau. (2002). *Annual demographic supplement to the March 2002 current population survey.* Washington, DC: Author.

U.S. Census Bureau. (2003). Nearly 1-in-5 speak a foreign language at home. *U.S. Census Bureau News, Report CB03-157.* Washington, DC: Author.

Van Lancker, D., and Pachana, N. A. (1998). The influence of emotions on language and communication disorders. In B. Stemmer and H. A. Whitaker (Eds.), *Handbook of neurolinguistics* (pp. 301-311). San Diego: Academic Press.

Wallace, G. L. (1997). Treatment of individuals from diverse backgrounds. In G. J. Wallace (Ed.), *Multicultural neurogenics* (pp. 103-114). San Antonio, TX: Communication Skill Builders.

Walters, J. (2005). *Bilingualism: The sociopragmatic-psycholinguistic interface.* Mahwah, NJ: Lawrence Erlbaum.

Zecker, L. B. (2004). Learning to read and write in two languages: The development of early biliteracy abilities. In C. A. Stone, E. R. Silliman, B. J. Ehren, and K. Apel (Eds.), *Handbook of language and literacy: Development and disorders* (pp. 248-265). New York: Guilford.

Zentella, A.C. (1997) Spanish in New York. In O. Garcia and J. Fishman (Eds.), *The multilingual apple: Languages in New York City* (pp.167-201). Berlin: Mouton de Gruyter.

Zentella, A. C. (2005). Introduction. In A. C. Zentella (Ed.), *Building on strength: Language and literacy in Latino families and communities* (pp. 1-12). New York: Teachers College Press.

In: Speech and Language Disorders in Bilinguals ISBN 978-1-60021-560-5
Editors: Alfredo Ardila and Eliane Ramos, pp. 213-234

Chapter 12

BILINGUALISM AND COGNITION: THE GOOD, THE BAD, AND THE UGLY OF BILINGUALISM

Alfredo Ardila and Eliane Ramos
Department of Communication Sciences and Disorders
Florida International University
Miami, Florida 33199 USA

"He who knows no foreign language does not truly know his own."
Goethe

The relationship between bilingualism and cognition has been controversial (e.g., Ben-Zeev, 1977; Diaz, 1983; Hakuta. 1986; Haugen, 1956; Hu, 1999; Padilla et al, 1990). Until the 1960s it was generally assumed that bilingual individuals underperformed in a variety of verbal ability tests. For example, Darcy (1953) stated that research supported the conclusion that bilinguals suffered from a language handicap when measured by verbal tests of intelligence. Supposedly, bilingualism had a detrimental effect on language abilities. Similar negative opinions were expressed by other authors. In spite of generalized opinions about the negative effects of bilingualism in verbal tests before the 1960s, other authors argued that bilingualism did not affect cognitive development and performance in verbal ability tests. For instance, Weinreich (1953) denied the supposedly detrimental effect of bilingualism on mental development.

In 1962 Peal and Lambert published a seminal paper analyzing the relationship between bilingualism and intelligence. Using French-English bilinguals in Canada, they found that if social class were taken into account, true bilingualism was associated with higher scores in a variety of cognitive tests. This research was particularly influential because it emphasized the diversity of potentially confounding variables that may affect cognitive test scores. If those variables are not appropriately controlled (e.g., SES and educational level), they may obscure test results. Positive correlations between academic achievement and bilingualism were later documented (e.g., Fernandez and Nielsen, 1986). At approximately that same time, different studies supported the opposite point of view: the simultaneous knowledge of two different languages can positively affect performance in a diversity of not only verbal but also nonverbal tasks. For instance, Rumbaut and Ima (1988) showed significant differences between true bilinguals and monolinguals, and true bilinguals and semibilinguals among high school students in San Diego. True bilingualism showed a positive effect on academic performance.

Progressively, the idea that bilingualism has a positive effect in cognitive test performance has prevailed (e.g., Craik and Bialystok, 2005). This positive effect has been reported not only in verbal, but also in non verbal ability tasks (e.g., Bialystok and Shapero, 2005; Gorrell et al., 1982).

Positive and Negative Effects of Bilingualism

Some positive, but also negative effects of bilingualism have been reported in contemporary literature. Positive effects include metalinguistic awareness (e.g., Lombardi, 1986), increased cognitive control (enhanced executive functioning) (e.g., Bialystok et al., 2005), and mental flexibility (e.g., Bialystok and Shapero, 2005). Negative effects include decreased verbal fluency (e.g., Gollan, Montoya, and Werner (2002), and slower language development (e.g., Topprlberg et al., 2002).

Positive Effects

Using two different languages may result in developing new cognitive strategies, providing some potential advantages to the bilingual individual. It can be conjectured that bilingualism advantages in cognitive ability can be related with, (a) learning new cognitive strategies, (b) getting a better insight of one's own language, and (c) increasing cognitive control.

(A). Learning New Cognitive Strategies

Learning new cognitive strategies may be relate to the different components of language (phonologic, lexical/ semantics, grammatical, and pragmatics). Advantages, nonetheless, may be more evident at the grammatical and lexical/semantic levels. Grammar represents types of "logics" (i.e., how to organize sequences of ideas) and lexicon/ semantics provides a classification system (i.e., how elements are grouped and distinguished). The bilingual may use two logical reasoning systems (grammar), and an extended classification system (lexical/semantic). Furthermore, the bilingual may have an extended phonological knowledge, potentially associated with increased phonological awareness and auditory discrimination. Pragmatics (i.e., how to use language) is not usually mentioned in the bilingualism literature. Pragmatics has been generally approached in the context of cross-cultural communication (e.g., Chick, 1996). Nonetheless, pragmatics not only refers to the social and cultural rules governing the use of the language. It also has to be taken into account that each language contains certain implicit pragmatic rules. For instance, some languages (such as English) distinguish only one second person pronoun ("you"); whereas others (such as Spanish) distinguish two ("*usted*"=formal, polite, indicating distance and/or respect; and "*tú*" = indicating closeness). As a matter of fact, a diversity of possibilities in the number and use of pronouns are found that will indicate how to address people in specific contexts. Using two languages requires the correct use of these pragmatic rules. Bilinguals may possess an increased flexibility and awareness in the use of language pragmatics. It is not surprising that this enlarged language knowledge (phonologic, lexical/ semantic, grammatical, and pragmatic) may lead to stronger metalinguistic awareness.

Pavlenko (2005) argued that bilingual individuals can significantly contribute to the understanding of linguistic relativity and the interactions between language and thought. Departing from the new developments in the Sapir-Whorf linguistic relativity hypothesis, she examined linguistic differences in different areas (color, object and substances, numeric systems, space, motion, time, emotions, personhood, discourse, and autobiographical memory) to find that language may indeed create different worlds for their speakers. Bilinguals draw on distinct conceptual representations when speaking their respective languages. Pavlenko concluded that "...bilingualism could be extremely beneficial for enriching the speakers' linguistic repertoires and offering them alternative conceptualizations crucial for flexible and critical thinking" (p. 447).

(B). Getting a Better Insight of His/Her Own Language

Learning a second language may also result in getting a better understanding of the native language ("metalinguistic awareness"). Learning a second language may be the most direct way to understand that our language represents just a specific and particular way to organize the reality and our personal experiences, not the only way to conceptualize the world. Bilingualism has been found to be associated with higher metalinguistic and metacognitive abilities (Lombardi, 1986).

(C). Increasing Cognitive Control.

During recent years, some research studies have approached the question of cognitive control in bilinguals. Bilingualism has been associated with more effective controlled processing in children. Furthermore, it seems that the simultaneous management of two competing languages potentially enhances executive functions (e.g., Craik and Bialystok, 2005).

Negative Effects

Some negative effects of bilingualism have also been reported. These supposedly negative effects frequently have been controversial. They depend upon a diversity of variables, and different studies often present inconsistent results. Using two languages, for instance, may also result in interference and decreased verbal ability. Diverse studies have illustrated that bilingualism may be associated with slower language development in children (when children are tested in each one of the languages separately), decreased verbal fluency, and interference. These negative effects of bilingualism are usually reported when both languages are active languages, and permanent switching is required.

It can be conjectured that bilingualism disadvantages in cognitive ability can be related to (a) increased language difficulties in children with language impairments; (b) increased probability of certain psychopathological conditions, particularly emotional/behavioral problems; (c) decrease in verbal fluency; and (d) interference between both languages.

(A). Bilingual Children with Language Impairments

In a retrospective case study of medical records, Cheuk, Wong and Leung (2005) selected 326 children with specific language impairment and 304 controls in Hong Kong. These children had been assessed by their pediatricians using the Griffiths Mental Developmental Scale (GMDS), which was standardized in the United Kingdom and includes a subtest for language development. Children who scored below one standard deviation from the mean in the language domain and within normal levels in the other domains tested were classified as having a specific language impairment. The mean ages of cases and controls were 2.56 and 2.89 years respectively. Boys predominated in both groups. The children were exposed to between one and four languages at home, the major ones being Cantonese Chinese followed by English. Multivariable linear regression was applied to examine the effects of covariates on the language comprehension and expression standard scores. A significant linear dose-response relationship was found for each additional language to which the child was exposed. Male gender, positive family history of language impairment, lower education levels of parents and lower occupational status of fathers were also risk factors for specific language impairment. Multilingual exposure also significantly reduced the language quotient and language comprehension standard score of children with specific language impairment, but not of normal children. It was concluded that multilingual home environment is associated with specific language impairment with a dose-response relationship. The authors suggested that even though exposure to multiple languages does not cause language impairment, it may represent an additional burden to children who have this disability and further interfere with language learning. This conclusion may be premature because of the many limitations of this study. Most importantly, the use of a standardized test that has not been validated for use with this population and the classification of such young children as having a specific language impairment. In general, children are not given this diagnosis until the age of 4, because many of them turn out to be late talkers and outgrow their language difficulties.

Salameh, Nottelbladt and Gullberg (2002) in Sweden analyzed risk factors for language impairment relative to degree of severity in bilingual and monolingual children. Two groups of children with language impairments were compared, 252 bilinguals whose parents were both non-Swedish speakers and 446 monolinguals. A multivariate linear regression for both groups showed that two risk factors were the same: parental distress, and short attention span. Male gender was an additional predictor for LI relative to degree of severity in the monolingual group. Specific risk factors for LI relative to degree of severity in the bilingual children were maternal arrival within 1 year in relation to birth and parental need for an interpreter after more than 5 years in Sweden. It was concluded that risk factors for language impairment relative to degree of severity in this study seemed to apply to both groups, although they sometimes appeared in another form in the bilingual group. Gender and possibly also hereditary factors seemed to need to interact with environmental factors to appear as risk factors for the bilingual children in this study.

In a more recent study, Salameh, Hakansson, and Nottelbladt (2004) studied 20 Swedish-Arabic bilinguals aged 4 to 7 years over a 12 month period. Ten subjects had severe language impairments and 10 had no language impairments. The two groups of children developed both languages in the expected order, with the only difference being that children with language impairments showed slower development, which was comparable to what is expected of monolingual speakers of each language with language impairments.

It is extremely difficult to study bilingual children with language impairments and draw conclusions about their ability to learn two languages or more. Confounding variables such as amount of exposure to each language, age of introduction of the second language, parental proficiency in each language, and language of schooling, to name just a few, are constant in this population. Paradis et al. (2003) were able to control most of these variables by studying eight 7-year-old French-English bilingual children with specific language impairment in Canada. This group of children was fairly homogenous because they were all exposed to both languages from birth from native speakers of each language and lived in a community where both languages were used socially and educationally, and neither is considered a minority language. The authors studied aspects of grammars such as verb forms and object pronouns that often pose difficulty for these children. As expected, the children showed difficulties in both languages, but their difficulties were comparable to those shown by monolingual speakers of each language who also have specific language impairment. Apparently, in this population, learning a second language did not present an extra burden, and while these children may never become completely proficient in both languages (just as monolingual speakers with specific language impairment may never become completely proficient in their one language), they are likely to enjoy many of the benefits of being bilingual in their community.

(B). Bilingualism and Psychopathology

Topprlberg et al. (2002) investigated (1) the prevalence of language deficits and disorders and (2) the relationship of bilingual language skills and psychopathology, in Spanish-English bilingual children referred for child and adolescent psychiatry service. Bilingual language skills, emotional/behavioral problems, sociodemographics, immigration variables, and nonverbal IQ were studied in 50 consecutively referred children. Estimated prevalence for language deficits and disorders was high (between 40 and 50%), with most cases (>79%) being of the mixed receptive-expressive type. This prevalence is comparable to those found in studies of monolingual children. In children with clinically significant emotional/behavioral problems, bilingual language skills were strongly and inversely correlated with problem scores, particularly global problems; social, thought, and attention problems; as well as delinquency and aggression. These correlations remained significant after IQ adjustment. The authors assumed that their results supported prior findings, namely (1) the high prevalence of mixed receptive-expressive and other language disorders and delays and (2) the close tie between poor language skills and emotional/behavioral problems. It seems that bilingualism does not increase the risk for psychopathology. Rather, language deficits may lead to social isolation and maladjustment in both monolingual and bilingual children. Therefore, it is important to assess language skills in bilingual children to avoid attributing psychopathology to bilingualism.

(C). Decrease in Verbal Fluency

Rosselli et al (2000) observed equal performance of bilingual and monolingual Spanish-English participants in different verbal fluency tests except that of semantic verbal fluency:

Number of animal named in one minute (semantic verbal fluency task) was decreased in a similar way for both languages with regard to the monolingual participants. Gollan, Montoya, and Werner (2002) found similar results. The authors selected Spanish-English bilinguals and English monolinguals to complete 12 semantic, 10 letter, and 2 proper name fluency categories. Bilinguals produced fewer exemplars than monolinguals on all category types, but the difference between groups was larger (and more consistent) on semantic categories. It can be concluded that semantic verbal fluency may be decreased in bilingual individuals, probably related with the extra time required to select the language and/or to decide if a particular item belongs to L1 or L2

Interesting to note, bilinguals have more tip-of-the-tongue states (a condition where we cannot remember the word we want to find, but we have the feeling of knowing it, and even some characteristics can be mentioned, such as how it begins or how long it is) than monolinguals (unless the target word had translatable cognate names, such as *flower/flor*) (Gollan and Acenas, 2004).

(D). Interference Between Both Languages

Interference depends upon a diversity of variables. Interference increases when both languages are active languages. Interference may be higher when L1 and L2 are close languages. Interference may partially account for the decreased verbal fluency sometimes reported in bilinguals. Interference may also result in code switching and code mixing. Continuous code switching and code mixing may eventually result in a hybrid inter-language, such as so-called Franglais (French and English), Chinglish (Chinese and English), Portuñol (Portuguese and Spanish), Spanglish (Spanish and English), etc. Ardila (2005) proposed that in a hybrid interlanguage such as Spanglish, two different types of linguistic phenomena can be distinguished: "superficial", including borrowing and code-switching; and "deep", including lexical-semantic, grammatical, and the "equalization to English" phenomenon.

Controlling interference has been interpreted as an executive function depending on frontal lobe activity. Bilingual individuals need effective mechanisms to prevent interference between their languages. Using event-related brain potentials (ERPs) and functional magnetic resonance imaging (fMRI), Rodriguez-Fornells (2005) presented evidence for interference of phonological information from the nontarget language in German-Spanish bilinguals. Bilinguals showed phonological interference when compared with monolinguals, which was evident in their performance, ERPs, and fMRI patterns. Nonlanguage specific brain areas such as the left middle prefrontal cortex were found to be crucial for the control of interference. Noteworthy, it is generally accepted that language switching and selecting/maintaining a language represents an executive function; using functional neuroimaging techniques, an increased activation of the left dorsolateral prefrontal area is usually reported (Hernandez, Dapretto, Mazziotta, and Bookheimer, 2001).

Executive Control

Bilingualism in children has been associated with some advantages in using cognitive processes (Bialystok, 2001, 2005; Bochner, 1996). Information about potential advantages of bilingualism in adults, nonetheless, is more limited. Bialystok, Craik, Klein, and Viswanathan (2004) reported that bilingualism may attenuate the negative effects of aging on cognitive control (metacognition). They observed that executive control is more effective in bilinguals and that bilingualism helps to attenuate age-related losses in certain executive processes. Bialystok et al. (2005) have even suggested that the management of two language systems leads to systematic changes in frontal executive functions. Craik and Bialystok (2005) have further proposed that the advantage shown by bilinguals in levels of control may lie in their greater ability to maintain a task-relevant set in working memory, and perhaps also in their greater responsiveness and flexibility in both set formation and translation of stimuli into appropriate responses. Indeed, using two different languages may require different levels of cognitive control, depending on the specific linguistic characteristics and the particular situation. For instance, having a single, active, primary and dominant language, and possessing a second, late and dormant language requires a minimal of cognitive control, whereas simultaneous interpretation (requiring that language comprehension and production take place simultaneously) probably represents the most complex and control-demanding bilingual task (Christoffels and de Groot, 2005).

Mohamed et al. (2004) examined the functioning of inhibitory mechanisms (an executive function) in younger and older bilinguals using a bilingual version of the Stroop test.[1] Older unbalanced bilinguals showed greater interlingual interference when they responded with their second language to visual stimuli written in their dominant language. Balanced bilinguals showed equivalent interference effects between all conditions. The authors suggested that manipulating two languages may enhance the efficiency of inhibitory mechanisms. Rosselli et al. (2002a) also analyzed the performance of Spanish-English bilinguals in the Stroop test. In bilinguals, the Stroop Test was administered in English and in Spanish. Overall, performance was slower in bilinguals than in monolinguals. No significant differences were observed in color reading but bilinguals did not score as well in the naming color condition. Within the bilingual group, the Stroop Test scores were similar in both English and Spanish. Age of acquisition of the second language and language proficiency did not predict the Stroop Test performance, but subject's age significantly correlated with performance.

Rosselli et al. (2000) examined the impact of bilingualism on verbal fluency and repetition tests in older Spanish/English bilinguals. Bilinguals who learned English before age 12 performed significantly better on the English repetition test and produced a higher number of words in the description of a picture than the bilinguals who learned English after age 12. The authors suggested that variables such as task demands, language interference, linguistic mode, and level of bilingualism may impact fluency and repetition skills in bilinguals.

Strategies in reasoning styles and categorization can differ across languages. For instance, bilingual Chinese subjects organize objects in a more relational and less categorical

[1] One of the best-known procedures to study response interference and inhibition is the Stroop Test (ST) (Stroop, 1935). ST has frequently been used as an executive functioning task. The ST requires participants to name/read colors as fast as they can under three conditions. In one control condition, participants are presented a list of color words printed in black ink and requested to read them. In a second control condition, participants are presented with a list of XXXX's printed in different colors and are required to name the color of the ink. In the last condition (Color-Word) participants are presented with a list of color words printed in ink of an incongruent color and are required to name the color of the ink while ignoring the written word. In this last condition the subjects need to inhibit the automatic response of reading the word (e.g. when presented with the word *RED* written in green they are supposed to answer "green"). Ink color naming is faster when the two dimensions of the stimulus are congruent (e.g. *RED* written in red) than when they are incongruent (e.g. *RED* written in green). That is, the irrelevant, to-be-ignored dimension interferes with processing the relevant dimension. This pattern of response is called the Stroop effect.

way than Europeans and Americans, whether tested in English or in Chinese (Ji , Zhang and, Nisbett, 2004). Nevertheless, language also may affect some Chinese bilinguals' categorization. It was observed that the responses of Chinese from the Mainland and Taiwan were more relational when tested in Chinese than when tested in English. Responses of Chinese from Hong Kong and Singapore were equally relational when tested in Chinese and in English. Rosselli et al. (2002b) using verbal fluency tests observed that English monolinguals generated significantly more grammatical words than Spanish monolinguals, and bilinguals produced a significantly higher number of grammatical words in English than in Spanish. There is no explanation to account for why English speakers include a significant amount of grammatical words in fluency tests, whereas Spanish speakers do not. Bilinguals behave more as English speakers when performing the test in English and more as Spanish speakers when performing the test in Spanish. Animal subcategories and semantic associations, however, were similar in both languages for all groups. The authors proposed that different cognitive strategies were available with the use of each language, and bilinguals may possess extended cognitive strategies taken from the two languages.

Tanako and Noda (1993) suggested that the use of a second language may result in a temporary decline of thinking ability because of the heavier processing load imposed by a foreign language. Using a divided-attention experiment with Japanese/English and English/Japanese adult bilinguals they observed that subjects' performance on a thinking task (calculation) declined when a concurrent linguistic task (question-answering) had to be performed in the foreign language. This decline is distinguishable from foreign-language processing difficulty per se because the thinking task involved no foreign-language use. The same effect was found when using spatial reasoning problems adapted from intelligence tests.

Solving mathematical problems can be considered as a paradigm of thinking. It requires not only the understanding of the conditions of the problem, but also developing an algorithm for solving it, and the application of some specific arithmetical procedures. It has been observed that the ability to solve numerical problems may be better in L1 than in L2. Bernardo (2002) analyzed the ability to understand and solve word problems in arithmetic when using L1 and L2. Filipino-English bilinguals were selected, and divided into two subgroups: students whose 1st language was Filipino and students whose 1st language was English. The results indicated a 1st-language advantage; that is, the students were better able to understand and solve problems in their 1st language, whether the 1st language was English or Filipino. Ardila et al (2000) using Spanish-English bilinguals also found that calculation ability accuracy was higher in the participant's native language. Solving mathematical problems was also easier in L1 than in L2.

Ben-Zeev (1977) analyzed the influence of bilingualism on the ability to use different cognitive strategies. He hypothesized that mutual interference between the bilingual child's two languages forces the child to develop particular coping strategies which may accelerate cognitive development. Two groups of Hebrew-English bilingual children and two groups of monolingual children were selected. It was found that in spite of lower vocabulary level, bilinguals showed more advanced processing of verbal material, more discrimination of perceptual distinctions, more propensity to search for structure in perceptual situations, and more capacity to reorganize their perceptions in response to feedback.

Controlling attention represents a major executive function. Segalowitz and Frenkiel-Fishman (2005) investigated the relationship between attention control and proficiency in a complex cognitive skill. The participants were English-French bilinguals with varying degrees of second-language (French) proficiency. Attention control was operationalized as the shift cost obtained in a linguistic version of the alternating runs task-switching paradigm. Hierarchical regression revealed that, overall, attention control accounted for 59% of the variance of proficiency and that second-language attention control alone accounted for 32% of the unique variance of proficiency, indicating a high degree of skill domain (second language) specificity in the relationship between attention control and proficiency. Bialystok (2005) Examined three cognitive domains: concepts of quantity, task switching, concept formation, and theory of mind. The major conclusion was that bilinguals are more advanced than monolinguals in those cognitive tasks requiring the inhibition of irrelevant information. In consequence, bilingualism facilitates the development of those cognitive functions concerned with attention and inhibition. The positive effect of bilingualism will be more evident in those processes and tasks requiring controlling attention and the inhibition of irrelevant information.

Creativity is a type of higher cognitive process not frequently analyzed in bilingualism literature. Okoh (1980) hypothesized that the bilingual person should have an advantage over the monolingual in "creativity" since s/he would presumably have a greater repertoire of cognitive cues, signs, meanings, and relationships on which to draw. Two samples of primary school pupils in Nigeria and Wales (N = 289, aged 9 to 11 years) were selected. A battery of tests of verbal and nonverbal creativity, verbal intelligence, and language proficiency was administered to both groups. Results showed that bilingual children scored significantly higher on the verbal creativity test than monolinguals, but there was no significant difference between the two groups in the nonverbal creativity tests.

Bilingualism and Memory

Any human activity is carried out in a particular context and is associated with a specific type of cognition. Language is the major instrument of cognition. The language used in different human activities is one of the elements (or the instrument) of the cognition required to carry out that activity. Bilinguals can potentially code their experiences into different systems provided by the two languages. It is not surprising that memory is dependent on the language in which the information was initially acquired. Marian and Neisser (2000) studied autobiographical memory in Russian/English bilinguals exploring the hypothesis that memories become more accessible when the linguistic environment at retrieval matched the linguistic environment at encoding. A group of Russian/English bilingual participants retrieved more experiences from the Russian-speaking period of their lives when interviewed in Russian and more experiences from the English-speaking period of their lives when interviewed in English. The authors concluded that the language at the time of retrieval, like other forms of context, played a significant role in determining what would be remembered. Similarly, Schrauf and Rubin (2000) found that older Hispanic immigrants who had arrived in the United States as adults internally retrieved autobiographical memories in Spanish for events in the country of origin and in English for events in the United States. Bilinguals encode and retrieve certain autobiographical memories in one or the other language according to the context of encoding the experience, and these linguistic characteristics are stable properties of those memories over time.

Cabeza and Lennartson (2005) selected a group of 30 English-French bilingual university students. Participants studied lists of converging associates using the Stadler, Roediger, and McDermott's paradigm. Each list consisted of the 12 strongest associates (e.g., pin, haystack, etc.) to a "critical lure" (e.g., needle). Some lists were presented in English and some in French. The participants further performed a recognition test containing studied list items and nonstudied critical lures whose language matched or mismatched the language at study. Participants were instructed to answer only if the test cue was in the same language as the studied word. The results yielded a robust false memory rate both within-language and across-languages. The effect of the study-test language shift was much larger for list items than for critical lures. Findings suggested that memory representations for critical lures contain primarily semantic gist traces and little surface information, and hence is more consistent with the fuzzy trace view than with the implicit associative response view. In sum, the study demonstrated the existence of false memory across languages, and provided information about the memory traces underlying veridical and illusory recognition.

The concept of "working memory" (Baddeley, 1986, 1992) has become notoriously influential. It refers to a temporary processing and storage of information. It has been proposed that working memory is involved in a diversity of cognitive processes, including language comprehension, planning, reasoning, problem solving and even consciousness. Working memory has been assumed to be related with second language acquisition as well. In 1988 Baddeley, Papagno, and Vallar reported the case of a 26 year-old Italian woman with a very pure deficit in short-term memory after a left-hemisphere stroke. A series of experiments comparing the subject's learning capacity with that of matched controls showed that her capacity to learn pairs of meaningful words in her native Italian language was within the normal range. The subject, however, was incapable of learning to associate a familiar word with an unfamiliar item from another language (Russian) through auditory presentation. The authors concluded that short-term phonological storage is important for learning unfamiliar verbal material, but is not essential for forming associations between meaningful items that are already known. It was proposed that one of the working memory functions accounts for the learning of new phonological material, and consequently plays a fundamental role in the acquisition of a second language. Similarly, Hummel (2002) noted that there is a significant relationship between working memory as measured by an L2 reading span task and L2 proficiency.

Papagno and Vallar (1995) studied polyglot and non-polyglot Italian subjects. Tests assessed verbal (phonological) memory as well as visuospatial short-term and long-term memory, general intelligence, and vocabulary knowledge in their native language. Polyglots had a superior level of performance in verbal short-term memory tasks (auditory digit span and nonword repetition) and in a paired-associate learning test, which assessed the subjects' ability to acquire new (Russian) words. By contrast, the two groups had comparable performance levels in tasks assessing general intelligence, visuospatial short-term memory and learning, and paired-associate learning of Italian words. The authors suggested a close relationship between the capacity of phonological memory and the acquisition of a second language. Conversely, dyslexia has been found to be associated with shorter digit span, difficulties in reading and repeating pseudowords, and difficulties in learning foreign languages (Ganschow et al., 1991). The term "foreign language learning disability" was even proposed to refer to those subjects unable to repeat pseudowords, decreased digit span, history of reading difficulties, and deficits in acquiring a second language. By the same token, the ability to repeat words ("pseudowords") in an unknown language significantly correlates with the ability to succeed in learning that language (Service, 1992).

It has been conjectured that the ability to learn a second language is a function of (1) Language analytic capacity ("metalinguistic" ability); (2) Phonetic coding ability (phonological awareness in L2); and (3) Memory ability (working memory: the ability to get a phonological store using an articulatory loop) (Mikaye and Friedman, 1998; Skehan, 1989). It has been established that the length of the words and the phonological similarity affect learning words in a second language (Papagno and Vallar, 1992). Phonological discrimination effort in a second language may decrease the capacity of working memory, affecting second language learning and understanding.

Speed of presentation of the verbal information represents a poorly studied variable in bilingualism research. Everyday observation clearly suggests that with increasing rate of speech, language understanding in L2 significantly decreases, even approaching zero. With very high rates, *language understanding in L2 usually ceases not immediately but after a few sentences.* So, the question of working memory in a second language does not only refer to the amount of verbal information that can be stored, but also to the speed with which that information can be stored (Ardila, 2003). Processing L2 takes longer than processing L1, as in general, language processing requires an increased effort, correlated with a broader cerebral activation (Perani and Abutalebi, 2005; Rodriguez-Fornells et al., 2002). In lexical decision tasks, a significant correlation is observed between reaction time and word frequency ("frequency effect"). That is, it takes longer to find the meaning of low frequency words. Obviously, words in L2 may function as low frequency words, and finding the meaning takes longer. Language processing is slower for L2 and semantic search is less efficient.

Several studies have approached the question of brain activation and working memory in bilinguals. Kim (2002) used positron emission tomography (PET) in 14 normal subjects in order to identify the neural correlates selectively involved in working memory of native (Korean) and second (English) languages. All subjects were poorly proficient in the second language. Cognitive tasks were a two-back task for three kinds of visually presented objects: simple pictures, English words, and Korean words. The anterior portion of the right dorsolateral prefrontal cortex and the left superior temporal gyrus were activated in working memory for the native language, whereas the posterior portion of the right dorsolateral prefrontal cortex and the left inferior temporal gyrus were activated in working memory for the second language. It was proposed that the right dorsolateral prefrontal cortex and left temporal lobe may be organized into two discrete, language-related functional systems. The authors concluded that internal phonological processing seems to play a predominant role in working memory processing for the native language (high proficiency), whereas visual higher order control does so for the second language (lower proficiency).

Rinne et al. (2000) measured brain activation (PET) in professional interpreters during simultaneous interpreting (SI) vs. repetition (shadowing) of auditorily presented text. SI into the native language (Finnish) elicited left frontal activation increases. SI into the non-native language (English) elicited much more extensive left-sided fronto-temporal activation increases. SI activates predominantly left-hemispheric structures (particularly the left dorsolateral frontal cortex) related to lexical search, semantic processing and verbal working memory. Brain activation patterns were clearly modulated by direction of translation, with more extensive activation during translation into the non-native language, which is often considered to be the more demanding task.

In a recent paper, Chee (2005) reported differences in the patterns of brain activation and deactivation in bilinguals with different levels of proficiency in their second language. The author suggested that a more readily available working memory system might correlate with the attainment of superior proficiency in a second language.

Verbal Abilities in Bilinguals

Verbal abilities in bilinguals have been the focus of disagreement and polemic for a long time. The major concern refers to how to evaluate verbal skills in bilinguals: from the perspective of each one of the languages? Or rather, assuming that the bilinguals have a different language organization, and hence, cannot be evaluated using the monolingual strategies and norms? If the second perspective is taken, there are two problems very difficult to overcome: (1) norms for bilinguals are usually unavailable; and (2) bilinguals represent a tremendously heterogeneous population, and hence comparisons are difficult It is illustrative, however, to keep in mind that when the bilingual is allowed to use both languages during language testing, scores are higher than when testing is carried out independently in each one of the languages (e.g., Colon-Papazoglou, 1999). Perfectly balanced bilinguals are extremely rare (if they exist!) and usually bilinguals have a better mastery of L1 in certain topics and contexts, and a better L2 verbal ability in other topics and contexts. Most frequently, there is a common core knowledge that can be accessed both from L1 and L2 but there are also other types of knowledge in which L1 or L2 is dominant. As Grosjean (1989) clearly pointed out, the bilingual is not two monolinguals in one person.

Currently, the idea that verbal abilities in bilinguals depend upon the degree of mastery of the two languages seems to prevail. Low levels of proficiency in either language result in no significant advantage in general language ability, and can even be interfering if both languages are active languages. High levels of bilingualism, on the other hand, have a positive effect not only in verbal but also in general cognitive abilities. This point of view is usually referred to as the "Threshold Hypothesis" (or Threshold Theory) (Cummins, 1978, 1984, 1991). The threshold hypothesis was advanced to account for apparently contradictory research data concerning the effects of bilingualism on cognition. It suggested that the levels of proficiency bilinguals attain in their two languages may act as an intervening variable in mediating the effects of bilingualism on their cognitive functioning. Different studies have in general supported this proposal (e.g. Lee and Schallert, 1997; Ricciardelli, 1992). For instance, recently Andreou and Karapetsas (2004) investigated native language verbal skills among low and highly proficient bilinguals, using the WISC III verbal subtests. Highly proficient bilinguals showed superiority for almost all verbal subtests. The authors assumed that this finding lends support to the Threshold Theory. They also suggested that verbal ability underlying proficiency in the native language can be generalized to a foreign language.

An important question refers to the mutual interfering or facilitating effects of two languages. Using L1 may create a specific "mental set" that can result in the tendency to use certain utterances or grammatical structures if switching to L2. Hartsuiker, Pickering, and Veltkamp (2004) approached the question of the extent to which grammatical information is shared between languages. They investigated whether syntactic information is shared during testing if syntactic priming occurs between languages. For example, Spanish-English bilingual participants described pictures to each other in a dialogue game. It was found that a participant who had just heard a sentence in Spanish tended to use the same type of sentence when describing the next picture in English.

The same phenomenon has been found with regard to the lexicon: when the phonological form of a word is similar between L1 and L2, a facilitating effect is found. Kohnert (2004) trained a 62-year-old Spanish-English bilingual man with severe non-fluent aphasia. The patient was trained with cognates (cross-linguistic word pairs that are similar in meaning and form, such as rosa/rose) and non-cognates (cross-linguistic word pairs with shared meaning but different forms, such as mesa/table). Treatment 1 resulted in modest gains in both Spanish and English. Treatment 2 resulted in improved naming for non-cognates as well as cognates within each language. However, the generalization of gains from Spanish to English was apparent only for cognate stimuli. Costa , Santesteban , and Cano (2005) emphasized that a word's cognate status is an important dimension affecting the naming performance of bilingual speakers.

METALINGUISTIC AWARENESS

Supposedly, one major result of using two different languages is the ability to understand how language is organized (metalinguistic awareness). Results in general have been conflicting, though the majority of the studies have reported an advantage of bilinguals over monolinguals (e.g., Ben–Zeev, 1977; Cummins, 1978; Edwards and Christophersen, 1988; Galambos and Goldin–Meadow, 1990; Smith and Tager–Flusberg, 1982).

Ianco-Worrall (1972) suggested that bilinguals were able to make judgments based on meaning much earlier than monolingual children aged 4-6 years. Learning a second language provides an opportunity for developing an understanding of *the* arbitrary nature of *the* relationship that exists between words and meanings ("nominalism"). For example, it takes time for a child to learn that *the* particular sounds found in *the* English word 'house' are not inherently related to *the meaning* of *the* word 'house'. However, a child who learns that another collection of sounds, such as those found in Spanish (*casa*) or Russian (*dom*) can also mean 'house', has learned that the relationship between words and meaning are arbitrary, increasing the metalinguistic awareness.[2]

Lombardi (1986) proposed a similar point of view arguing that a child who acquires more than one language in either a simultaneous or sequential manner develops higher metalinguistic awareness than a monolingual child. Fluent bilingualism results in higher metalinguistic and metacognitive abilities that facilitate reading acquisition.

Rubin and Turner (1989) analyzed phonological awareness on children just beginning to learn a second language. They compared English-speaking first-grade children in English programs to those in French immersion programs. Children in the immersion group, who were only minimally bilingual, performed better than their peers in the English program in the phonological awareness tasks. Yelland et al. (1993) studied kindergarten and Grade 1 children; the bilingual children were native speakers of English who had limited exposure to

[2] Vygotsky tells of a Russian peasant in conversation with an eminent astronomer. After the astronomer had explained to the peasant about the distance of different stars, the peasant observed. "I think I understand how we found out how far away the stars are", says the peasant, "but what I can't fathom is how we discovered their names".

Italian. Children were required to make judgments of the sound structure of words by determining whether simple pictures depicted an object that had a long name (polysyllabic) or a short name (monosyllabic). The authors found an initial advantage for bilinguals that disappeared by the end of Grade 1. They also found that the Grade 1 bilinguals maintained an advantage over monolinguals in word recognition.

Bruck and Genesee (1995) compared monolingual English-speaking children with other Anglophone children attending French schools. Thus, French was a second language for the bilingual children and their only exposure to this language was at school. The children were followed from kindergarten through first grade in several tasks. An advantage was found for the children in the French programs in kindergarten, but it disappeared in Grade 1. Nicoladis and Genesee (1996) examined word awareness comparing bilingual and second-language learners with monolingual preschool children. Diverse tasks were used, including word segmentation, name manipulation, and word judgment. Results indicated that preschool bilingual or second-language children were not more lexically aware than monolingual children, especially in word segmentation and word judgment tasks. The authors concluded that second-language acquisition does not promote increased word awareness in children.

More recently, Bialystok, Majumder and Martin (2003) carried out three studies directed to assess the development of phonological awareness in monolingual and bilingual children between kindergarten and second grade. In the first study, monolingual and bilingual children performed equally well on a complex task requiring phoneme substitution. The second study replicated these results and demonstrated a significant role for the language of literacy instruction. The third study extended the research by including two groups of bilingual children and a range of phonological awareness and reading tasks. Spanish–English bilinguals performed better than English-speaking monolinguals on a phoneme segmentation task, but Chinese–English bilinguals performed worse. Other measures of phonological awareness did not differ among the three groups.

The general conclusion can be that bilingualism promotes phonological awareness in small children, but the gains tend to disappear when advancing through school. Phonological awareness is just one element in language awareness. Bilingualism seems to promote language awareness in general.

Bilinguals' Performance in General Cognitive Tests

The question about the performance of bilinguals in intelligence tests, particularly in verbal intelligence tests, has been polemic (e.g., e.g., Ben-Zeev, 1977; Diar, 1983; Hakuta. 1986; Haugen, 1956; Hu, 1999; Padilla et al, 1991). Some authors, particularly during the first half of the 20th century, reported decreased scores in verbal intelligence tests (e.g., Darcy, 1953). Further research has challenged these initial conclusions (e.g., Bialystok, 2001). It is not surprising to find that verbal intelligence may be decreased in bilinguals, considering that verbal intelligence is usually measured using vocabulary tests –or at least, vocabulary tests are considered the most informative verbal intelligence tasks. The bilingual can have an extended vocabulary if considering the total number of words, but a decreased vocabulary if considering only one of the languages (Pearson, Fernandez, and Oller, 1993). Usually, intelligence tests are administered to bilingual individuals in either L1 or L2. However, it has been observed that scores in intelligence tests are higher when intelligence tests are administered in a bilingual way (Colon-Papazoglou, 1999).

School performance can have a certain association with the child's general intellectual level, particularly with verbal abilities, considering that our current educational system is heavily biased on verbal learning. Bochner (1996) examined the hypothesis that bilingual students have a cognitive advantage over comparable monolinguals. Using 496 children aged 14 and 16, the author showed that the learning strategies of the bilingual male students were superior to those of their monolingual cohorts. Results were interpreted as consistent with predictions that bilingualism has a positive effect on school children.

Nonetheless, the impact of bilingualism on non verbal abilities may be more informative than the impact on verbal abilities in pinpointing the potential association between bilingualism and general cognitive functioning. Some studies have approached this question. Gorrell et al. (1982) selected a group of bilingual first graders (N = 10 Vietnamese-English, 10 Spanish-English) and compared their performance with a group of monolingual children (N = 20) on the Wechsler Intelligence Scale for Children-Revised Block Design and on spatial role-taking tasks of increasing complexity. It was hypothesized that the cognitive flexibility of bilinguals would lead to significantly higher scores than the control groups on both types of task. Analysis of variance yielded main effects for bilingualism and for culture. No significant interaction was found. For all spatial role-taking tasks no significant main effects were found. Significant interactions were found for the two most complex role-taking tasks.

Bialystok and Shapero (2005) reported two different studies using monolingual and bilingual children, approximately 6 years old, who attempted to identify the alternative image in a reversible figure. In both studies, bilingual children were more successful than monolinguals in seeing the other meaning in the images. In consequence, the effect of bilingualism may go beyond the performance of purely verbal tests. Some increased "mental flexibility" may be conjectured, that is also reflected in the performance of nonverbal tests.

When is Being Bilingual an Advantage and a Disadvantage?

From the previous sections, it is evident that bilingualism can have both, positive (e.g., increased cognitive control) and negative (e.g., decreased verbal fluency) effects in different cognitive tasks. The obvious question is, when does bilingualism have a positive effect and when does it have a negative effect? It could be hypothesized that it depends upon the particular type of relationship between both languages. The "threshold theory" (Cummins, 1978, 1984, 1991), -stating that the levels of proficiency bilinguals attain in their two languages may act as an intervening variable in mediating the effects of bilingualism on their cognitive functioning, can provide a potential answer to this question. However, other factors, such as the similarity between both languages ("linguistic distance") can also be involved. It is well established that one of the most detrimental effects of bilingualism is the potential inter-linguistic interference, resulting in decreased language performance. Interference is clearly inversely related with the similarity existing between both languages. Another obvious factor refers to the active/passive dimension of bilingualism. When both languages are active, the likelihood of interference is highest. When only one language is activated in everyday life, probability of interference is minimal. Interference can also be observed between two late languages, because they share the characteristic of being L2 languages.

The paper "*Cognitive Factors Associated with the Attainment of Intermediate Levels of Bilingual Skills*" (Cummins, 1977) represented a seminal study in the understanding of the conditions that make bilingualism advantageous or disadvantageous. In his research study, Cummins examined differences in cognitive performance between three 6th graders in a French-English bilingual education program in Canada who had attained balanced bilingual skills and students who had attained only intermediate levels of bilingual skills. The following cognitive abilities were measured: Verbal ability, general reasoning, verbal divergence, and nonverbal divergence. For students from French and mixed French-English speaking home backgrounds bilingual balance was positively related to both reasoning and divergent thinking skills. Within the English home background group, those who had attained balanced bilingual skills were superior to those who failed to attain balance on verbal measures of divergent thinking; no differences between groups on reasoning measures were found. The author suggested that these results could be interpreted in two different ways: either divergent thinking is correlated with the ability to become functionally bilingual within a bilingual education program, or, differences are a result of different levels of bilingual skills attained by balanced and nonbalanced children. However, a comparison of divergent thinking performance of these groups with a unilingual group matched on IQ and SES indicated that verbal fluency and cognitive flexibility of the nonbalanced group may have been negatively affected and verbal originality skills of the balanced group positively affected by the program. These general results have been replicated during the following years (e.g., Lasagabaster, 1998; Ricciardelli, 1992). As an illustration, it has been found in Spanish-English bilingual Mexican-American students that Spanish proficiency significantly correlates with academic achievement (Garcia-Vazquez et al., 1997). According to Cummins (1984) "limited bilingualism" may have negative consequences (e.g., Duncan and De Avila, 1979) but solid bilingualism has positive consequences on a diversity of intellectual ability tests.

The specific effect of bilingualism on cognition can depend on the individual's age. Initially, bilingualism can have a detrimental effect on language abilities, but after a certain age, positive effects are found. Nonetheless, advancing age may be associated with better learning of L2 and hence the crucial factor is the level of bilingualism. Goncz (1988) investigated the relationship between early Hungarian-Serbo-Croatian bilingualism and cognitive development using a diversity of verbal and nonverbal cognitive tests at the age of 6 and 10 years. Results showed that bilingualism was negatively associated at age six, with the volume of passive vocabulary in the first language and with the ability to derive relations and correlatives. At age 10, differences in passive vocabulary disappeared, and there was a positive association of bilingualism with the ability to derive relations and correlatives. Interestingly, a similar positive effect of bilingualism has been found in subjects with mental retardation (Whitaker, Rueda and Prieto, 1985).

As stated by Cummins and Corson (1998), the research is unambiguous in relation to three issues: (a) the distinction between conversational and academic skills in a language; (b) the positive effects of bilingualism on children's awareness of language and cognitive functioning; and (c) the close relationship between bilingual students' academic development in their first and second languages (L1 and L2) in situations where students are encouraged to develop both languages.

CONCLUSIONS

To speak two languages is obviously more demanding than speaking only one. It is not surprising to find that a second language requires an extended brain pattern of activation. That is related with the increased effort and demand that the second language requires. Language switching, and language selection requires additional attentional resources. Nonetheless, the specific pattern of brain activity for each language depends upon the mastery of each one of the languages, and probably, on a diversity of situational conditions.

Traditionally, the bilingualism literature has emphasized the negative consequences of bilingualism, such as, delayed language acquisition, increased interference, and decreased vocabulary for each language. During the last decades, however, the emphasis has moved to the positive consequences of bilingualism, including metalinguistic awareness, cognitive flexibility and cognitive control. These positive consequences are observed not only in verbal but also in non verbal tasks. Bilinguals may score higher in a diversity of verbal and non verbal cognitive tests.

Some factors influence the positive or negative effects of bilingualism. When both are active languages and frequent switching is required, interference and decreased verbal fluency can be anticipated. Conversely, language represents the major instrument of cognition (Vygotsky, 1962) and the possibility to use two different languages may increase the individual's cognitive resources. The "Threshold Hypothesis" represented an attempt to integrate the reported positive and negative effects of bilingualism. Educational consequences, particularly with regard to the natural or societal bilinguals (i.e., those individuals living in a bilingual environment, such as Hispanics in the USA) are enormous: a poor learning of one or both languages can be detrimental, but a solid learning of **both** languages may result in significant cognitive and academic advantages.

REFERENCES

Andreou, G. and Karapetsas, A. (2004). Verbal abilities in low and highly proficient bilinguals. *Journal of Psycholinguist Research, 33*, 357-64.

Ardila, A. (2003). Language representation and working memory with bilinguals. *Journal of Communication Disorders, 36*, 233-240.

Ardila, A. (2005). Spanglish: An anglicized Spanish dialect. *Hispanic Journal of Behavioral Sciences, 27*, 60-81.

Ardila, A., Rosselli, M., Ostrosky-Solis, F., Marcos, J., Granda, G., and Soto, M. (2000). Syntactic comprehension, verbal memory, and calculation abilities in Spanish-English bilinguals. *Applied Neuropsychology, 7*, 3-16.

Baddeley, A.D. (1986). *Working memory*. Oxford: Oxford University Press

Baddeley, A.D. (1992). Working memory. *Science, 255*, 556-559.

Baddeley, A. D., Papagno, C., and Vallar, G. (1988). When long-term learning depends on short-term storage. *Journal of Memory and Language, 27*, 586-595.

Ben-Zeev, S. (1977). The influence of Bilingualism on cognitive strategy and cognitive Development. *Children Development, 48*. 1009-1018.

Bernard, A.B. (2002). Language and mathematical problem solving among bilinguals. *Journal of Psychology, 136*, 283-97.

Bialystok, E. (2001). *Bilingualism in development: Language, literacy, and cognition*. New York: Cambridge University Press.

Bialystok, E. (2005). Consequences of bilingualism for cognitive development. In: J.F. Kroll and A.M.B de Grood (eds.), *Handbook of bilingualism. Psycholinguistic approaches* (pp. 417-432). New York: Oxford University Press.

Bialystok, E., Craik, F.I., Klein, R., and Viswanathan, M. (2004). Bilingualism, aging, and cognitive control: evidence from the Simon task. *Psychology and Aging, 19*, 290-303.

Bialystok, E., Craik, F.I., Gray, C., Chau, W., Ishii, R., Gunji, A., and Pantev, C. (2005). Effect of bilingualism on cognitive control in the Simon task: evidence from MEG. *Neuroimage, 24*, 40-9.

Bialystok, E., Majumder, S. and Martin, M.M. (2003). Developing phonological awareness: Is there a bilingual advantage? *Applied Psycholinguistics, 24*, 27–44

Bialystok, E. and Shapero, D. (2005). Ambiguous benefits: The effect of bilingualism on reversing ambiguous figures. *Developmental Science, 8*, 595-604

Bochner, S. (1996). The Learning Strategies of Bilingual versus Monolingual Students. *The British Journal of Educational Psychology, 66*, 83-93

Bruck, M., and Genesee, F. (1995). Phonological awareness in young second language learners. *Journal of Child Language, 22,* 307–324.

Cabeza, R. and Lennartson, E.R. (2005). False memory across languages: Implicit associative response vs fuzzy trace views. *Memory, 13*, 1-5.

Chee, M.W. (2005). Brain differences between bilinguals of differing proficiency: An empirical look at an emotional issue. *Singapore Medical Journal., 46*, 49-53.

Cheuk, D.K., Wong, V., and Leung, G.M. (2005). Multilingual home environment and specific language impairment: A case-control study in Chinese children. *Paediatric Perinatal Epidemiology, 19*, 303-14.

Chick, J. K. (1996). Intercultural communication. In S. L. McKay and N. H. Hornberger (Eds.), *Sociolinguistics and language teaching,* (pp. 329-348). Cambridge: Cambridge University Press.

Colon-Papazoglou, A.A. (1999). The Relationship of Bilingualism, Language of I.Q. Test Administration and Maternal Acculturation on the Intellectual Performance of Bilingual Puerto Rican-American Children. *Dissertation Abstracts International*, B: Sciences and Engineering, 60, 1, July, 381-B IS.

Costa, A., Santesteban, M. and Cano, A. (2005). On the facilitatory effects of cognate words in bilingual speech production. *Brain and Language, 94*, 94-103

Craik, F. and Bialystok, E. (2005). Intelligence and executive control: Evidence from aging and bilingualism. *Cortex, 41*, 222-224

Christoffels, I.K. and de Groot, A.M.B. (2005). Simultaneous interpretation: A cognitive perspective. In: J.F. Kroll and A.M.B de Grood (eds.), *Handbook of bilingualism. Psycholinguistic approaches* (pp. 445-479). New York: Oxford University Press.

Cummins, J. (1977). Cognitive Factors Associated with the Attainment of Intermediate Levels of Bilingual Skills. *The Modern Language Journal, 61*, 3-12

Cummins, J. (1978). Bilingualism and the development of metalinguistic awareness. *Journal of Cross-Cultural Psychology, 9*, 131-149.

Cummins, J. (1984). *Bilingualism and special education: Issues in assessment and pedagogy*. Clevedon England: Multilingual Matters.

Cummins, J. (1991). Interdependence of first- and second-language proficiency in bilingual children. In E. Bialystok (Ed.) *Language processing in bilingual children*. (pp. 70-89). Cambridge: Cambridge University Press.

Cummins, J. and Corson, D. (Eds.). (1998). *Bilingual education*. Dordrecht, The Netherlands: Kluwer Academic Publishers.

Darcy, N. T. (1953). A review of the literature on the effects of bilingualism upon the measure of intelligence. *Journal of Genetic Psychology, 82*, 21-57.

Diaz R. M. (1983). Thought and two languages: The impact of bilingualism on cognitive development. In E. Gordon (Ed.), *Review of Research in Education* (Vol. I, pp. 23-54). Washington: American Educational Research Association.

Edwards, D., and Christophersen, H. (1988). Bilingualism, literacy and meta-linguistic awareness in preschool children. *British Journal of Developmental Psychology, 6,* 235–244.

Fernandez, R., and Nielsen, F. (1986). Bilingualism and Hispanic scholastic achievement: Some baseline results. *Social Science Research, 15,* 43-70.

Duncan, S. and De Avila, Ed. (1979). Bilingualism and cognition: Some recent findings. *NABE Journal 4*, 15-50.

Galambos, S. J., and Goldin–Meadow, S. (1990). The effects of learning two languages on levels of metalinguistic awareness. *Cognition, 34,* 1–56.

Ganschow, L., Sparks, R.L., Javrosky, J., Pohlman, J. and Bishop-Mabury, A. (1991). Identifying naïve language difficulties among foreign learners in college: A "foreign language learning disability?". *Journal of Learning Disabilities, 24*, 530-541.

García-Vázquez, E., Vázquez, L.A. and López, I.C. (1997). Language proficiency and academic success: Relationships between proficiency in two languages and academic achievement among Mexican American students. *Bilingualism Research Journal, 21*, 395-408

Gollan, T.H. and Acenas, L.A. (2004). What is a TOT? Cognate and translation effects on tip-of-the-tongue states in Spanish-English and tagalog-English bilinguals. *Journal of Experimental Psychology: Learning Memory and. Cognition, 30*, 246-69.

Gollan, T.H., Montoya, R.I., and Werner, G.A. (2002). Semantic and letter fluency in Spanish-English bilinguals. *Neuropsychology, 16*, 562-76.

Goncz, L. (1988). A Research Study on the Relation between Early Bilingualism and Cognitive Development. *Psychologische Beitrage, 30*, 75-91.

Gorrell, J. J., Bregman, N.J., McAllister, H.A., and Lipscomb, T.A. (1982). A Comparison of Spatial Role-Taking in Monolingual and Bilingual Children. *The Journal of Genetic Psychology, 140*, 3-18.

Grosjean, F. (1982). *Life with two languages*. Cambridge, MA: Harvard University Press.

Grosjean, F. (1989). Neurolinguists, beware! The bilingual is not two monolinguals in one person. *Brain and Language, 36*, 3-15.

Hakuta, K. (1986). *Mirror of language: The debate on bilingualism.* New York: Basic books.

Hartsuiker, R.J., Pickering, M.J., and Veltkamp, E. (2004). Is syntax separate or shared between languages? Cross-linguistic syntactic priming in Spanish-English bilinguals. *Psychology Sciences,.15*, 409-414.

Haugen (1956). The Effect of bilingualism on Intelligence. Bilingualism in the Americas. A Bibliography and Research Guide. *American Dialect Society*. No. 26. Montgomery: University of Alabama Press.

Hernandez, A.E., Dapretto, M., Mazziotta J., and Bookheimer, S. (2001). Language switching and language representation in Spanish-English bilinguals: an fMRI study. *Neuroimage, 14*, 510-520.

Hu, G. (1999). Review of Studies of Bilingualism and Intelligence. *Foreign Language Teaching and Research, 3*, 28-36.

Hummel, K.M. (2002). Second language acquisition and working memory. In: F. Fabbro (Ed.), *Advances in the neurolinguistics of bilingualism*. (pp. 95-117). Udine (Italy): Forum.

Ianco-Worral, A. (1972) Bilingualism and Cognitive Development. *Child Development, 43*, 1390-1400.

Ji, L.J., Zhang, Z., and Nisbett, R.E. (2004). Is it culture or is it language? Examination of language effects in cross-cultural research on categorization. *Journal of Personality and Social Psychology, 87*, 57-65.

Kim, J.J., Kim, M.S., Lee, J.S., Lee, D.S., Lee, M.C., and Kwon, J.S. (2002). Dissociation of working memory processing associated with native and second languages: PET investigation. *Neuroimage, 15*, 879-891.

Kohnert, K. (2004). Cognitive and cognate-based treatments for bilingual aphasia: a case study. *Brain and Language, 91*, 294-302.

Lasagabaster, D. (1998). The threshold hypothesis applied to three languages in contact at school. *International Journal of Bilingual Education and Bilingualism, 1*, 119-133.

Lee, J., and Schallert, D. L. (1997). The relative contribution of L2 language proficiency and L1 reading ability to L2 reading performance: A test of the threshold hypothesis in an EFL context.*TESOL Quarterly, 31*, 713-739.

Lombardi, J. (1986). The Metalinguistic Abilities of Bilingual Subjects Le abilita metalinguistiche nei soggetti bilingui *Rassegna Italiana di Linguistica Applicata, 18*, 103-114.

Marian, V. and Neisser, U. (2000). Language-dependent recall of autobiographical memories. *Journal of Experimental Psychology: General, 129*, 361-368.

Mikaye, A. and Friedman, N.P. (1998). Individual differences in second language proficiency: Working memory as language aptitude. In: A.F. Healy and L.E. Bourne (Eds.), *Foreign language learning: Psycholinguistic studies in training and retention* (pp. 339-364). New Jersey: Lawrence Erlbaum.

Mohamed, Z.K., and Phillipe, A., Pinon, K., Havet-Thomassin, V, Aubin, G., Roy, A., Le Gall. D. (2004). Bilingualism and adult differences in inhibitory mechanisms: Evidence from a bilingual Stroop task. *Brain and Cognition, 54*, 254-256.

Nicoladis, E. and Genesee, F. (1966). Word Awareness in Second Language Learners and Bilingual Children. *Language Awareness, 5*, 80-90.

Okoh, N. (1980). Bilingualism and Divergent Thinking among Nigerian and Welsh School *Children Journal of Social Psychology, 110*, 163-170.

Pavlenko, E.. (2005). Bilingualism and thought. In: J.F. Kroll and A.M.B de Grood (eds.), *Handbook of bilingualism. Psycholinguistic approaches* (pp. 433-453). New York: Oxford University Press.

Padilla, A. M., Fairchild, H.H., Valdez, C.M. (Eds.) (1990). *Bilingual Education: Issues and Strategies*. Newbury Park, CA: Sage Publications.

Papagno, C. and Vallar, G. (1992). Phonological short-term memory and the learning of new words: The effect of phonological similarity and item length. *Quarterly Journal of Experimental Psychology, 44A*, 47-67.

Papagno C, Vallar G. (1995). Verbal short-term memory and vocabulary learning in polyglots. *Quarterly Journal of Experimental Psychology, 48*, 98-107.

Paradis, J., Crago, M., Genesee, F., and Rice, M. (2003). Bilingual children with specific language impairment: How do they compare with their monolingual peers? *Journal of Speech, Language, and Hearing Research, 46*, 1-15.

Peal, B., and Lambert, W. (1962). The relation of Bilingualism to intelligence. *Psychological Monographs: General and Applied. 76*, (27) 1-23.

Pearson, B. Z., Fernandez, S. C., and Oller, D. K. (1993). Lexical Development in Bilingual Infants and Toddlers: Comparison to Monolingual Norms. *Language Learning, 43*, 99-120.

Perani, D. and Abutalebi, J. (2005). The neural basis of first and second language processing. *Current Opinions in Neurobiology, 15*, 202-206.

Ricciardelli, L. (1992). Bilingualism and cognitive development in relation to threshold theory. *Journal of Psycholinguistic Research, 21*, 301-316.

Rinne, J.O., Tommola, J., Laine, M., Krause, B.J., Schmidt, D., Kaasinen, V., Teras, M., Sipila, H., and Sunnari, M.. (2000).The translating brain: cerebral activation patterns during simultaneous interpreting. *Neuroscience Letter, 294*, 85-88.

Rodriguez-Fornells, A., Rotte, M., Heinze, H.J., Nosselt, T., and Munte, T.F. (2002). Brain potential and functional MRI evidence for how to handle two languages with one brain. *Nature 415*, 1026 – 1029.

Rodriguez-Fornells, A., van der Lugt, A., Rotte, M., Britti, B., Heinze, H.J., and Munte, T.F. (2005). Second language interferes with word production in fluent bilinguals: brain potential and functional imaging evidence. *Journal of Cognitive Neurosciences, 17*, 422-433.

Rosselli, M., Ardila, A., Araujo, K., Weekes, V.A., Caracciolo, V., Padilla, M., and Ostrosky-Solís, F. (2000). Verbal fluency and repetition skills in healthy older Spanish-English bilinguals. *Applied Neuropsychology, 7*, 17-24.

Rosselli, M., Ardila, A., Santisi, M.N., Arecco, M.R., Salvatierra, J., Conde, A., and Lenis, B. (2002a). Stroop Effect in Spanish-English Bilinguals. *Journal of the International Neuropsychological Society, 8*, 819-827.

Rosselli, M., Ardila, A., Salvatierra, J., Márquez, M., Matos, L., and Weekes, V.A. (2002b). A cross-linguistic comparison of verbal fluency tests. *International Journal of Neurosciences, 112*, 759-776.

Rubin, H., and Turner, A. (1989). Linguistic awareness skills in grade one children in a French immersion setting. *Reading and Writing: An Interdisciplinary Journal, 1*, 73–86.

Rumbaut, R.G. and Ima, K (1988). *The Adaptation of Southeast Asian Refugee Youth: A Comparative Study*. Washington, DC: U.S. Office of Refugee Resetlement.

Salameh, E.K., Nettelbladt, U., and Gullberg, B. (2002). Risk factors for language impairment in Swedish bilingual and monolingual children relative to severity. *Acta Paediatrica, 91*, 1379-1384.

Salameh, E.K., Hakansson, G., and Nettelbladt, U. (2004). Developmental perspectives on bilingual Swedish-Arabic children with and without language impairment: A longitudinal study. *International Journal of Language and Communication Disorders, 39,* 65-91.

Segalowitz, N., and Frenkiel-Fishman, S. (2005). Attention control and ability level in a complex cognitive skill: attention shifting and second-language proficiency. *Memory and Cognition, 33*, 644-653.

Service, E. (1992). Phonology, working memory, and foreign language learning. *Quarterly Journal of Experimental Psychology, 45A,* 21-50.

Schrauf, R.W. and Rubin, D.C. (2000). Internal languages of retrieval: the bilingual encoding of memories for the personal past. *Memory and Cognition*, *28*, 616-23.

Skehan, P. (1989). *Individual differences in second language learning*. London:Edward Arnold.

Smith, C. S., and Tager–Flusberg, H. (1982). Metalinguistic awareness and language development. *Journal of Experimental Child Psychology, 34,* 449–468.

Stroop, J.R. (1935). Studies of interference in serial verbal reactions. *Journal of Experimental Psychology, 18*, 643-662.

Takano, Y. and Noda, A. (1993). A Temporary Decline of Thinking Ability during Foreign Language Processing. *Journal of Cross-Cultural Psychology, 24*, 445-462.

Toppelberg, C.O., Medrano, L., Pena Morgens, L., and Nieto-Castanon, A. (2002). Bilingual children referred for psychiatric services: associations of language disorders, language skills, and psychopathology. *Journal of the American Academy of Child and Adolescence Psychiatry, 41*, 712-722.

Vygotsky, L.S. (1962). *Thought and language.* Cambridge, MA: MT Press

Weinreich, U. (1953), *Languages in Contact*, The Hague, Mouton

Whitaker, J. H. and Rueda, R., and Prieto, A. (1985). Cognitive Performance as a Function of Bilingualism in Students with Mental Retardation. *Mental Retardation, 23*, 302-307.

Yelland, G. W., Pollard, J., and Mercuri, A. (1993). The metalinguistic benefits of limited contact with a second language. *Applied Psycholinguistics, 14,* 423–444.

INDEX

A

B

C

D

E

F

G

H

I

J

K

L

M

Q

R

S

T

U

V

W

Y